Parkinson's Disease
A Self-Help Guide

Parkinson's Disease

A Self-Help Guide

Marjan Jahanshahi
BSc, MPhil (Clin Psychol), PhD

C. David Marsden
MRCPsych, DSc, FRS

With contributions from
Richard G. Brown, BA, MPhil (Clin Psychol),
Brigid McCarthy, BA, Dip Clin Psychol (BPS), MSc,
and Lanny E. Perkins and Sara D. Perkins

Demos Medical Publishing, Inc., 386 Park Avenue South, New York, New York 10016

Library of Congress Cataloging-in-Publication Data

Parkinson's disease : a self-help guide / Marjan Jahanshahi, C. David Marsdan ; with contributions from Richard G. Brown. ... [et al.].
     p. cm.
   Includes index.
   ISBN 1-888799-38-2
   1. Parkinson's disease—Popular works.   2. Self-care, Health.
 I. Jahanshahi, Marjan.   II. Marsden, C. David.
RC382.P253   2000   00-035859
616.8′33—dc21

Printed in Canada

Contents

Part III: Coping with Parkinson's Disease

Part IV: Epilogue

Acknowledgments

We have spent many years treating people with Parkinson's disease and conducting research on the illness. During this period, many of those people have shared their experiences with us, and in so doing have been instrumental in teaching us what we know. Others have been generous with their time, participating in studies evaluating the impact of Parkinson's on daily living, or in more experimental tests. We see this book as a way of repaying our debt of gratitude. We will find it rewarding indeed if it goes some way toward making living and coping with Parkinson's disease easier for those who have the illness, their caregivers, and their families.

Marjan Jahanshahi
David Marsden

Preface

Parkinson's disease is one of the most common neurologic disorders. One person in every thousand of the population has it. Although young adults can develop the illness, it is usually a disorder of old age. In Western countries, increased life expectancy means that the proportion of elderly will also increase. Since the risk of developing Parkinson's increases with age, there will be more people with it.

What is Parkinson's disease?

What is the cause?

Is there a cure?

Can it be treated?

What other symptoms will I get?

How quickly will I deteriorate?

Can I carry on working?

Will it affect my mind?

Will I be confined to a wheelchair?

Is there anything I can do to alleviate my symptoms?

Will my children get Parkinson's disease?

These are some of the questions that will be asked by someone who has been diagnosed as having Parkinson's disease. In the limited time available in an initial visit, most doctors can provide only minimal information about the nature of the disorder and its drug treatment. Some of these questions may not come to mind when a person is first told that he or she has Parkinson's disease. It is usually during the following days and weeks that some of the questions will surface. The subsequent medical management of the illness mainly focuses on adjusting the level of medication to control the symptoms. The person with Parkinson's disease and his or her family are often left unaided to anticipate and adapt to the long-term social implications.

The aim of our book is to fill this gap in patient–doctor communication and to provide the individual and his or her family with the essential information about the nature of the illness, its diagnosis and medical treatment, its implication for their daily lives, and about how best to cope with the changes brought about by it.

A number of informative books about the experience of living with Parkinson's disease have been written by people who have it, and there are some excellent books by health professionals providing information about the illness and its management. Our book differs from these publications in three main ways.

1. We provide much more detailed information about the symptoms of the disease, its possible causes, the process of diagnosis, and its medical treatment. We have tried to collate in a single book all the information that people with Parkinson's disease and their caregivers may want to access. By its nature, much of this information is very technical, but we have assumed that our average intelligent reader will find it enlightening.

2. The symptoms of Parkinson's disease, the associated disability, and its progression vary from person to person. We have tried to portray these varied experiences. The lives of the spouse or partner and of the family who live with and care for the person with Parkinson's are also affected by the illness, so we also consider their experiences and needs, which are often overlooked.

3. In addition to medical treatment, there are many other ways in which the person with Parkinson's disease and his or her family can soften the impact of the illness on their lives. We describe a range of self-

help strategies that can help people cope better with disability and reduce its effects on their daily activities, mood, and social relationships.

The book is organized into three main parts. The first, "Parkinson's Disease: The Medical Facts," provides up-to-date medical information about the symptoms, what is known about the possible causes, the aims and procedures of different tests used in diagnosis, and treatment with medication or surgery. In this era of modern health care, the individual is considered an active participant in his or her health care rather than a passive recipient of treatment. "Patient education"—or providing the person with a chronic illness with information about the disorder and its medical treatment—is beneficial in two main ways. First, it can alleviate the anxiety and anticipation experienced when an individual faces the unknown. By creating a sense of familiarity, information can generate a sense of choice and control. Second, it provides the individual with the opportunity to actively participate in his or her own health care. The person diagnosed with Parkinson's disease has to travel many novel and personally uncharted waters in the course of the illness. The general medical information provided in Part I may provide signposts to guide the person with Parkinson's disease and his or her family on this journey. Informed decisions are often more rational, and their consequences easier to live with, and we hope that the information provided in Part I will facilitate such informed decisions.

The onset and development of a progressive and disabling illness such as Parkinson's constitute a traumatic life crisis that can have a major impact on the psychological well-being and social functioning of both the person with the disorder and his or her family. The knowledge that one's experiences are not unique, that they are shared by others in the same situation, can be reassuring and take the edge off the threatening aspects. The experience of Parkinson's disease is shared by approximately 500,000 people in the United States. As the great variability of symptoms across individuals would imply, there is no one form of the disorder. This, combined with the very individual way in which each person responds to stress and change, means that no standard experience of the illness exists either. Nevertheless, by portraying some of the common experiences of living with it, we aim to offer some assurance to those who have to experience it.

Part II, "Living with Parkinson's Disease," deals with the impact of chronic illness on the individual. His or her feelings and reactions to the illness are traced from the shock and anger experienced in the early acute phase, through the sense of loss and mourning, to the ensuing acceptance and adjustment that occur in the later, more chronic, stage. The effect of Parkinson's disease is considered in terms of the changes brought about in the various spheres of life, ranging from everyday activities, work and finance, to family, marital, sexual, and social relationships. These psychosocial changes are considered from the perspective both of the person with the disorder and of the family. Although, as we noted, it is in the majority of cases a disorder of old age, it can develop before the age of 40. A minority, approximately 15 percent to 20 percent of people with Parkinson's disease, will develop impaired memory and intellectual abilities. The special needs of the person with Parkinson's disease and cognitive impairment and of the "young-onset" patient are considered in Chapters 7 and 8.

Faced with the challenge of a chronic illness such as Parkinson's, the individual has to overcome the effects of the symptoms on his or her mobility and health and strive to preserve his or her identity, lifestyle, and social relationships from the assault of the illness. Part III, "Coping with Parkinson's Disease," focuses first on various external sources of help. It describes a multitude of health professionals, as well as outside agencies and voluntary organizations, and details the kind of help that they can offer. Strategies that can be used by the patient for controlling the symptoms and reducing the associated disability are proposed in Chapter 10. In human terms, the main impact of the disease may be on the individual's identity. Self-help techniques are suggested to help him or her come to terms with the reality of the illness, to optimize his or her coping with its effects, to prevent depression and anxiety, and to maintain emotional well-being. The ultimate goal, of course, is to ensure that the individual possesses the necessary resources to meet the many challenges and to achieve the best quality of life possible within the confines of the illness. To ensure a good quality of life, the physical and psychological well-being of the caregiver is as important as that of the patient. Also considered in Part III are methods that can be used by the caregiver to minimize and cope with the stresses produced by the illness.

In the last part of the book, a history of the illness and of the research that has been carried out on it provides the background for a discussion of future horizons. The outstanding questions yet to be answered and the directions for future research are considered. The book ends with an Appendix containing a list of of useful organizations and other publications that readers may find of interest. Because Parkinson's disease may produce extensive and disruptive financial burdens on the family, this issue is addressed in detail, as are the resources available to deal with these problems.

As neither of us nor our co-authors has Parkinson's disease, our writing about living and coping with the illness is undoubtedly second-hand, gained by treating, working with, and talking to many patients and their relatives over many years. But by quoting people with Parkinson's disease and their relatives, we have been able to reflect first-hand experiences of what it is like to live with the illness. These quotations come from two sources: from patients we have known, treated, or worked with ourselves, and from books by people who have the illness. When reproducing the words of people known to us, we have changed details such as names, professions, and so on to protect their identities and to ensure confidentiality. When we have used quotations from books or other texts, we have, of course, referred directly to the authors.

We hope that the particular order we have imposed on the information gathered here will be perceived as a logical way of conveying it. However, this does not mean that the book necessarily has to be read from page 1 to the end, chapter by chapter. We hope that most of our readers will have the interest and the time to do so, but for those who haven't, each chapter has been written to stand alone, without the need to read preceding or subsequent ones in order to understand the information. This also provides the reader with the option of referring to specific chapters as the need arises or of refreshing his or her memory on any particular aspect.

It would be difficult indeed to find two people with identical symptoms of Parkinson's and consequently two people with very similar experiences of the illness. One might say that there are as many experiences of living with Parkinson's disease as there are people with the disorder. Although we use case examples to illustrate and clarify certain issues, inevitably much of the book is written in general terms that may not be easily applicable to any individual person. But we hope that everyone with Parkinson's disease and every caregiver who reads this book will find in it something of value.

We would like to thank all the individuals who have over the years shared with us their experiences of living and coping with Parkinson's disease. Our special thanks go to Paul Rayner and Colin Moat, who have been indispensable volunteers for our research studies, who read through the text and indicated places where we had been overzealous in our use of medical jargon. Last but not least, we would like to thank our co-authors for their significant contributions.

Marjan Jahanshahi and David Marsden

PART I

Parkinson's Disease:
The Medical Facts

What Is Parkinson's Disease?

Parkinson's disease is a neurologic illness, meaning a disease caused by a dysfunction of the brain or the spinal cord—the two main parts of the central nervous system—or of the peripheral nervous system and muscles. The major symptoms are tremor, slowness in starting and carrying out movements (bradykinesia), rigidity or muscle stiffness, and problems with balance and walking. The disorder is named after James Parkinson, the British doctor who first described it in 1817 (the history of the discovery of Parkinson's disease and the research into its causes and treatment are outlined in Chapter 14). Our aim in this first chapter is to provide you with the basic medical information.

HOW COMMON IS IT AND WHO GETS IT?

One person in every thousand develops Parkinson's disease. As it is commonly a disorder of old age, the risk of contracting it increases with age. Among those over 65, the incidence rises to 1 in 100. For those over the age of 80, 1 person in 50 develops Parkinson's disease. The illness starts between the ages of 50 and 60 in 40 percent of cases, which makes the sixties the average age of onset. However, approximately 1 in 7 of those with Parkinson's have developed the symptoms before the age of 40. In so-called young-onset Parkinson's disease, the illness develops between the ages of 21 and 40. Chapter 8 focuses on the special needs of those with young-onset Parkinson's disease. "Juvenile parkinsonism," in which the illness starts before the age of 21, is relatively rare.

Men and women are equally likely to develop Parkinson's disease, although some studies have suggested that men are slightly more prone to it. The illness is not selective in terms of either socioeconomic status or occupation—all ethnic groups and occupations are about equally affected. This is reflected in the varied professions of the famous people who have had Parkinson's disease: Sir John Betjeman (Poet Laureate), Chairman Mao Tse-tung (Chinese Communist leader), General Douglas MacArthur (American military leader), Michael J. Fox and Sir Michael Redgrave (actors), A. J. P. Taylor (historian), and Janet Reno (U.S. Attorney General). The only exceptions to the nonselectivity of the disease is boxers, who, over many years of receiving blows to the head, are more likely to get it—witness Muhammad Ali.

Evidence suggests that the prevalence of Parkinson's disease has not substantially changed over the years. In general, distribution figures in various countries demonstrate that, with a few exceptions, the disorder is not limited to a particular part of the world.

One intriguing finding is that, in studies of large samples of people with Parkinson's disease, there are many who have never smoked and very few current smokers. In other words, people who have never smoked are overrepresented and smokers are underrepresented. This has led to the proposal that perhaps cigarette smoking in some way protects against the disease. The reasons for the association between cigarette smoking and lower vulnerability to Parkinson's disease are not known. One possibility is that people with Parkinson's disease who have smoked die earlier of illnesses associated with smoking, but this cannot be the full explanation. The fact that few people with Parkinson's disease are smokers is also true of people who develop the disease at an early age. Of course, once the illness has started, smoking is unlikely to be of benefit. So don't start now!

Since the 1970s, when levodopa therapy became the main symptomatic treatment for Parkinson's disease, the life expectancy of patients has been about the same as for the general population, particularly during the first five years of the illness. After 10 to 15 years, the life expectancy of people with Parkinson's disease drops to about 75 percent to 65 percent of the general population. People with Parkinson's disease die of the same causes as do other people of the same age, except that there is a negative association between Parkinson's disease and cancer. In other words, people with Parkinson's disease are less likely to die of cancer, perhaps because they are less likely to smoke.

THE SYMPTOMS

The symptoms of Parkinson's disease are listed in Table 1-1. Each symptom is described in more detail in the following pages. When looking at the list, it is important to remember a number of facts.

❖ Doctors usually distinguish between major and minor symptoms of a disease, and Table 1-1 observes this distinction. The major symptoms are those present in the majority of people with Parkinson's disease, and one or more have to be present before a person is said to have the illness. The minor symptoms are not encountered in every case. But this distinction overlooks the fact that which symptoms are experienced as major or

Table 1-1. The symptoms of Parkinson's disease

Major symptoms	Minor symptoms
Tremor	Dysphonia (low soft voice)
Rigidity (muscle stiffness)	Micrographia (small size of and
Bradykinesia (slowness	difficulty with handwriting)
of movement)	Masked facies (loss of facial
Akinesia (poverty or absence	expression, "poker face")
of movement)	Seborrhea (excessive greasiness
Balance and walking problems	and scaliness of the skin)
	Dysphagia (difficulty in swallowing, and dribbling)
	Autonomic symptoms (postural hypotension, urinary urgency, sweating)
	Pain and other sensory symptoms
	Fatigue
	Cognitive dysfunction and dementia
	Depression
	Sleep disturbance
	Sexual problems

minor may be different for each individual. For example, for someone who has mild tremor or bradykinesia, the symptom of dribbling may be major in the sense of causing the most distress and embarrassment. For an actor, the major symptoms may be the dysphonia, or soft and monotonous voice, whereas for an architect it may be the tremor. Nevertheless, this medical differentiation between major and minor symptoms is useful when talking in general terms, particularly when considering the effectiveness of treatment.

❖ Not everyone with Parkinson's disease will necessarily develop all the symptoms.

❖ No two cases are alike. There are great differences between people with Parkinson's disease in terms of (1) what the first symptom is; (2) the order in which, and precise time after onset of the first symptom that, other symptoms develop; and (3) the severity of the symptoms. The course of the disorder can vary from slowly progressive with relatively little disability to a more aggressive form with faster progression and earlier decline and disability.

❖ The symptoms may show daily fluctuations in severity. Some people with Parkinson's disease report a period in the early morning when the symptoms are less evident or milder. In his book *Ivan: Living with Parkinson's Disease,* Ivan Vaughan describes this morning benefit:

For a long time I had noticed an extraordinary boost in muscular fluency which flooded my body some time around dawn.

❖ As the symptoms are not static across time and fluctuate even in the course of a day, it may be difficult to ask the person with Parkinson's disease to give a clear picture of his or her symptoms.

❖ It is important not to confuse the symptoms with the side effects of the medication used to control those symptoms. After a number of years of levodopa therapy, most patients develop dyskinesias, or involuntary movements of the limbs and face. These dyskinesias are a side effect of levodopa therapy and not a symptom of the disease. The distinction between the symptoms and the side effects of medication may sometimes be difficult to make because some of the symptoms may be made worse by certain types of medication. For example, constipation is a symptom of the disease that can also be a side effect of anticholinergic medication. The side effects of medication are listed for each type of drug in Chapter 3.

❖ In most cases, as already noted, Parkinson's disease is a disorder of old age. An elderly person may also have other illnesses, such as arthritis or heart or lung disease, each of which has its associated symptoms. So in some cases, some symptoms may be related to these other disorders and not to Parkinson's disease.

The history of two people with the illness illustrates the large individual differences in the type, severity, and time of onset of the symptoms, and in the course of the illness and the efficacy of treatment. Susan was fortunate, as her Parkinson's disease remained mild and well controlled for many years. In contrast, Helen's illness progressed relatively rapidly and after a while medication failed to produce symptomatic control, bringing on moderate to severe disability within a relatively short time.

Susan is a 70-year-old married woman who at the age of 57 noticed the first symptoms of Parkinson's disease, which were tiredness and a general feeling of awkwardness, together with a slight tremor of the left hand. She was diagnosed as having the illness two years later. Although her symptoms remained relatively mild and were well controlled with medication, Susan took early retirement from her job as a hospital nurse because of her increased susceptibility to fatigue. Her symptoms remained well controlled on Sinemet and selegiline for eight to ten years, and were associated with mild to moderate disability. During this period, she was a very willing and cooperative volunteer, giving generously of her time to participate in many experimental studies and research programs on Parkinson's disease. During the last two to three years, her illness had progressed and the associated disability had increased mainly as a result of "end-of-dose deterioration" and the development of dyskinesias. She put it this way: "The period of time when medication controls my symptoms is growing shorter, and the involuntary movements are unpleasant. I still manage to give myself a short 'on' period, but I am caught by the unpredictable 'running out of steam.'"

Helen, married with two young children, developed Parkinson's disease at the age of 42, a few years after opening her own beauty salon. With a lot of hard work, she had built up a busy and successful business in the span of two years, employing two other stylists. She had been aware of feelings of tiredness and being generally "run down" for many months before a slight tremor of her right hand appeared. She ignored this for a while, hoping it would go away. When it persisted, she consulted her internist, who referred her to a neurologist who diagnosed Parkinson's disease and started her on medication. For the next three years, the medication controlled her symptoms well. During this period, she carried on with her work at the salon, although she was slower and could see fewer clients. The medication gradually stopped controlling her symptoms, and the involuntary movements made shampooing, cutting, and setting her clients' hair impossible tasks. She was persuaded by her husband to take on a less active role in the salon and to employ a third stylist to stand in for her. This eased the pressure on her and she continued in her managerial role for the next 18 months. With further progression of the illness and worsening of the symptoms, even dressing and leaving the house in the morning became difficult. Six years after the first appearance of tremor, she was forced to sell the salon. Having spent most of her adult life working outside the home, she welcomed her new role of housewife and focused on busying herself with household chores, with a little help from her mother, who visited daily, and some input from her teenaged daughter after school hours.

The Major Symptoms

Tremor

Tremor is the symptom by which Parkinson's disease is known to most people. It is the first symptom in approximately 50 percent of cases. On the other hand, approximately 15 percent of people with the illness never develop it. Tremor in Parkinson's disease has a number of typical features that allow a doctor to distinguish it from forms of tremor present in other movement disorders.

❖ The tremor in Parkinson's disease is mainly a *resting tremor.* This means that it is only or mostly present when the individual is at rest, not using or moving the part of the body that has the tremor. For example, the resting tremor of the hands is most noticeable when the hands are resting in the lap. In fact, in some cases the resting tremor of Parkinson's disease tends to be reduced, or even disappears completely, when the individual moves the hand or uses it to reach toward an object or to grasp the object. This is a blessing in a way because it means that tremor often does not interfere too much with active movements. However, in approximately 40 percent to 50 percent of cases, in addition to resting tremor there may also be some *action tremor* and *postural tremor.* These are the types of tremor that become evident when one is moving a limb or keeping it in a particular position, respectively.

❖ The second typical feature of the Parkinson's tremor is that it is regular and rhythmic and occurs at a particular rate, approximately four to six beats per second. In other words, the affected hand or leg shakes or trembles about five times in a second.

❖ In Parkinson's disease, tremor can affect either a few or many different parts of the body, and can be either mild or severe. For example, at one extreme it may be limited to a single finger of one hand, whereas at the other extreme it may be present in both hands and legs and even in the muscles of the chest, jaw, tongue, and lips. The head and voice are rarely affected by tremor. The tremor usually is unilateral—that is, it starts on one side of the body—and the other side is affected later (the tremor becomes bilateral), as the disease progresses. Not only the extent but also the severity of the tremor varies considerably from person to person. It may be so mild that it is only noticeable to the patient. Tremor of the chest or abdomen often is felt as an internal quivering or shaking that cannot be seen by others. At the other extreme, the tremor can be so severe as to result in violent shaking of the limbs and body. When the tremor of the hands is severe, the thumb may move back and forth in front of the fingers. To the early physicians who used to mix and prepare their own medication by hand, this to-and-fro movement gave the impression of rolling a pill, which gave rise to the label *pill-rolling tremor.*

❖ The fourth characteristic of tremor in Parkinson's disease is that it is quite variable and can change considerably with the person's circumstances. It disappears when he or she is sleeping deeply and is reduced when he or she is very relaxed or sedated. It often becomes worse when the individual is anxious or under stress, or has to concentrate hard. Some people can suppress the tremor for a limited period of time through an effort of will.

Dyskinesias, the involuntary movements associated with medication, can be a cause of embarrassment later in the illness. In the early stages, tremor is probably the symptom that is most noticeable, and that can be embarrassing. As a result, the patient may go to great lengths to hide it. Some people sit on the affected hand. Others hide it in a trouser pocket or coat pocket, or behind a newspaper. Still others cover the trembling hand with the unaffected one.

Rigidity, or Muscle Stiffness

At least in the earlier stages, rigidity—in contrast to tremor—is often a symptom that people with Parkinson's disease are not too aware of. Only relatively later in the course of the illness will rigidity be experienced by the patient as muscle stiffness, and be evident to others as a stooped posture, with the knees and arms bent at the joints. Earlier on, rigidity becomes apparent only during clinical examination by a doctor. It can be brought out by having the patient move one arm while the other arm is moved passively by the doctor. When the doctor passively moves the joints in order to stretch the affected muscles, he or she encounters increased resistance to the movement. This resistance has been compared to bending a lead pipe—hence it is called *lead-pipe rigidity.* Also, during the clinical examination the resistance to passive movements may have a regular jerking characteristic, which has been labeled *cogwheel rigidity.* The extent and severity of rigidity vary considerably and can affect one arm or one leg or all four limbs. With the progression of the disorder, rigidity can become so severe that the muscles look and feel tense even when they should be relaxed—for example, when the individual is at rest. Rigidity gives rise to aches in the shoulder and neck, back pain resulting from the stooped and forward-leaning posture, muscle cramps in the legs or feet, and sometimes even chest pain.

Slowness of Movement—Bradykinesia and Akinesia

The word *bradykinesia* is of Greek origin, *brady* from a word for slowness and *kinesia* from a word meaning movement. It refers to the slowness in initiating and executing movement. In Parkinson's disease, when a movement is repeated several times, it becomes gradually slower and "smaller." The slowness affects all forms of movement, but slowness in initiating and executing movement is more evident in certain types of movement. Activities that involve *repetitive movements*, such as brushing the teeth, stirring a saucepan, and polishing shoes, are particularly affected. So is the performance of *fine movements,* such as changing a plug, turning the page of a newspaper, or fastening buttons. *Bimanual movements* (movements carried out with both hands) are usually slower than are movements with one hand. *Doing two things at once,* such as getting up from a chair while talking, may become difficult or almost impossible. Activities that involve *sequential movements,* such as fastening buttons, are also slowed down because there is an increased pause between the individual movements in a sequence, which slows down the whole process. Certain movements, such as walking, swinging the arms when walking, blinking, and swallowing, are normally done automatically without paying attention to their performance. But in Parkinson's disease, such *automatic movements* are more affected than are *learned* ones, so that the person may still be able to perform previously learned dance steps or play the piano.

Rigidity, or muscle stiffness, can add to slowness of movements but is not the cause of it. Slowness can be present even when there is no rigidity. The severity of bradykinesia may vary from situation to situation. Normally, slowness is evident during movements such as getting out of a chair or walking in and out of a room, and can become worse with increased fatigue. However, under certain circumstances the person with Parkinson's disease can overcome the slowness. The extreme example of this is *akinesia paradoxica*, when an individual who is ordinarily unable to move unassisted from his chair or bed moves at normal speed—for example, when in danger. Paradoxic kinesis reportedly happened in the case of a usually wheelchair-using and immobile man with Parkinson's disease who jumped into the water and saved a drowning man! In general, movements that are triggered by external stimuli are less affected than are movements initiated by the individual under his or her own steam. For example, despite experiencing problems walking on flat surfaces, the person with Parkinson's disease can climb stairs remarkably well because each stair acts as a stimulus for taking a step.

A related symptom is *akinesia*, which means absence or poverty of movement, and in Parkinson's disease refers to the reduction of spontaneous movements. Akinesia is particularly noticeable in the lack of automatic movements such as blinking and swallowing—in other words, movements that are normally carried out without the individual paying attention to them or expending any effort in doing them. For example, in Parkinson's disease, the arm swing is lost during walking; when sitting still, the individual moves very little; while he or she talks, there is little gesturing with the hands or change in facial expression or blinking; the reduced rate of swallowing results in the accumulation and drooling of saliva. The effect of the reduced rate of blinking is that the normal lubrication of the eyes fails to occur, and the eyes become irritated, dry, red, crusted, and sore.

The loss of automaticity in performing movements is a particularly disturbing aspect of akinesia and bradykinesia. The person with Parkinson's disease has to consciously think about each phase of the simplest movement.

"Freezing"—that is, an inability to move that lasts a few seconds or longer—is another example of akinesia. It occurs during walking, so that the person feels glued to the spot and unable to lift the feet to take steps. Freezing often happens when he or she approaches a doorway or other confined area, or when trying to turn. Sudden freezing while walking can lead to falls—the feet stick to the ground, but the momentum of the body continues, so that the person falls forward.

One of the reasons bradykinesia and akinesia occur may be that in Parkinson's disease the muscles are not sufficiently activated at the appropriate moment. As a result, movements are not only slow but also are often "smaller" than is necessary. For example, when reaching for an object such as a cup, the individual undershoots and the hand falls short of the target, so that the normally smooth and rapid aiming movement is replaced by a slow, stepwise approach to the cup. These problems affect not only the muscles of the hands, arms, and legs, but also all muscles. The coordination of the muscles that move the eyes may be impaired, resulting in difficulty in focusing on nearby objects or slowness in shifting the gaze.

Slowness can be frustrating for the person with Parkinson's disease. Subjectively, bradykinesia is experienced as a sort of a block between willing a movement and its actual performance. People often feel that they are no longer the masters of their own muscles. Movements previously performed automatically become difficult, and this often calls for a great input of will in order to start them and to overcome what sometimes appears to be a counterforce preventing them. This is partly the cause of the excessive fatigue.

As well as producing difficulty with the kind of daily activities previously described, bradykinesia and akinesia are at the root of communication problems arising from the expressionless face, the monotonous voice, and the absence of gesturing.

Balance and Walking Problems

People with Parkinson's disease have problems controlling the balance of their bodies. These problems are evident when the individual is sitting or standing, as well as when walking and moving about. When he or she is standing, the balance deficits are seen as a stooped posture, with the body bent slightly forward. This is a result of rigidity as well as problems with balance control. In an attempt to compensate for the balance problems, the legs are bent at the knees and the arms at the elbows, and the arms are often held in front of the body. The person may tilt to one side while sitting and be unable to correct this without help. The person with Parkinson's disease has problems getting out of a chair or bed or in and out of a car because he or she cannot bring about the necessary changes of balance and shifting of body weight to achieve these movements.

Balance problems are particularly evident during walking and turning. In Parkinson's disease, walking (or gait) has a number of characteristic features.

❖ The individual has difficulty starting to walk. This is called start hesitancy. He or she has problems lifting the foot in order to start walking and takes a few small uncertain steps before walking at a steady pace.

❖ The automatic swinging of the arms during walking is lost.

❖ The individual walks by taking a series of small, short steps, known as a *shuffling gait*. This derives from the reduced length of the stride, in which the feet are not raised high enough while walking.

❖ The individual walks with the bulk of the body weight on the front part of the feet so that there is no striking of the heels.

❖ These last two features result in the so-called *festinant* (or hurried) *gait,* in which walking consists of a series of small, short, shuffling steps that become increasingly rapid.

❖ Propulsion and retropulsion (literally, forward-pushing and back-ward-pushing) are the effects of the festinant gait. *Propulsion* occurs when the individual starts walking faster and faster with shorter and shorter steps while leaning forward, until he or she falls forward or is stopped by an obstacle. The tendency to lean backward and take a few hurried backward steps is called *retropulsion*.

❖ The individual has difficulty turning while walking. The body turns in one piece without the head twisting first, followed by the trunk and legs. There is also some hesitation when turning is carried out in a number of steps rather than smoothly.

❖ The loss of righting reflexes—that is, reflexes that compensate for an unexpected loss of balance—causes problems that result in falls. Approximately one third of people with Parkinson's disease fall rel-atively frequently. They flex their knees to prevent themselves from falling forward.

❖ When falls occur, people with Parkinson's disease cannot quickly throw out their arms to correct their balance or even to protect them-selves. For this reason, falls often cause injuries.

❖ *Freezing* can occur during walking. As mentioned previously, this mainly happens in doorways. A freezing episode lasting 10 minutes is very clearly described by Miss D., a woman with postencephalitic parkinsonism whose case history figures in Oliver Sacks' book, *Awakenings:*

It's like they [her feet] had a will of their own. I was glued there, you know. I felt like a fly caught on a strip of fly-paper. . . . I have often read

about people being rooted to the spot, but I never knew what it meant—
not until today.

❖ The festinant gait, propulsion, and retropulsion are partly brought on
   by the fact that, as a result of the stooped, forward-leaning posture,
   the center of gravity is not over the feet, and because the arms are
   not moved during walking, the appropriate stabilization is not provided.

The Minor Symptoms

Speech Problems: Dysphonia

Dysphonia in Parkinson's disease is an inability to raise the voice, which
results in a very low-volume soft voice that is barely audible to others. It
is caused by bradykinesia and rigidity affecting the many muscles of the
chest and throat that are involved in the production of speech by regu-
lating air flow through the larynx. The reduction in the volume of the
voice is often first noticed by the spouse or by colleagues, who may complain that the individual is mumbling. Dysphonia is sensitive to the individual's emotional and physical state and may become worse when he or
she is tired, depressed, or anxious. In the early stages of the illness,
however, he or she may be able to raise the volume through conscious
effort or when feeling emotional. With time, not only is the voice of low
volume, but also its normal modulation and rising-and-falling intonation,
the familiar sing-song of speech, are lost, and it becomes more
monotonous.

In addition to dysphonia, speech may show a number of other abnormalities, some of which mirror the problems seen during walking. There
may be hesitation in starting to talk or when answering questions, and
inappropriate silences in the middle. The person may get stuck on the first
word of a sentence and repeat it several times. Additionally, the "festina-
tion," or hurrying, experienced during walking may be present when
talking, so that the speech may speed up toward the end of a sentence.
There also may be some slurring. These changes in speech affect communication with other people—for example, they can cause problems when
the individual is using the telephone.

Writing Problems: Micrographia

Micrographia, a reduction in the size of handwriting, becomes evident when current and previous samples of a patient's handwriting are compared. The letters are well formed but small, and the script becomes smaller as writing continues. The alteration in size may be accompanied by cramps in the muscles of the hand and arm during writing—known as "writer's cramp." Writing problems generally improve with treatment.

Skin Problems: Seborrhea

This excessive oiliness and scaliness of the skin is especially noticeable around the forehead and nose, which appear shiny, and in the eyebrows, which may be full of dandruff. Another aspect of seborrhea is excessive sweating; sudden drenching sweats may occur for no apparent reason, requiring frequent changes of clothing.

Loss of Facial Expression: Masked Facies

Masked facies (pronounced fayshees), or an immobile and expressionless face, is often combined with a fixed stare. The failure to produce the variations of facial expression that normally accompany speech or emotional change results from the poverty of action and rigidity of the face muscles. Nonverbal cues are thus lost, making communication with the person with Parkinson's disease difficult. On the positive side, the immobility of the face muscles may give him or her a wrinkle-free and youngish-looking skin.

Swallowing Problems: Dysphagia

Dysphagia, a problem with swallowing, is caused by the reduced ability to transfer food from the mouth to the throat and by a reduced motility of the muscles of the esophagus, the tube that connects the throat to the stomach. As a result, saliva is not swallowed frequently enough, which causes dribbling. The disturbance of posture that tilts the head forward so that the chin points down makes the dribbling worse.

Autonomic Symptoms

Autonomic symptoms are produced by dysfunction in the autonomic nervous system, the part of the nervous system that controls the involuntary functions of the body, such as blood pressure, heartbeat, breathing rate, and movements of the stomach and intestines, the bowel and the bladder, and the sexual organs. The main autonomic symptoms of Parkinson's disease are postural hypotension, flushing, excessive sweating, urinary frequency and urgency, and constipation.

People with Parkinson's disease often have low blood pressure, particularly when standing; the pressure tends to fall when they stand up from a sitting position. This drop in blood pressure with change of body posture from sitting to standing is called *postural hypotension* and may be experienced as feelings of dizziness and light-headedness.

The bladder may not be properly emptied, so that several visits to the bathroom may be necessary instead of one. In addition, an urgent need to empty the bladder, even when only small volumes of fluid have accumulated, may result from a tendency for the bladder to be irritable. Such frequency and urgency can disturb sleep at night. Constipation, a frequent complaint, arises from the reduced motility of the bowels and is made worse by the general lack of physical activity and by treatment with anticholinergic drugs.

Pain and Other Sensory Symptoms

Although Parkinson's disease is a motor disorder, approximately 40 percent of people also experience sensory symptoms, such as pain, numbness, and tingling. However, on clinical examination or investigation these sensory symptoms are not found to be accompanied by any sensory deficits, and sight, hearing, and touch remain normal, although the sense of smell is affected in approximately 90 percent of people.

The pain that is frequently experienced by people with Parkinson's disease is partly a result of rigidity and reduced movement of the joints. A dull aching in a limb may be felt many months or even years before the first appearance of tremor or other symptoms. A number of people also report a burning sensation. Pain is experienced mostly in the neck, shoulders, and arms, and sometimes in the legs. The forward-leaning stooped posture during sitting, standing, and walking can also give rise to back pain.

Fatigue

Fatigue, or excessive tiredness resulting from a relatively small amount of physical activity, is common in Parkinson's disease. Everyday tasks that call for physical exertion, such as cleaning or gardening, require more effort to carry out. The person with Parkinson's disease may need frequent periods of rest to be able to complete such tasks. The fatigue is not purely physical, and some people talk of a sort of mental fatigue, or lethargy. The exaggerated fatigue reaction means that the individual often feels that both physical and mental activity require excessive exertion. This may lead to avoidance of many activities over time, so that in the later stages of the illness he or she may spend many hours at a stretch simply sitting idle.

Cognitive Deficits and Dementia

Cognitive functions include intellectual abilities and other activities concerned with perceiving, remembering, thinking, reasoning, language, and speech. Most people with Parkinson's disease do not show any intellectual decline or major cognitive deficits. However, more subtle cognitive change may be noticeable over time, such as difficulty in remembering, inability to concentrate or to keep attention focused on a task, and sluggishness in thinking and talking. Some of these problems were expressed by Steve, who had had Parkinson's disease for seven years:

I am less alert and more forgetful and unable to express my thoughts. I know what I want to say but the words just don't come out properly.

In general, people with Parkinson's disease show cognitive deficits when the tasks they have to deal with are difficult and require effort. Such cognitive impairment seems to be magnified when the individual has to plan and do intellectually demanding tasks in his or her own head without any external aids or reminders.

The age of onset of the disease is an important determinant of cognitive decline. Those who develop it after the age of 65 tend to be more cognitively impaired. Those with a mainly tremulous Parkinson's disease tend to be less cognitively impaired than people for whom bradykinesia and rigidity are the core symptoms.

Cognitive deficits are by no means universally present, as is evident in the case of Michael, a 71-year-old man who had had Parkinson's disease since the age of 61. He reported:

Between the ages of 65 and 70, I undertook two years' A level study at a college and three years at the University of the Third Age, where I have graduated with a BA degree. I found the mental stimulus of studying helped alleviate my symptoms.

A small number of people with Parkinson's disease develop *dementia*, which is a syndrome of intellectual decline and memory impairment severe enough to interfere with one's occupational and social functioning. Approximately 15 percent to 20 percent of Parkinson's patients develop dementia, compared with about 7 percent to 10 percent of the elderly population as a whole. This means that the risk of dementia is approximately 10 percent to 15 percent higher than the expected risk in the general population of the same age. Age of onset and rate of progression of the illness predict the likelihood of dementia; it is more likely when the disease first develops at a later age and when it progresses more rapidly. The nature of dementia in Parkinson's disease, and particularly the special needs of the Parkinson's patient who has developed this condition, are discussed in more detail in Chapter 7.

THE CAUSES

Understanding the cause or causes of the disease may be the first step in designing a cure for it. For this reason, questions about its cause or causes have always been a primary focus of medical research. Unfortunately, the cause of Parkinson's disease has not yet been discovered. We know that it develops in the aftermath of a drastic reduction of *dopamine*, one of the chemical messengers in the brain, as a result of the degeneration of the neurons, or nerve cells, that produce it in a little part of the brain called the substantia nigra. What we do not know is what causes the degeneration of the neurons in this area. To explain it, a number of different theories have been suggested. Although none of these has yet proved correct, we describe some of them in more detail later.

First, in considering the causes of Parkinson's disease, a distinction is usually made between primary and secondary parkinsonism.

Primary and Secondary Parkinsonism

What has become clear since the 1960s is that the core symptoms of parkinsonism—rigidity and bradykinesia—can have many causes and be present in a number of disorders other than Parkinson's disease. Approximately 76 percent of those who were diagnosed as having primary or *idiopathic*—that is, without a known cause—Parkinson's disease in life are found on postmortem examination to have a specific abnormality in the brain. This abnormality is a degeneration of the dopamine-producing neurons in the substantia nigra, accompanied by the presence in the remaining nerve cells of inclusions called Lewy bodies. Idiopathic Parkinson's disease is diagnosed when three of the five main symptoms (resting tremor, rigidity, bradykinesia, postural difficulty, and walking problems) are present, when there is no history of injury or illness or any other known cause of the symptoms, and when there is a good response to levodopa therapy.

For the remaining 24 percent, there are other causes, and they are therefore considered to have parkinsonism secondary to another illness or known cause. These various types of parkinsonism are listed in Table 1-2.

We now briefly consider the most common causes of secondary parkinsonism; in addition to those listed here, it may, very rarely, be caused by a tumor or head injury.

Postencephalitic Parkinsonism

Between 1916 and 1926 there was an epidemic of a viral infection, identified first in Vienna and other European cities, which subsequently spread throughout the world and which, among a host of other symptoms, also produced parkinsonism. The neurologist von Economo called this illness encephalitis lethargica, or sleeping sickness. The name derived from the fact that it involved inflammation of the brain (encephalitis) and one of the first symptoms was sleepiness (lethargica).

Many of the patients died in the early phases of the illness. In countries across the world a number survived but were severely disabled and confined to long-term care. The traumas of these patients and their short-lived periods of "awakening" with levodopa were movingly portrayed by Oliver Sacks in his book *Awakenings*, which was later dramatized on film.

Table 1-2. The various types of parkinsonism

1 IDIOPATHIC OR PRIMARY PARKINSON'S DISEASE

2 SECONDARY PARKINSONISM

Postencephalitic parkinsonism
Drug-induced parkinsonism

(a) Major tranquilizers, e.g., chlorpromazine
(b) Medication to reduce high blood pressure, e.g., reserpine

Parkinsonism caused by toxins, e.g., MPTP, carbon monoxide, manganese
Parkinsonism as part of other neurodegenerative disorders

(a) Multiple-system atrophy
　　Olivopontocerebellar atrophy
　　Striatonigral degeneration
　　Shy-Drager syndrome
(b) Steele-Richardson-Olszewski syndrome
(c) Corticobasal degeneration
(d) Wilson's disease
(e) Guam disease
(f) Vascular parkinsonism
(g) Parkinsonism associated with dementia, e.g., Alzheimer's disease
　　and diffuse Lewy body disease

Parkinsonism due to other causes: boxing, other head injury, hydrocephalus
Other causes of juvenile Parkinson's disease

Few survivors of the epidemic are alive today. New cases of postencephalitic parkinsonism have rarely been documented, and encephalitis lethargica is no longer a major cause of parkinsonism.

Drug-Induced Parkinsonism

Approximately 7 percent of people with parkinsonism have developed the movement disorder following chronic treatment with a particular medication. Any drug that blocks the action of dopamine—referred to as a *dopamine antagonist*—is likely to cause parkinsonism. Major tranquilizers used to treat schizophrenia and other psychotic disorders can cause it, as can drugs such as reserpine and methyldopa (Aldomet) used to treat high blood pressure, and some drugs used to treat indigestion, such as metoclopramide, or dizziness, such as prochlorperazine. The major characteristic of drug-induced parkinsonism is that it usually disappears when the medication is stopped. It may take a month or more after withdrawal of the drugs for the symptoms to disappear.

Parkinsonism Caused by Toxins

Environmental toxins also can cause parkinsonism. The condition sometimes develops following carbon monoxide or manganese poisoning, although this is very rare. The most intriguing demonstration of the ability of a toxin to produce parkinsonism is the "MPTP story." In 1982 there were reports from California that a number of young drug addicts had developed symptoms of parkinsonism virtually overnight. Further investigation by the neurologist J. William Langston and his colleagues revealed that all those affected had taken a "designer drug," synthesized to produce effects similar to those of heroin. The development of the classic symptoms of parkinsonism—tremor, rigidity, and bradykinesia—was related to the presence of a substance called MPTP (1-methyl-4-phenyl-1,2,3,6-tetrahydropyridine) in the drug, which in the body was converted to MPP+. MPP+ acted as a specific toxin, causing the death of the dopamine-producing neurons in the substantia nigra, the part of the brain that is affected in classic Parkinson's disease.

Parkinsonism as Part of Other Neurodegenerative Disorders

Since the mid-1960s, a number of other related disorders have been recognized that have the parkinsonian features of slowness and rigidity. In addition, these disorders have numerous other symptoms, underlying disease processes, and courses that are different from those of classic Parkinson's disease. A distinction is made between these "parkinsonism plus" syndromes and idiopathic Parkinson's disease. The parkinsonism plus disorders include various types of multiple-system atrophy, or MSA (striatonigral degeneration, olivopontocerebellar atrophy, Shy-Drager syndrome), Steele-Richardson-Olszewski (SRO) syndrome (also known as progressive supranuclear palsy or PSP), Wilson's disease, other causes of juvenile parkinsonism, and Guam disease. Postmortem studies have shown that MSA and SRO account for approximately 20 percent of all cases of parkinsonism encountered.

As some of these disorders are described in the next chapter, only Guam disease needs to be mentioned here.

Guam disease was recognized after reports of a higher than usual incidence of a parkinsonism and dementia together with motor neuron disease among the Chamorro natives of Guam. This was subsequently traced to the increased use of cycad seeds as part of their diet. These seeds contain a neurotoxin that causes parkinsonism.

Finally, there is the question of whether a stroke or a disorder of the blood vessels supplying the brain can cause parkinsonism. When a blood vessel is blocked by a clot, or bursts, the blood supply to an area of the brain is cut off, brain cells are deprived of oxygen and nutrients, and these brain cells die. The resulting area of dead tissue is known as an infarct. The basal ganglia have a rich blood supply, and rupture of the blood vessels rarely occurs there. In an elderly population, vascular or arteriosclerotic parkinsonism may be due to the overlap of cerebrovascular disease and parkinsonism, in which symptoms appear after a number of small strokes, perhaps as a result of sclerosis, or hardening, of blood vessels. Because of this possible overlap, vascular parkinsonism, which probably accounts for about 1.5 percent of all cases of parkinsonism, is sometimes called pseudo-parkinsonism.

Dopamine, the Substantia Nigra, and the Basal Ganglia

The brain is our most complex organ. It is made up of many hundreds of millions of cells. Neurons, or nerve cells, are designed in such a way as to maximize communication with other neurons. As shown in Figure 1-1, each neuron has a cell body, a long axon, and many shorter dendrites. The dendrites allow cross-talk between adjacent neurons. Dendrites receive messages from neighboring neurons and pass them on to the cell body, which sends a response down the axon and to the terminal buttons. Here a neurotransmitter (a chemical signal) is released, which transmits the message to another neuron via a synapse (shown in Figure 1-2), which is a cleft between two neurons that forms a communication bridge between neighboring neurons.

Classic Parkinson's disease—the type for which no apparent cause is found in the course of taking the history, in clinical examination, or from laboratory tests—develops when there is a degeneration of

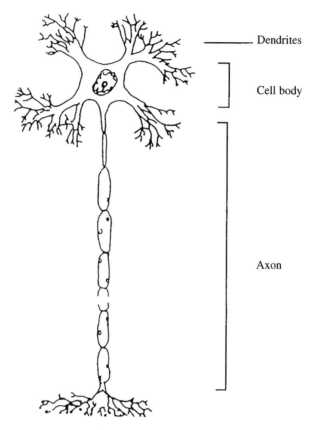

Figure 1-1.   A neuron

dopamine-producing neurons in that small area at the base of the brain called the *substantia nigra* (literally meaning "black substance"). It is called this because it contains black-pigmented neurons—neurons that normally are black because they contain a pigment called neuromelanin. These neurons normally produce the chemical dopamine, which is a neurotransmitter—that is, a chemical in the brain that helps convey messages between neurons. When the brains of people with Parkinson's disease have been examined after death, the substantia nigra is not black because it has lost its melanin-containing neurons. The cause of this degeneration of dopamine-producing neurons is not known.

The substantia nigra is connected to other groups of neurons located at the base of the brain, called the *basal ganglia*. The location of the basal ganglia in relation to other parts of the brain such as the *frontal cortex* (front section of the brain), the *thalamus* (the relay station connecting the basal ganglia to the frontal cortex), and the *cerebellum* (another area of the brain involved in motor function, located at the back of the skull) is shown in Figure 1-3. The basal ganglia consist of two parts, the striatum and the globus pallidus. The striatum is further subdivided into the caudate nucleus and the putamen. Reduction of dopamine in the substantia nigra results in reduction of dopamine in the striatum, particularly in the putamen. The symptoms of Parkinson's disease become manifest when nearly half of the neurons in the substantia nigra have degenerated and the amount of dopamine in the brain is reduced by 80 percent. For this reason, Parkinson's disease is considered a dopamine-deficiency syndrome. Another pathologic hallmark of the disorder is the presence of smooth spherical "bodies" with a pale halo called Lewy bodies (named after Frederick Lewy, who first described them) in the remaining neurons of the substantia nigra.

Besides the dramatic reduction of dopamine in the striatonigral (from "striatum" and "substantia nigra") system, dopamine is also dimin-

Figure 1-2. Communication between two neurons across a synapse through release of a neurotransmitter

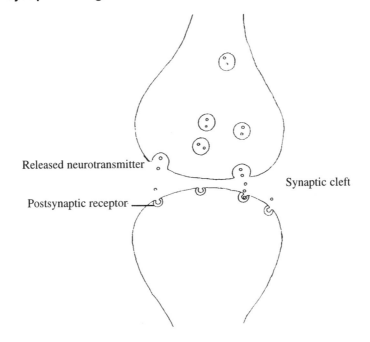

Released neurotransmitter

Postsynaptic receptor

Synaptic cleft

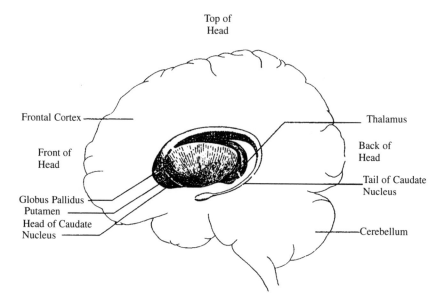

Figure 1-3. The location of the basal ganglia in relation to other parts of the brain (relative sizes do not represent the real scale)

ished in other areas of the brain. Neither is it the only chemical messenger, or neurotransmitter, that is affected in Parkinson's disease; others include *noradrenaline, acetylcholine,* and *serotonin.* Acetylcholine is another important neurotransmitter that is present in the striatum and in all other parts of the brain. Dopamine and acetylcholine seem to have a see-saw relationship, affecting each other in a reciprocal manner so that a decrease of dopamine is associated with an increase of acetylcholine. This is the case in Parkinson's disease, so that the pharmacologic treatment of the illness centers on substances that enhance the action of dopamine *(dopaminergic medication)* or inhibit the action of acetylcholine *(anti-cholinergic medication)*

Possible Causes of Classic Parkinson's Disease

From a scientific perspective, Parkinson's disease is important. It was the first neurologic disorder in which a specific chemical dysfunction in the brain was demonstrated. But although we know that the symptoms are due to the degeneration of dopamine-producing neurons, what we do not know is what causes this degeneration and the subsequent dopamine depletion in the basal ganglia. A number of factors have been considered as possible causes.

Inheritance

The question of whether Parkinson's disease is an inherited or a genetic disorder has been addressed in several ways. First, it was determined what percentage of identical twins both have Parkinson's disease. Because they are the product of the splitting of a single fertilized egg, identical twins have an identical genetic makeup. Similar rates of Parkinson's disease in identical twins would support the notion that genetic factors play a part in the disease. For comparison, nonidentical twins are also studied—that is, twins born of two separate eggs fertilized at the same time and so bearing as much genetic similarity as ordinary sisters and brothers. Recent studies have found 17 percent of identical and 10 percent of nonidentical twins to be concordant—that is, both twins in these instances have Parkinson's disease. These rates are higher than the respective rates of 8 percent and 5 percent reported by earlier investigators.

The second line of evidence concerns the percentage of people with Parkinson's disease who have an affected relative, with whom they share some genetic material and would therefore have a greater genetic similarity than with nonfamily members. Approximately 10 percent to 15 percent of people with Parkinson's disease report that they have a relative with similar symptoms. When these relatives have been examined by a neurologist, only about half of them are found to have Parkinson's disease, and the rest have other disorders such as essential tremor. This actual percentage, approximately 5 percent to 7 percent, is no higher than what we would expect from chance alone. On the other hand, in cases of familial Parkinson's disease—that is, families with many members having the disorder over several generations—also extensively studied, the evidence suggests that heredity does play a part. However, the weight of the evidence favors the proposition that in the majority of cases the genetic contribution to Parkinson's disease is not of primary importance.

Viral Infection

The postencephalitic parkinsonism of the 1920s epidemic was caused by a viral infection. The existence of this version of the illness has led to the hypothesis that Parkinson's disease may be a result of a slow-acting virus that could have invaded the brain early in life, many years before the onset of the symptoms. During the intervening years a slow degeneration of the dopamine-producing cells might have occurred, which is compensated until a level is reached beyond which compensation is no longer possible, at which point the symptoms become manifest. So far, the search for a viral agent has been fruitless, but if the pathologic process giving rise to Parkinson's disease *does* start many years before the appearance of the symptoms, risk factors arising much earlier in life need to be examined.

Environmental Toxins and Endogenous Toxic Processes

The current interest in environmental and endogenous (internally generated) toxins as possible causes of Parkinson's disease has been sparked by two events: first, the report of parkinsonism in drug addicts induced by MPTP; second, the report of parkinsonism as an aspect of Guam disease among the Chamorro natives. These two phenomena have led to the suggestion that Parkinson's disease might result from a toxin that gradually accumulates in the brain, causing the degeneration of particular neurons in the substantia nigra. This toxin could build up either through exposure to an environmental, or external, toxic source or as a by-product of an endogenous, or internally generated, process in the brain. Alternatively, it is possible that the disorder arises from exposure to a toxin in early life, together with the later natural aging of the striato-nigral system.

With regard to the *environmental toxin* hypothesis, the focus has been on finding a toxin that generates substances known as free radicals—oxygen molecules missing an electron that are attracted to other substances from which they can derive one. Free radicals can kill neurons by interfering with the fundamental metabolic processes that take place in mitochondria, tiny vesicles contained in all cells. Mitochondria are powerhouses of living cells where material is metabolized, or broken down, to generate energy. No such environmental toxin has yet been discovered. Again, there may be some difficulty in detecting the possible effects of environmental toxins if they had their causal effect early in an individual's life.

The suggestion that an environmental toxic material such as industrial pollutants, herbicides, and pesticides may cause Parkinson's disease has led to a search for variations in prevalence in different parts of the world and between rural and urban areas. No firm evidence has been obtained from these studies. Furthermore, the fact that the prevalence of the disorder has not altered significantly during the last hundred years, and that it is not confined to areas of the world in which industrial or agricultural pollutants and toxins may be more prevalent, makes it unlikely that a modern industrial pollutant or an agricultural herbicide is the culprit.

As far as the *endogenous toxic mechanism* hypothesis is concerned, there is evidence that the number of neurons in the substantia nigra declines as part of the natural aging process. Elderly people exhibit in mild form some symptoms that are reminiscent of Parkinson's disease, such as slowness of movement, a stooped posture, shorter strides, and a greater number of falls. This raises the question of whether the degeneration of the striatonigral dopaminergic system in Parkinson's disease represents an accelerated aging process. More specifically, it has been suggested that in Parkinson's disease the by-products of dopamine metabolism may act as endogenous toxins in the brain and may be the root of the degenerative process in susceptible neurons. The breakdown of dopamine produces free radicals and hydrogen peroxide, which can have toxic effects by interfering with normal oxidative metabolism in mitochondria and by damaging the membranes of neurons. That "oxidative stress" might be a possible mechanism of neuronal degeneration in Parkinson's disease is partly supported by studies that have shown mitochondrial abnormality in the disease. In addition, in the course of postmortem study, iron, which catalyzes (mediates) oxidative reactions has been found in increased concentrations in the brains of people with Parkinson's disease, even in the early stages of the illness. This also supports the notion of increased oxidative stress being a possible mechanism of neuronal degeneration. However, the nature of the trigger that sets off this chain of oxidative stress in Parkinson's disease is not known. Neither is it clear whether these changes are primary and causal or a consequence of the disease, or even a result of medication. Future research is needed to throw light on these alternatives.

Other Factors

As conscious beings with the ability to reflect on our experiences, we try to make sense of our lives and of what happens to us, so the tendency to seek reasons for or to identify the causes of our ills is quite natural. Because the precise cause of Parkinson's disease is not known, doctors cannot provide any causal explanations. However, this does not stop most people with the disease from searching for causes of their illness. Helen Rose, the author of *An Old-age Pensioner at Eighteen: or My Life with Parkinson's Disease,* exemplifies such attempts at causal attribution:

> *Who can I blame? Can I blame my parents? They both contracted polio when they were young children and were left with severe disability. But polio is an infectious disease—Parkinson's disease is not. So of course it is not their fault. Was it my own fault for banging my head when I fell from a railing that I was sliding down? No. There is no medical evidence to prove that theory. Is it because I was an unmarried mother? What a ridiculous idea. When I pull myself together, I give myself a thorough telling-off. How can anyone be to blame? But as yet, there are no explanations as to why the disease occurs. So, for the time being, I blame the operator on the assembly line for letting me through Quality Control.*

Most people with Parkinson's disease sometimes worry that any one of a number of other factors may have caused their illness, such as stress, diet, their personality, a tumor, or head injury. As mentioned previously, tumors or head injury very rarely cause parkinsonism. With regard to stress, some patients when questioned, report experiencing some form of stress or trauma before the start of the illness, such as loss of a loved one, undergoing an unwanted divorce, or loss of employment. But such events are also reported by people who suffer from other illnesses, so they cannot be considered as playing a specifically causal role. It *is* possible, however, that stress or trauma just before the first symptoms appear in fact precipitate those symptoms in individuals already predisposed to developing the illness.

With the current emphasis on the importance of diet and the popularity of the idea that "we are what we eat," it is not surprising that some people worry about the role that diet may have played in their illness. But with the exception of the cycad seeds consumed by the Chamorro Indians, evidence shows that diet does not play a part in the development of Parkinson's disease. People who eat the same food over long periods, such as husbands and wives and people living in institutions such as prisons, show rates of Parkinson's disease no higher than those in the general population.

The notion that this particular disease was in some way brought on by the individual's personality will not bear scrutiny either. Personality consists of the habitual patterns of thinking, feeling, and behaving that make each of us a unique individual. Our personality is shaped by the temperament we are born with and our subsequent life experiences. There have been some suggestions that certain "premorbid" personality types— those marked by rigidity, inflexibility, punctuality, precision, and obsessionality—are predisposed to Parkinson's disease. But there is little evidence to support this. Retrospective assessment of the premorbid personality—that is, of the personality before the start of the illness—is virtually impossible. Furthermore, any similarities that are observed in the personalities of people with Parkinson's disease are more likely to be the effects of common experiences of living with a chronic, progressive, and disabling illness. This is borne out by the fact that some people with other chronic illnesses such as essential tremor or dystonia (another movement disorder) are also found to have similar personality characteristics, indicating that such personality traits are in no way specific to any particular disorder.

KEY FACTS 1

What is Parkinson's disease?

Parkinson's disease is a neurologic illness—that is, a disease that affects the functioning of a small part of the brain. Its main symptoms are slowness of movement, tremor, rigidity, and problems with balance and walking.

How common is it?

It is a relatively common disorder. Approximately 1 in 1,000 people get it.

Who gets it?

Age is the only known risk factor. Symptoms usually appear after the age of 50 and the risk of getting the illness increases with age. However, in some cases it starts before the age of 40. Smoking is the only factor that shows a reverse association with Parkinson's disease—people who smoke seem less likely to develop it.

What causes it?

The symptoms of the disorder develop when dopamine-producing neurons in the substantia nigra degenerate and dopamine in the striatonigral pathways are reduced by approximately 80 percent. In classic Parkinson's disease, the causes of this degeneration and of dopamine deficiency are not known. We do know that the illness does not result from something the individual has done, from his or her diet, or from stress. With the exception of people with familial Parkinson's disease, heredity does not play a major causal role. What *is* possible is that some individuals have a genetic susceptibility to develop Parkinson's disease—for example, by being unable to deal with infectious agents or toxic material, whether induced by environmental factors or by some endogenous internal mechanism. There are numerous theories about the possible causes of the illness, but none is yet proved. Most investigators believe that the cause is likely to be multifactorial—that is, that many factors may play a role.

Is Parkinson's disease life-threatening?

Parkinson's disease is not a "killer disease." Treated with medication for its symptoms, it is to be feared no more than hypertension or diabetes when they are controlled with the appropriate medication. Parkinson's disease does affect the individual's daily activities and "quality of life."

Does it affect the intellectual faculties?

Only a minority of cases develop a true dementia—that is, intellectual decline and loss of memory. Many people with Parkinson's disease complain of isolated cognitive problems such as absent-mindedness, slowness of thinking, and difficulty with mentally effortful tasks. Others experience no noticeable change in their cognitive abilities.

2

Diagnosis and Prognosis

Diagnosis is the process by which a doctor decides what illness a person has. Diagnosis is important because it determines what the doctor does next—what advice he or she gives and the choice of treatment. The term we use is the "process of diagnosis," and we use it for two reasons. First, in most cases there is a delay between the first appearance of symptoms and their diagnosis, or labeling, by a doctor as Parkinson's disease. Second, it is not always possible to establish the diagnosis on the basis of a single consultation or test result. In some cases, the way the disease changes over time may alter the diagnosis.

A doctor diagnoses Parkinson's disease mainly by taking a history of the development of the symptoms from both the patient and a close relative, then making a clinical examination of the patient. A number of laboratory tests and scanning procedures are also carried out to exclude other causes of the symptoms. These tests are mainly for differential diagnosis—that is, to distinguish classic Parkinson's disease from other causes of parkinsonian symptoms. The *prognosis*, or prediction of the likely course of the illness, in any one individual is difficult. Nevertheless, there have been some attempts to identify factors that may predict the course or that may have prognostic significance.

In this chapter our aim is to provide you with information about the process of diagnosis and the factors that may affect the prognosis.

FIRST SYMPTOMS: THE PREDIAGNOSTIC PHASE

The symptoms of Parkinson's disease usually develop very gradually. The onset can be so gradual that a person may have difficulty recollecting precisely when the symptoms first appeared. This slow onset means that he or she may be aware of something being wrong for years before the symptoms are noticeable to family or friends, or evident enough to warrant a diagnosis of Parkinson's disease by a doctor. This early phase may be marked by periods of worry interspersed with self-reassurance, denial, and minimization of the significance of the perceived change.

The initial symptoms noticed by the individual vary from person to person. As mentioned in Chapter 1, tremor is the most commonly reported symptom. A number of less well defined symptoms usually precede the first appearance of tremor. A sense of weakness, slowness, or clumsiness of one arm or leg is commonly reported. The person may notice loss of manual dexterity or difficulty in using one arm during writing or daily activities such as shaving, fastening buttons, and putting on makeup. Getting out of chairs and cars or rolling over in bed may have become difficult. Some people complain of a sense of internal trembling before the development of resting tremor. Others remember feeling generally tired and being unable to perform tasks such as gardening or cleaning the house for long periods without taking a rest. The voice may lose its power and become inaudible to others. Pain, especially in the neck and shoulders, may be a common early complaint and may lead to a misdiagnosis of cervical spondylosis or arthritis.

The symptom or change in function that is perceived first and that brings the individual to medical attention probably also depends on his or her profession. For example, for an architect, slowness of hand movements or muscle rigidity that interferes with the ability to draw may be most noticeable. For a teacher or a singer, a lower voice may be noticed first, although it may not necessarily have been the first symptom to have developed.

Early changes in posture and balance, or loss of facial expression, occasionally are evident in photographs taken a number of years before the diagnosis of Parkinson's disease. Sometimes it is someone close to the individual who first notices that there is a change or that there is some-

thing wrong; slowness of movement or change in posture may be perceived by relatives. Alternatively, it may be someone who has not seen
him or her for some time who first comments on changes such as lack of
facial expression, sluggishness of action, or a change in posture. Gradual
change may go undetected by those who see us daily.

In the majority of cases, the symptoms of the disorder start on one
side of the body and progress to the other side over time. In some cases,
the asymmetry may persist, and one side may be affected more severely
than the other for the duration of the illness. In the early presymptomatic
phase, the change may be so mild that a doctor may be unable to detect
anything amiss in the course of the neurologic examination. Or, the clinical examination may reveal one noteworthy change that on its own does
not indicate a problem and would be insufficient for a diagnosis, but
which the doctor may record but not mention to the patient so as not to
cause unnecessary alarm. Or again, at this presymptomatic phase when
the initial symptoms are often only noticeable to the patient, it is possible
for doctors to dismiss them and write them off as being neurotic—in the
individual's mind rather than real.

Alternatively, the process of diagnosis may take multiple referrals
over years, as illustrated by the following comments:

*It took a long time for me to be diagnosed, although I think my symp-
toms were obvious.*

*My initial symptom was slowness of movement of my fourth finger. I
went to see my GP. The first diagnosis was pinched nerve. Later on, the
second diagnosis was arthritis. On a subsequent visit I was referred to a
rheumatologist, who finally referred me to a neurologist.*

FIRST CONTACTS WITH THE MEDICAL PROFESSION

The disease eventually will progress, and one or more of the symptoms
will become significantly noticeable. This brings the individual to medical
attention and a doctor diagnoses the illness. When the symptoms appear,
most people are likely to go first to see an internist, who either makes the

diagnosis or refers the individual to a neurologist or occasionally, if he or she is elderly, to a geriatrician. The majority of those referred to a neurologist are seen in the physician's office. Some may initially, or at a later stage, be admitted to a hospital for assessment. Here we briefly describe the first contact with your own physician and the procedures followed during neurologic consultations, focusing on what you can expect during an office visit or during a hospital stay.

The Internist/Primary Care Physician

Apart from his or her role in arranging a referral to a consultant neurologist, contact with your internist or family physician is very important in the management of Parkinson's disease in several ways:

- ❖ He or she is the doctor with whom you have probably been in contact for a considerable length of time, and who therefore knows the most about you and your general health and is best suited to discuss your specific needs.

- ❖ Your family physician will be concerned with the management of any other problems that you may have, whether an ear infection, arthritis, or heart trouble.

- ❖ Increasingly, access to most other sources of local help is usually arranged through referral by your primary care physician.

- ❖ Also increasingly common with "managed care," repeat prescriptions of medication may be obtained from your primary care physician.

- ❖ Most importantly, as Parkinson's disease is a chronic illness, continuity of care from a single doctor or personnel of an HMO has many advantages, not the least of which is the possibility of developing a warm and personal patient–doctor relationship that overcomes the need to explain afresh the history of your symptoms and your circumstances at each consultation.

In her book *Living Well with Parkinson's Disease*, Glenna Wotton Atwood lists her expectations of both specialists and primary care physicians:

Will listen to me, will treat me as a whole person, will not rush me, will respect my feelings, will explain his findings and will answer my questions, will educate me about my illness, will respect my intelligence and have me take an active role in decision-making, will be willing to refer to other doctors if their expertise might help me, will write up my visit and send me a copy for my records, will be available or will have an alternate who will be available after office hours in case of emergency, will be a person with whom I can feel comfortable.

These qualities would probably match what most people expect of any good doctor, and two of them are particularly important. First, the person with Parkinson's disease should be actively involved in the management of his or her illness, because he or she is the best person to inform the doctor about the benefits and side effects of any treatment. Second, doctors should be aware that besides needing medical treatment of the symptoms, the patient and his or her family also need emotional and practical support. There is much to recommend a holistic approach—that is to say, an approach that, in addition to treating the illness and its symptoms, considers the whole person and his or her circumstances and needs, while also attempting to manage the personal, emotional, and practical problems associated with the illness.

However, a good patient–doctor relationship depends on the patient's behavior as well as the doctor's. If you need more time to discuss your worries, try to do so even if the doctor seems pressed for time. If you do not understand a particular term or piece of information, ask for clarification. Clearly state your preferences about possible medical and complementary treatments. Many primary care physicians are likely to have a few patients with Parkinson's disease, so he or she should know something about it. If, over time, because of your personal interest you find that you have become more knowledgeable about the illness than is your physician, don't let it overshadow your relationship. Remember that every physician must deal with many disorders and that he or she handles the day-to-day management of many types of problems. Material is available from the many Parkinson's disease groups about the details of treating and managing the disease. If you believe that you are not getting the best care from your physician or that there is simply a personality clash, you may wish to see another physician.

The Neurologist

A neurologist specializes in the diagnosis of neurologic illness and its management. The type of neurologist involved in the diagnosis and care of Parkinson's disease has a special interest in movement disorders. Most people with Parkinson's disease will be initially diagnosed by a neurologist. There may then be follow-up contacts with the neurologic team for a number of years to tailor medication so as to achieve optimal control of symptoms and minimize disability. When complications arise, or when close monitoring of response to or alteration of medication is required, admission to a hospital may be arranged by the neurologic team.

The Neurologic Outpatient Clinic

The team in a neurologic outpatient clinic is headed by a neurologist and may include a number of other professionals. If the team works in a multidisciplinary fashion, it may include a nurse clinician, a psychologist, a physical therapist, a speech therapist, an occupational therapist, and a social worker. The neurologist has overall clinical responsibility for the patients, and each member of the team plays a particular role in patient care. Where such multidisciplinary teams exist, not all members necessarily become involved in each individual case—the involvement of particular team members will be dictated by the needs of each individual person.

The first visit is likely to take several hours. As with many physician appointments, prepare yourself for a wait and do not expect to be seen at the time specified for your appointment.

On your first visit to a neurologist who practices as part of a multidisciplinary team, you are likely to be first seen by a nurse clinician who will take down the history of the development of your symptoms and ask additional questions about your health since childhood and the health of your family; then there will be a neurologic examination. This procedure can take up to an hour. A waiting period may ensue, during which the nurse will discuss your case with other members of the team, and provide them with a summary of your history and the results of the clinical examination. While you are waiting, you may be asked to have a number of blood and urine tests or X-rays. Later, you will see the neurologist, who may ask further questions and carry out a clinical examination. At this stage you will usually be given a diagnosis by the neurologist. Some general information about the illness and a broad outline of what to expect in the coming years will be provided, often by the nurse clinician, together with suggestions about possible medical treatments.

Receiving the Diagnosis

Early diagnosis is important for several reasons. First, delay in diagnosis delays effective management and treatment of the disorder. Second, a delay in diagnosis may be demoralizing both for the person with Parkinson's disease and for his or her family. Knowing the correct diagnosis brings the reality of the illness home. It allows everyone involved to start the process of acceptance and adjustment and to consider the implications for their work, their finances, their daily lives, and their future prospects; and to start preparing and planning. After being given the diagnosis, some people obtain a second opinion from a second neurologist, usually one with a special interest in Parkinson's disease and other movement disorders. This seeking of a second opinion is further confirmation of the reality of the diagnosis, and it may in fact be this that finally brings the truth home.

For most people, contact with a neurologic team has a number of shortcomings. These include:

❖ Medical visits often involve rather one-sided communication. Most of the conversation centers on answering specific questions asked by the neurologist. For this reason, the patient and any accompanying relatives may feel frustrated that they have not had a chance to ask any questions or express their worries.

❖ The neurologist may know very little about the individual's life circumstances and about him or her as a person. The doctor often relies on what he or she is told by the patient, before arriving at diagnostic or therapeutic decisions. Research studies suggest that about 40 percent of people who are hospitalized with neurologic disorders have psychiatric problems such as depression, most of which (about 70 percent) remain undetected by neurologists. It appears that most neurologists simply don't ask about, and patients fail to report, any emotional or adjustment problems. So you and your family should be alert to this fact and bring any feelings of depression or anxiety to the attention of the neurologist.

In addition, many people are unhappy with the manner and circumstances in which they were first given the diagnosis. People can be upset by such things as the length of time taken for a final diagnosis to be arrived at and by the detached and sometimes rather unsympathetic manner in which diagnosis is given.

At the time of diagnosis, I did not feel that I was given any support. I was given very little information.

In retrospect, my initial diagnosis, which lasted five minutes, was pretty brusque. As I was, at that time, only marginally affected it didn't upset me. However, to someone more incapacitated it could have been very traumatic.

The neurologist who gave me the diagnosis did so in a very abrupt manner and responded to my devastation and disbelief with a flippant "You have at least five good years ahead," and appeared very dismissive of my "It's a life sentence" response! However, an hour later when I saw him again, he did put a very comforting arm around my shoulder. I think he realized then how shocked I was. I then spent some time having tests and coffee with a nurse—I'll never forget her, she was so caring and kind. I also wrote down many questions, as I was to see the neurologist again. This second discussion was well timed and conducted, as many decisions about taking medication, work and family had to be made eventually. The information gathered that day set me in motion, and concentrated my thoughts really well on those aspects which were of most importance.

Supposing Parkinson's disease to be a "killer," my very first reaction was one of horror, but once the consultant explained some of the basics of the condition and suggested I join the Parkinson's Disease Society, I quickly accepted the situation. I find the PDS literature of tremendous help to the "newcomer," and for consumption by friends and family too.

Despite the potentially negative impact that the diagnosis may have on the individual and the accompanying friend or relative, it is important for doctors to portray a realistic picture. Therefore, the question is not whether to tell the patient or not, but rather *how* to tell him or her, and what and how much information to convey. The manner in which information is conveyed about the illness early on may have paramount and lasting effects. A true expert diagnostician is a doctor who has up-to-date medical knowledge and astute powers of observation that enable him or her to diagnose even rare and unusual cases, combined with an understanding of the needs, hopes, and fears of the patient that allow him or her to communicate with that patient with sympathy and tact. That this is possible is reflected by the following experiences:

I found some doctors were very caring and absolutely marvelous, whereas others were hardly interested.

I cannot speak too highly of the way in which both my own GP and the neurologist dealt with me. If anyone could make such an occasion a pleasant experience, this particular neurologist could.

The manner in which the news was first broken to me was very professional and sympathetic.

Telling an individual that he or she has a chronic and progressive neurologic illness amounts to conveying unpleasant and sometimes devastating news. Clearly, this is not an easy task, and doctors may have difficulty in communicating the diagnosis in an empathic and caring manner for several reasons. First, like all other professionals, individual doctors differ widely in their personal manners and communication skills. Second, it is only relatively recently that the social nature of medicine has been emphasized in medical schools and the need to specifically train doctors in the art of communication has been recognized. Third, there is the inevitable process of becoming accustomed to dealing with trauma that occurs in the course of medical training and practice. Fourth, diagnosis is not always a straightforward exercise. Doctors, especially younger ones, can get so engulfed in the task of history-taking, clinical examination, and recording their observations that they forget the important interpersonal aspect of dealing with people.

These reasons may help explain the shortcomings of some doctors in the field of good communication, but they should not serve as excuses. The purpose of medical training at all stages, and the duty of each individual doctor, should be to cultivate such interpersonal and communication skills. Caring communication means being sensitive to the needs of each patient. People differ in the extent to which they want information, and with sensitivity the doctor can pick this up. The information should be tailored to the capacity of the individual. The truth should not be hidden, but neither should it be thrust upon someone who is indicating that he or she is not ready to deal with it. People come to terms with the reality of illness at their own pace. Obviously, communication is a two-way process and the person with Parkinson's disease and/or an accompanying relative need to be assertive enough to air their concerns if they don't want to leave the doctor's office in a bewildered state and full of unvoiced questions. In his book *Ivan: Living with Parkinson's Disease,* Ivan Vaughan, a psychologist, writes about both his immediate and his delayed reactions to being told by a neurologist that he had the illness:

I tried to remain casual and got up to leave, remembering the Marx brother's joke: "I've got Parkinson's disease, and he's got mine."

But shortly later:

As I passed through the doorway on my way out at the end of the interview a host of unasked questions began to crowd into my mind.

What is often overlooked by the doctor in the course of a busy day is that it is essential to *make* the time to convey information, to deal with worries, answer questions, and reassure the patient and his or her family.

THE NEUROLOGIC EXAMINATION AND THE DIFFERENTIAL DIAGNOSIS TESTS

No single test exists that can reliably lead to the diagnosis of Parkinson's disease. This particular diagnosis is a clinical decision arrived at by a doctor on the basis of his or her observation of the patient's appearance and behavior, from clinical examination, and from consideration of the history of the development of the disease in the case concerned. In addition, the patient may be referred for a number of laboratory tests, which are usually carried out in order to exclude other diseases. We briefly describe here what these various procedures entail.

The Neurologic Examination

The neurologic consultation has three major components: observation, history-taking, and neurologic examination. By the time the patient has walked through the door, said hello, and sat down, the neurologist will have made a number of important observations about his or her posture and gait, about the presence or absence of arm swing, and the tone of voice. In the course of the appointment, the doctor continues to observe the patient's behavior—noting, for example, the presence or absence of spontaneous changes of posture, crossing and uncrossing of the legs, automatic hand gestures during talking, blinking, changes of facial expression.

The neurologist combines this observation with taking the history of the illness from the patient and the accompanying relative. This account covers a number of topics, such as the course of the illness from the onset to now—what were the first symptoms noticed? when did they develop? what happened subsequently? any previous medical consultations, tests, or treatments?—plus any history of other illnesses or hospitalizations or medication taken, any periods of psychological trauma and stress or physical injury, any family history of similar symptoms or disorders. Questions of a more personal nature may also be asked—about marital status, occupational history, social and leisure activities.

Then comes the neurologic examination, which may first concentrate on assessment of the functioning of the sensory organs: the eyes, ears, and senses of touch and sometimes smell. The doctor may move on to examine the functioning of the muscles and of the nerves that connect them to the spinal cord and the brain. He does this by asking you to tense particular muscles or to move parts of your body against resistance. The doctor assesses muscle tone by passively moving each body part while it is relaxed, to determine if rigidity is present. A special hammer is used to test reflexes. To bring out any slowness in initiating and executing movements and any worsening of bradykinesia with certain types of movement, the doctor will ask you to carry out different movements. You are asked to perform these movements with both the right and the left hands, in order to determine whether bradykinesia is bilateral or confined to one side of the body. As mentioned in Chapter 1, tremor is a symptom of other disorders besides Parkinson's disease: it can be present in essential tremor, cerebellar disease, anxiety states, and thyroid disease. The doctor may spend some time doing a differential diagnosis (see next section) of tremor in order to distinguish the Parkinson's tremor from the other forms.

Posture while standing, walking, sitting, and getting out of a chair is noted. Balance is tested by recording the effects of a gentle push on your stability. Also, you will be asked to write a short sentence as a sample of your handwriting. To bring out any writing tremor, you will be asked to draw a number of concentric circles. The body temperature may be taken and the pulse and blood pressure assessed while sitting as well as while standing. The neurologic examination usually includes a number of quick tests of mental state. General orientation in time and place will be assessed by asking you the date and the name and location of the hospital. Ability to do mental tasks may be evaluated with the "serial sevens" test, which involves asking you to count backwards from 100 in steps of seven. Memory is tested by asking you to retain and then recall after a few minutes a series of words.

The Laboratory Tests Used for Differential Diagnosis

To rule out other illnesses, the neurologist may recommend a number of laboratory tests such as a blood test, urinalysis, and tests of autonomic function; recording the electrical activity of the brain (the electroencephalogram, or EEG) or of the activity of muscles and nerves (the electromyogram or, EMG; and nerve conduction studies, or NCS); and maybe one or more types of brain scan (computed tomography, or CT; magnetic resonance imaging, or MRI). Occasionally, a lumbar puncture to examine the spinal fluid may be required. These tests, which are described in more detail below, allow the doctor to arrive at the diagnosis of classic Parkinson's disease (cause unknown) by a *process of exclusion.*

The first purpose of these tests is to exclude any treatable cause for the observed symptoms. For example, low levels of the hormone thyroxine produced by the thyroid glands located at the front of the neck can result in hypothyroidism, which can also slow down movements. A blood test will reveal such a deficiency, which can then be easily treated. As we said in Chapter 1 and as is evident from Table 2-1, the symptoms of Parkinson's disease can be an integral part of a number of disorders other than classic Parkinson's disease. The second purpose of the tests is to allow the doctor to distinguish among the various syndromes that can cause the symptoms of parkinsonism.

According to standard diagnostic criteria, a person is considered to have classic Parkinson's disease when bradykinesia is present together with at least one other symptom, which can be muscular rigidity, resting tremor, or postural instability. Other positive criteria that would support the diagnosis are unilateral onset or persisting asymmetry of symptoms, the progressive nature of the disorder, an excellent initial response to levodopa lasting five or more years, severe levodopa-induced abnormal movements, and a clinical course of ten or more years.

As mentioned previously, there is no test on a living patient that will result in a definite diagnosis of classic Parkinson's disease; the clinical diagnosis of the disorder can be confirmed only by post-mortem pathologic examination. Nevertheless, despite being largely based on clinical judgment, the accuracy of such a diagnosis is relatively high. Studies have shown that in about 80 percent of those diagnosed during life as having Parkinson's disease the diagnosis is confirmed post-mortem. In such cases, in addition to degeneration of the substantia nigra, the presence of Lewy bodies (spherical bodies surrounded by a halo), mentioned earlier, is a characteristic pathologic finding. The remaining 20 percent of cases are found to have other causes for their symptoms. Multiple-system atrophy, Steele-Richardson-Olszewski syndrome (progressive supranuclear palsy), and corticobasal degeneration account for the majority of the misdiagnoses. These disorders are called akineto-rigid or parkinsonism-plus syndromes, because akinesia and rigidity are their symptoms; they also have a number of additional symptoms not seen in classic Parkinson's disease.

Multiple-system atrophy, progressive supranuclear palsy, and corticobasal degeneration are distinguished from Parkinson's disease in three major ways:

1. Unlike Parkinson's disease, the parkinsonism-plus syndromes are rarely responsive to levodopa therapy; even if it seems to help a little at first, its long-term efficacy is relatively limited. In contrast, in Parkinson's disease, once the symptoms have become disabling, the introduction of levodopa produces a clear beneficial effect that persists for many years before the appearance of complications such as on–off fluctuations and dyskinesias.

2. Parkinsonism-plus syndromes show additional symptoms and signs that are atypical of Parkinson's disease. For example, in Steele-Richardson-Olszewski syndrome a downward-gaze palsy (inability to move the eyes down), and a more frequent and certain occurrence of dementia, are additional features. The presence of apraxia (inability to carry out symbolic movements on command such as blowing a kiss or waving goodbye) and alien limb phenomenon (not feeling in control of the activities of an arm or leg) are characteristic of corticobasal degeneration. Early and severe autonomic symptoms (such as fainting and urinary incontinence) and the presence of cerebellar ataxia (uncoordinated movement) or pyramidal signs (spastic muscles and brisk tendon reflexes) are the distinct features of multiple-system atrophy.

3. Two other features can also help in the differential diagnosis. The absence of resting tremor and frequent falls early in the course of the disorder are usually indicative of a diagnosis other than Parkinson's disease.

Distinguishing these parkinsonism-plus syndromes from classic Parkinson's disease is not always easy, because some abnormalities of eye movement or mild autonomic dysfunction can occur in idiopathic Parkinson's disease, and dementia, as noted in Chapter 1, is a late feature of the disorder in a small proportion of patients. Furthermore, it is usually only when the patient has been seen on a number of occasions over many years and when changes in symptoms during this follow-up period have been observed that it becomes possible to distinguish these disorders from each other.

We now describe some tests commonly used to distinguish classic Parkinson's disease from the parkinsonism-plus syndromes and to exclude other causes for the symptoms.

Blood and Urinalysis

Examination of the urine and blood can be useful indicators of the normality or abnormality of the levels of various chemicals secreted by the body's glands or organs and of the presence of infections. These analyses usually focus on tests of thyroid and liver function. There are no changes in blood count or blood chemistry that would help in the diagnosis of Parkinson's disease. The results of the blood and urine analysis are usually normal in Parkinson's disease, unless the individual is suffering from other disorders such as thyroid disease or diabetes.

X-rays of the Chest and Neck

The X-ray is a radiologic technique that uses small amounts of radioactive material to provide a picture of an internal part of the body. A chest X-ray provides an image of the lungs and the heart, while from an X-ray of the neck, the cervical spine (vertebrae of the neck) can be seen. The results of the chest X-ray are normal in Parkinson's disease, unless the individual has an infection or a cardiac or pulmonary disorder. In some people the neck X-ray is likely to reveal a degree of cervical spondylosis, or deformation of the neck vertebrae, that occurs as a result of age in a proportion of the population.

Electroencephalography

The brain emits electrical activity that can be detected with the right equipment. Electroencephalography, also referred to as EEG, is a method of measuring the electrical activity of the brain using sensors that are temporarily glued to the surface of the scalp. Tumors, strokes, and epilepsy can affect the EEG, which will show an abnormal pattern of activity in such cases. The EEG results are normal in Parkinson's disease.

Special kinds of EEG-recording, involving the presentation of certain light flashes or patterned visual stimuli, auditory tones or clicks, or small electrical stimuli applied to the skin, are used to assess the functioning of particular sensory areas in the brain and of the corresponding sensory pathways in the nervous system. These are called visual evoked potentials (VEPs), auditory evoked potentials (AEPs), and somatosensory evoked potentials (SSEPs), and respectively assess the visual, auditory, and somatosensory pathways in the nervous system. AEPs and SSEPs are normal in Parkinson's disease, while VEPs are reported as abnormal; this may be related to the reduction of dopamine normally present in the retina.

Electromyography

The electromyogram (EMG) is recorded to assess the functioning of the skeletal muscles (the muscles attached to the skeleton, including the spine, that produce movement). The electrical activity generated by the muscles is measured by means of special sensors placed over the muscles of the arms or legs. The EMG may reveal the presence of resting tremor before it becomes noticeable. In Parkinson's disease, the size of the first "muscle burst" that triggers the muscle into activity is reduced. This may be partly responsible for deficits in force generation and slowness of movement in the disorder.

The Measurement of Nerve Conduction Velocity

Here the aim is to measure the speed with which information is conveyed from the motor areas of the brain, via the motor neurons, to the muscles. To do this, a motor neuron is stimulated at two separate points along its course over the skin, and the time of the onset of activity (motor unit potentials) produced in an associated muscle is recorded. From this the delay between the stimulus and the start of the contraction of the muscle is measured, which allows the rate of conduction of the impulse along the motor neuron to be calculated. The stimuli used are usually small electrical shocks that can be perceived but are relatively painless. Nerve conduction velocity is normal in Parkinson's disease.

Computerized Tomography

The CT scan is a form of X-ray of the brain that reveals any abnormal changes in its structure. The head is placed in an X-ray tube containing many radiation detectors, which can rotate around the head and take pictures at various angles. A large number of measurements are taken, and from these a computer reconstructs a series of images that can reveal the presence of any tumors or other structural abnormalities such as signs of previous strokes. In Parkinson's disease, the CT scan may show a number of nonspecific changes—that is, changes that are also found in other disorders and may be partly associated with the normal process of aging.

Magnetic Resonance Imaging

The MRI scan is a more sensitive method of obtaining information about any changes in brain structure. (MRI does not involve radiation or the use of radioactive substances.) The head is placed in a tube that contains a powerful magnet, which aligns all the water molecules in the head with the magnetic force. In the presence of radio waves, the water molecules emit electromagnetic energy that is detected by special sensors; a computer then constructs images from these measurements. The MRI scan does not show any structural changes in the brain specific to Parkinson's disease, although some investigators have reported that the intensity of the signal received from the substantia nigra is reduced.

Positron Emission Tomography

The PET scan provides "functional" anatomic information about the brain. This means that with PET scans it is possible to assess the functioning of different parts of the brain while the individual is carrying out a particular movement or engaging in a specific mental activity. With PET it is also possible to examine the state of particular neurotransmitter receptor sites in the brain. PET scans require the use of radioactive material in very small quantities, usually equivalent to the radioactive exposure during a transatlantic flight. The dopaminergic systems in the brain can be assessed with PET scanning. Fluorodopa scans have shown that the capacity to take up levodopa and convert it into dopamine in the striatum is decreased in Parkinson's disease. This, in effect, has confirmed the specific dopamine deficiency of Parkinson's disease in living patients. Single-photon emission computed tomography (SPECT) is a cheaper but far less sensitive alternative to PET.

The Lumbar Puncture

The cerebrospinal fluid (CSF) is a clear and colorless liquid that fills the ventricles, or cavities, of the brain and the middle of the spinal cord and acts as a protective cushion for the brain and spinal cord against external pressure. The exchange of chemical material that occurs between the CSF can be of value in the diagnostic process. A specimen of the CSF and the blood allows the removal of metabolic waste products from the nervous system. Examination of the chemical contents of the CSF is obtained by a doctor carrying out a lumbar puncture. He or she will ask the patient to lie curled up in a fetal position, then insert a needle, under local anesthesia, into the lumbar region (lower back) below where the spinal cord ends. Microbiologic assessment and examination of the chemical contents of the CSF usually reveal no abnormalities in classic Parkinson's disease.

Autonomic Function Tests

These tests evaluate the functioning of the autonomic nervous system. Tests of autonomic function include assessment of blood pressure with changes in body position—from lying to tilting, to sitting, to standing. Changes in blood pressure are also assessed in a number of other situations: before, during, and after exercise, while doing mental arithmetic; while hyperventilating (taking fast and shallow breaths), or before and after putting one hand in ice-cold water for about two minutes. Autonomic disturbances such as excessive sweating and salivation, urinary urgency, constipation, and postural hypotension do occur in Parkinson's disease, as we noted earlier, but severe autonomic symptoms, particularly in the early stages of the illness, are usually indicative of multiple-system atrophy, one of the parkinsonism-plus syndromes.

Vestibular Function Tests

These tests assess the vestibular system located in the inner ear, which plays a role in the control of body balance. The main components of the vestibular system are three fluid-filled semicircular canals located at right angles to each other, which detect and compensate for changes in body position. Vestibular function is tested by maneuvers that stimulate these semicircular canals, such as quick changes of body position from standing to lying, or quick turning of the head to the right and left. Alternatively, caloric stimulation may be employed to assess vestibular function; during the caloric test, the right and left ears are in turn irrigated with cold and then warm water. This stimulation results in slow movements of the eyes that occur like the beating of a metronome, the duration and direction of which are noted. Vestibular function is not impaired in Parkinson's disease.

The Neuropsychological Assessment

People with Parkinson's disease are often referred to a clinical psychologist or neuropsychologist for a neuropsychological assessment. The main purpose of this is twofold. First, this kind of cognitive assessment may confirm the presence of dementia, which, particularly in the early stage of Parkinson's disease, would be considered atypical and would suggest a diagnosis other than classic Parkinson's disease. Second, mild cognitive dysfunction does occur in Parkinson's disease, and neuropsychological assessment establishes a baseline against which any future change can be assessed. Such an assessment usually takes between one and two hours, during which the patient performs a number of tests of cognitive function, including tests of intellectual ability, memory, attention, language, verbal fluency, and planning.

While, despite the various clinical and laboratory tests, no diagnostic marker of Parkinson's disease exists, the search for a specific test continues. This is outlined in more detail in Chapter 13.

Research-Related Tests

In addition to the clinical tests that are carried out to help in the diagnosis of Parkinson's disease, you may be asked to take part in studies for research purposes. This can happen while you are in the hospital or when you are being seen in the physician's office. The purposes and procedures of these research studies will be explained, so that you can decide whether to participate. Although they may be of no particular value to any one patient, it is important to remember that such research studies are the stepping-stones to our fuller understanding of Parkinson's disease, its causes, and its optimal treatment. All the same, you always have the option of declining to take part in them.

In his book *Parkinson's Disease: A Patient's View,* Sidney Dorros, who took part in the initial clinical trials to assess levodopa therapy, talks about the rewards of being a pioneer patient:

I've often been helped over difficult emotional periods by reflecting on my role as a pioneer experimental patient in the development of a medication that is helping thousands of fellow victims of parkinsonism. This satisfaction is enhanced by my recent discovery of the significance of some of the incidental basic research studies that were conducted on me while I was hospitalized six different times between 1970 and 1973. . . . During these few years, I estimate that I contributed hundreds of gallons of urine, dozens of quarts of blood, and a few pints of spinal fluid to the NIH [National Institute of Health] laboratories—all taken under special conditions designed to add to the basic information about the mechanisms of Parkinsonism, the drugs used to treat it, and the reactions of the body to both. Some of the information has been of direct help to me; some has led to improved treatment for Parkinsonism over a long time, sometimes indirect, route. . . .

PROGRESSION AND PROGNOSIS

What comes after diagnosis? Invariably one of the immediate concerns of the person who has been diagnosed as having Parkinson's disease is to find out what the course of the illness is likely to be.

Parkinson's disease is a progressive illness, which means that the symptoms gradually get worse over time. How quickly this progression occurs is difficult to determine. The only thing that can be said with any certainty is that it varies from person to person. For this reason, it is difficult to predict the likely course of the illness or to give a definite prognosis for any one individual. The symptoms may remain mild and unchanged for decades. Both before and after the levodopa era, a proportion of cases—about 5 percent to 10 percent—have been reported as following a mild course, with little disability during the first 10 years. Alternatively, the illness may rapidly progress to severe disability over a few years. Approximately 6 percent to 15 percent of cases show such a progression. The majority of cases lie somewhere between these two extremes.

Research studies have tried to determine whether the rate of progression and the prognosis are different for particular types of Parkinson's disease. The results of several research studies have suggested that three clinically distinct types of the illness can be distinguished in this respect.

1. *Classic type*   Most people with Parkinson's disease can be considered to have the "classic" disease, with akinesia, rigidity, and tremor. This type starts before or after the age of 60, is initially unilateral, then gradually develops into a bilateral disorder. Patients respond well to levodopa, and fluctuations do not develop until three to five years after starting such therapy.

2. *Akineto-rigid type*   This subgroup represents about 6 to 15 percent of all cases and tends to have a less favorable prognosis. Initial response to levodopa is not outstanding, and response fluctuations and involuntary movements may develop soon after starting treatment. Dementia and depression are also more common with this type of disease.

3. *Tremulous type*   Having tremor as the first presenting symptom and as the predominant symptom subsequently has been found to be prognostically favorable. This type of Parkinson's disease shows a slow progression and is less likely to be associated with depression and dementia. It probably constitutes about 5 percent to 10 percent of all cases.

Some evidence supports the distinction among these three subtypes. But there is also evidence that Parkinson's disease with tremor as the dominant feature and Parkinson's disease with predominantly akineto-rigid symptoms are not necessarily different in terms of prognosis. Furthermore, it may not be easy, whether immediately after the onset of the illness or in the early stages, to classify individual cases as being of one kind or another. Since the various symptoms develop at different times, classification may be possible only after observation of the clinical course of the disease. In addition, it is not clear whether the three subtypes of Parkinson's disease—the classic, the tremulous, and the akineto-rigid— differ in terms of the underlying disease process. A preliminary post-mortem study of small groups of people with Parkinson's disease did not find any pathologic differences between the akineto-rigid and tremulous types.

Progression has been examined in a number of ways. Various schemes for quantifying the severity of the illness over time have been developed. One such procedure involves the use of a stages-of-illness scale, devised by Drs. Hoehn and Yahr and their colleagues and subsequently known as the Hoehn and Yahr scale. This classifies Parkinson's disease into stages 1 to 5 (from mild to very severe).

Stage 1   The main symptoms—tremor, rigidity, bradykinesia, and postural abnormalities—are unilateral.

Stage 2   The disease has become bilateral, and other minor symptoms such as facial masking and swallowing and speech difficulties may have developed.

Stage 3   The same bilateral symptoms are present but may be somewhat worse. The important feature is that balance problems have appeared for the first time.

Stage 4   The patient has become increasingly disabled and needs help with some or all activities of daily living.

Stage 5   The patient is confined to a wheelchair or bed and needs complete assistance.

With the Hoehn and Yahr stages-of-illness scale, an index of progression was obtained by determining the average duration of the illness at each of the five stages, both for patients receiving levodopa therapy and those whose illnesses were untreated. At stage 2, the average duration of illness for treated cases was 9 years, compared to 6 years for untreated ones; at stage 3, it was 12 and 7 years, respectively, for treated and untreated cases; at stage 4, 12 years as opposed to 9 years; and at stage 5, 18 years compared with 14.

From these figures it is clear that levodopa delays progression through the stages by three to five years. However, levodopa therapy does not appear to alter the *rate* of progression of the illness. Many studies have tried to find out whether there are any associations between levodopa therapy and progression, but the results have been contradictory. Despite the controversy, however, comparison of data from the pre- and post-levodopa era suggests that treatment with levodopa has increased the life expectancy of people with Parkinson's disease. Some investigators argue that the prolonged life expectancy is dependent on starting levodopa therapy early in the course of the illness. Others disagree, reasoning that early levodopa treatment simply means that the drug will lose its efficacy and fluctuations will develop earlier in the course of the illness. The latter group propose that the primary guideline for starting levodopa therapy should be the indication that the symptoms in any given case are associated with moderate to severe disability that is interfering with the occupational and social life of the individual.

Selegiline has been approved by the Food and Drug Administration for use in the United States. Its suggested dose is 10 mg per day in two 5 mg doses taken before noon.

As is discussed in the next chapter, the use of a class of medication called monoamine oxidase inhibitors type B (MAO-B inhibitors) has been shown to "protect" laboratory animals against MPTP-induced parkinsonism. MAO-B type medication such as selegiline has therefore been used in the symptomatic treatment of Parkinson's disease, with the possibility that it may slow down the progression of the illness. The evidence at the moment is contradictory, and further investigations are required. The development of medication that can slow progression is a focus of current research.

KEY FACTS 2

What will the process of diagnosis involve?

Usually, the symptoms of Parkinson's disease develop gradually. The process of diagnosis usually starts when the individual consults his or her primary care physician, who will usually refer him or her to a neurologist or geriatrician. Besides taking the history of the development of the symp-

toms and conducting a neurologic examination, the neurologist may recommend that a number of laboratory tests be carried out, the results of
which will help in the process of differential diagnosis, to distinguish
classic Parkinson's disease from other conditions that produce parkinsonism. There is as yet no marker or specific test that helps in the diagnosis of the illness. It is diagnosed on the basis of clinical examination of
the patient by a neurologist and by exclusion of other causes for the symptoms.

How will the symptoms evolve over time?

Parkinson's disease is a progressive disorder, which means that the symptoms become more severe over time. However, the rate of progression
varies widely. The time between the onset of the symptoms and severe disability and dependency varies between three and thirty or more years. The
course can vary from a very mild disease that remains static for many
years to a more aggressive form of the disorder, with rapid progression
and severe disability within a few years.

Can the likely course of the illness be predicted?

It is not possible to predict the likely course of the illness in any one individual. However, there is some evidence that the predominance of tremor
may indicate a better prognosis, whereas the akineto-rigid form of the disorder may be associated with a less favorable one.

Can the progression be stopped or slowed down?

It cannot be stopped completely, but the development of medication that
can slow it down is a major focus of research.

Will the medication remain effective in controlling the symptoms?

Over time, most types of medication become less effective in controlling
the symptoms of Parkinson's disease. But once again, there are major
individual differences. Some patients require only minor changes in med-

ication, or in the timing of taking it, in the course of the illness. For others, frequent and major alterations of medication may become necessary to adequately control the symptoms.

Will I become totally incapacitated?

With progression of the illness and with the loss of efficacy of the medication after prolonged use, a proportion of people with Parkinson's disease become incapacitated, require a wheelchair, and become dependent on others for most daily activities. For most people, this is likely to happen, *if* it does, many years after first developing the illness.

3

The Medical and Surgical Treatment of the Symptoms of Parkinson's Disease

Although there still is no cure for Parkinson's disease, its medical treatment has come a long way since the first description of the disorder in 1817 by James Parkinson. In his *Essay on the Shaking Palsy*, Parkinson recommended that "blood should be first taken from the upper part of the neck, unless contraindicated by any particular circumstance. After which vesicatories should be applied to the same part, and a purulent discharge obtained." Although prescribing what was probably relatively standard treatment for most illnesses in the 1800s, Parkinson was acutely aware of the gaps in knowledge about the disorder; he also wrote, "Until we are better informed respecting the nature of this disease, the employment of internal medicines is scarcely warrantable." The difficulty in finding an effective treatment was also acknowledged by Jean-Martin Charcot, the famous French neurologist, who in the course of his lectures at the Salpêtrière Hospital noted: "Everything, or almost everything, has been tried against this disease."

This state of affairs changed only when a series of discoveries in the 1950s and 1960s revolutionized the symptomatic treatment of Parkinson's disease. In 1957 dopamine was discovered to be one of the neurotransmitters, or chemical messengers, in the brain. This was shortly followed by the demonstration that dopamine deficiency was a hallmark of Parkinson's disease. The new therapeutic era of the disorder dawned in the 1960s, when *levodopa* was administered to patients, and was found to control the symptoms effectively when given in large enough dosages. In the intervening years, experience of long-term therapy with levodopa has highlighted the possible complications that can occur and has led to further refinement of this form of drug treatment. Partly in response to the long-term complications of levodopa therapy, other avenues have been explored and developed, resulting in treatment with *dopamine agonists* (chemical substances having a similar effect to that of dopamine) and neuroprotective therapy, to slow down the progression of the disease. The 1980s and 1990s have been marked by other therapeutic explorations, mainly the development of a number of new surgical procedures for treating the symptoms of Parkinson's disease.

This chapter provides information about the two main forms of treatment currently used in Parkinson's disease: treatment with *medication* and treatment with *surgery*. Other therapies used to manage the illness are considered in Chapter 9.

MEDICATION

Medications are commonly available as tablets or capsules. Tablets have the advantage that they often have a groove on one side that makes it easy to break them in half for smaller doses; capsules are easier to swallow. More sophisticated methods of drug delivery have recently been developed. For example, controlled-release tablets of Sinemet (Sinemet CR) are manufactured in such a way that they are gradually broken down and absorbed in the stomach, making levodopa available to the brain for a longer period. Small portable pumps have also been used for the continuous delivery of dopamine agonists such as lisuride and apomorphine. The majority of drugs are available in several different strengths, or doses. The dose, 50 mg, say, refers to the amount of active ingredient contained in the tablet or capsule. For most medications there are recommended therapeutic doses, which are achieved by taking one or more tablets of a particular dose each day. This optimal daily amount may vary somewhat from person to person, depending on body weight and metabolism.

Most drugs have two types of label: a generic and a brand name. The generic name is the scientific name of the medication, sometimes referring to the composition of the drug—that is, the chemicals it contains. For example, trihexyphenidyl, the generic name for Artane, refers to its active contents. The brand name is the trade label given to the medication by the drug company that made it. Different companies give different brand names to the same drug, and the same drug is often produced under different names in different countries. The generic and brand names of the medications most frequently used in the symptomatic treatment of Parkinson's disease are given in Table 3-3.

General Principles

Because the cause of Parkinson's disease is not known, treatment is not aimed at eliminating the cause, but at controlling the symptoms. However, the aim of drug therapy is not to make the individual completely free from symptoms, but rather to prevent those symptoms from causing severe disability and handicap, so that he or she can continue living and working independently. More recently, as we noted in Chapter 2, medical treatment has also been aimed at slowing the progression of the illness—an aspect of therapy that is still in its infancy.

The aim of all medications currently used to treat Parkinson's disease is to normalize neurotransmitter function in the affected areas of the brain, particularly the striatonigral region (see p. 23). As we noted earlier, Parkinson's disease is characterized by a reduction in dopamine and a lesser reduction in another brain chemical, *acetylcholine*. As a result, the medical treatment of Parkinson's disease centers on substances that enhance the action of dopamine (*dopaminergic medication*) or inhibit the action of acetylcholine (*anticholinergic medication*). As the disorder is primarily a dopamine-deficiency syndrome, dopaminergic medications are much more effective than are the anticholinergics, which produce only about 25 percent symptomatic relief.

So the main focus of treatment is to boost dopaminergic transmission in the brain, which can be achieved by several different strategies:

❖ by increasing the synthesis of dopamine in the brain, which is achieved by administering levodopa in combination with a periph-

Table 3-3.   Medications commonly used in the treatment of Parkinson's disease

Type of medication	Brand name	Tablet dose (mg)	Daily dose (mg)
LEVODOPA			
levodopa	Levodopa	500	100–1,000
levodopa + carbidopa	Sinemet LS	levodopa 50, carbidopa 12.5	100–1,000
	Sinemet 110	levodopa 100, carbidopa 10	
	Sinemet-Plus	levodopa 100, carbidopa 25	
	Sinemet 275	levodopa 250, carbidopa 25	
	Sinemet CR	levodopa 200, carbidopa 50	
levodopa + benserazide (Not available in the U.S)	Madopar 62.5*	levodopa 50, benserazide 12.5	100–1,000
	Madopar 125	levodopa 100, benserazide 25	
	Madopar 250	levodopa 200, benserazide 50	
	Madopar CR	levodopa 100, benserazide 25	
	Madopar Dispersible		
DOPAMINE AGONISTS			
bromocriptine	Parlodel	1, 2.5, 5, 10	15–80
pergolide	Permax	50, 250 micrograms	2–5
apomorphine	Britaject (available in Canada)	2 or 5 ml ampule	
ANTICHOLINERGICS			
benzhexol/ trihexyphenidyl	Artane	2, 5	4–15
benztropine	Cogentin	2	1–4
orphenadrine	Disipal	50	100–300
procyclidine	Kemadrin	5	7.5–30

(continued)

Type of medication	Brand name	Tablet dose (mg)	Daily dose (mg)
MAO-B INHIBITOR			
selegeline Deprenyl/Jumex	Eldepryl	5	5–10
OTHER			
amantadine	Symmetrel**	100	200–300

* Madopar is available in all forms in Canada, but not in the United States.
** Generic also available in United States.

eral decarboxylase inhibitor such as carbidopa and benserazide, which prevent the conversion of levodopa into dopamine *outside* the brain

❖ by administering dopamine agonists such as bromocriptine, lisuride, pergolide, and apomorphine

❖ by inhibiting the breakdown of dopamine, the mode of action of selegiline

❖ by enhancing dopamine release, the mode of action of amantadine

❖ by blocking dopamine re-uptake at the synaptic terminals, the effect of other classes of medication such as tricyclics and of benztropine, sometimes used to treat Parkinson's disease symptoms.

The major and minor symptoms of the disease are differentially responsive to treatment. The various forms of medication produce their beneficial effects on different symptoms. In general, bradykinesia and akinesia respond well to treatment and are often much alleviated; rigidity is usually alleviated by levodopa therapy. Tremor also responds to medication, but it may not be completely eliminated. Balance and walking problems are usually the least improved. The more minor symptoms such as oiliness of the skin, sweating, aches and pains may also be relieved with medication.

All medications are chemicals that affect brain function. Ideally, they would only operate on and normalize function in the affected areas of the brain, but there is currently no way of restricting the action of any given medication to the affected areas. So most medications give rise to unwanted side effects as well as to the desired symptomatic relief. Usually the side effects are minor and outweighed by the benefits. But at times they can be so severe or disturbing that the patient cannot cope with them. In such cases the drug is discontinued or altered, whatever its beneficial effects might have been. The severity and the interfering nature of side effects differ from drug to drug. There are also some differences between people in terms of the severity and tolerance of the side effects. The aim of drug therapy is to strike a balance between obtaining maximal benefit and incurring minimal side effects.

It will by now be clear that there exists no specific recipe or formula for treating Parkinson's disease patients with medication. It is always necessary to tailor the precise kind of drug therapy, and the point at which it starts, to the symptoms of the individual patient. Treatment will not necessarily be started immediately after the diagnosis, especially in the case of levodopa therapy. And decisions about which drug to use and when to start it are ruled by the social and occupational circumstances of the individual, as well as by his or her particular symptoms. This means that comparing notes with other people about when treatment was first started and specific medication regimens is unhelpful and may be misleading. Clinical decisions about medication are not simply taken on the strength of a single consultation at the outset of the disorder. With the progression of the illness, the drug therapy may be revised, and adjustments may be necessary every six months or so to accommodate any changes in the symptoms and the associated disability. For this reason, continuity of care from your physician and other health care professionals is important.

But although the specific nature and timing of drug therapy are determined in each individual case, there are some general guidelines that doctors follow:

- ❖ When symptoms are so mild that there is no resultant disability, there is no need for medication.
- ❖ When the symptoms of tremor and akinesia become noticeable or interfere with daily activities or cause social embarrassment, anticholinergics or occasionally dopamine agonists may be introduced.
- ❖ When excessive stiffness or slowness appear, amantadine may be added to the anticholinergics. Temporary benefit may be produced

by amantadine, which has weak dopaminergic effects as well as anti-cholinergic properties.

❖ When walking and balance are affected and work and daily activities are disrupted, dopamine therapy is started. The choice will be between levodopa and a direct-acting synthetic dopamine agonist. Levodopa will be effective in most cases; a dopamine agonist such as bromocriptine will be of benefit in only one third of cases. Because of the major long-term drawbacks of levodopa therapy, when first introducing dopaminergic drugs most doctors rely on the strategy of using low dosages of levodopa (Sinemet or Madopar) with a dopamine agonist (bromocriptine or lisuride). Lisuride is not available in the United States. However, pergolide (Permax), pramipexole (Mirapex), and ropinirole (Requip) are now available.

❖ After long-term levodopa therapy, when the response becomes unreliable and on–off fluctuations and *dyskinesias* develop, the levodopa dosage will need to be modified, and various strategies for controlling these complications are introduced.

It is difficult to predict who will derive maximum benefit from a particular medication, because this changes with the stage of the illness and the severity of the symptoms. A degree of trial and error is involved in determining the optimal drug regimen, or drug dosage, for an individual patient. As a general rule, most medications start with the lowest possible dosage, which is then gradually increased to determine the optimal therapeutic dosage that will effectively control the symptoms without major side effects. When a drug is no longer effective in controlling the symptoms, it should be stopped. However, medication taken for Parkinson's disease, particularly levodopa, should not be stopped suddenly, but gradually withdrawn under medical supervision.

Although a variety of drugs is available to treat the disease, the aim is to achieve maximum control of symptoms and prevention of disability with the smallest possible number of drugs and the lowest dosages. Some people with Parkinson's disease may be taking more than one type of medication, but the number of tablets a person is taking is not an indication of the severity of the illness. Each individual has a set of specific symptoms that require treatment with particular types of medication. The medications that are prescribed for treating Parkinson's disease do not usually produce adverse reactions when taken together, and doctors are aware of those that might and so take it into account when prescribing. *You should always inform doctors and dentists about the types of medication you are taking.*

Levodopa Therapy

When it first became widely available as a symptomatic treatment for Parkinson's disease in the 1970s, levodopa produced such profound changes in symptoms that it was seen as a miracle drug. Even today, it is still the most effective drug available. In fact, it is so effective that one of the criteria for diagnosis of classic Parkinson's disease, as mentioned earlier, is that the symptoms improve with levodopa.

Levodopa treatment is a "replacement" therapy that aims to achieve symptomatic improvement by compensating for the dopamine deficiency. Only certain substances can get from the bloodstream into the brain, because the so-called blood–brain barrier acts as a selective filter, and dopamine is one of those substances that cannot cross it. For this reason it cannot be directly used in the treatment of Parkinson's disease. Levodopa, or L-dopa, is used instead, because it *can* cross the blood–brain barrier, where it is converted into dopamine in the brain. The dopa molecule exists in two forms that are mirror images of each other in three-dimensional space: an L-form (laevo, meaning left) and a D (dextro, meaning right) form. Only the L-form of dopa, or levodopa, occurs naturally and is effective in the treatment of Parkinson's disease. The full chemical name of L-dopa is L-3,4-dihydroxyphenylalanine. It is made up of hydrogen, oxygen, carbon, and nitrogen atoms. Levodopa is changed to dopamine by the action of dopa-decarboxylase, which is an enzyme (a substance that regulates chemical changes in the body). This conversion is not rate-controlled, which means that it is possible to increase the amount of dopamine in the brain by taking more L-dopa. L-dopa is an amino acid first discovered in the broad bean. It is also present in other plants, as well as in animal tissues. An amino acid called *tyrosine*, found in protein-rich foods, can be used in conjunction with the enzyme tyrosine hydroxylase to make L-dopa in the body. This mechanism is very strictly rate-controlled, so that eating more dietary tyrosine will not increase the amount of dopamine in the brain.

When levodopa is taken orally it passes from the mouth to the stomach and then to the small intestine. Dopa-decarboxylase, the enzyme that converts levodopa to dopamine, is present in the gut, liver, kidneys, and blood vessels, as well as in the brain. Levodopa is absorbed in the bloodstream from the lining of the intestines, then circulates around the body in the blood. Some of it is changed to dopamine and broken down in the kidneys, then excreted in the urine. Only about 1 to 10 percent of it reaches the brain. To prevent levodopa being converted into dopamine *peripherally*—that is, outside the brain—with the consequence that much of the resulting dopamine is wasted—the levodopa is combined with a *dopa-decarboxylase inhibitor* (a substance that inhibits the action of dopa-decarboxylase and thus the conversion process) that itself cannot get into the brain. In this way the amount of dopamine available to the brain is multiplied by a factor of 10, which in turn reduces the required oral dosage of levodopa. Also, side effects due to the action of dopamine outside the brain are reduced. Carbidopa and benserazide, peripheral inhibitors of dopa-decarboxylase, are combined with levodopa in the ratio of 10 to 1 or 4 to 1. Sinemet and Madopar contain levodopa and dopa-decarboxylase inhibitors, and are the medications most frequently used to treat Parkinson's disease patients.

When levodopa was first introduced, the general practice was to use the maximal tolerated dosage. Now, 25 years later, the experience gained from observing the effects of long-term treatment with levodopa has led to the minimal effective daily dosage being recommended; in other words, the optimal dosage is the smallest that will control the symptoms and the associated disability. Many doctors recommend that levodopa therapy is started with Sinemet LS or Madopar 62.5. Taking the drug with food or after a meal greatly decreases its benefit because all proteins (amino acids) in all food compete with brain receptors. For best results, take with soda crackers 45 to 60 minutes *before* meals. The dosage is then gradually increased to a 100 mg pill, taken three times a day. The patient should avoid the temptation to increase the dose in order to achieve complete relief of symptoms.

In 85 percent of those with classic Parkinson's disease, a marked alleviation of disability occurs with the start of levodopa therapy. All the main symptoms are relieved, with rigidity and bradykinesia responding the most. Tremor is less improved and, together with postural instability, may take some time to respond to the therapy. When levodopa treatment is first started, people with Parkinson's disease report that they are more alert and attentive, and can both move and perform daily activities more rapidly. But a feeling of restlessness and some problems in falling asleep may also be experienced. The period of action of the combined levodopa/decarboxylase inhibitor pills is about four hours.

In the initial phases of treatment, a relatively even response to levodopa therapy throughout the day is obtained. Some take their first dose of the day early, before getting washed or dressed. The best strategy is to try to time the doses so that the best benefit is obtained at times when it is important to be most mobile and physically active. For example, there is usually no point in taking one before going to bed or, for most people, in the evening, when they are most likely to be relaxing at home.

After taking a pill, there is a delay in the appearance of the benefits of levodopa because of the time-consuming digestive process that it undergoes when taken by mouth. It takes about twenty minutes for the drug to cross the barrier between the bloodstream and the brain. Acidity, or other factors that may delay the emptying of the stomach, can further delay the absorption of dopamine. Although, in order to reduce nausea, it is recommended that levodopa medication be taken with food to begin with, meals, particularly those with a high protein content, may delay its absorption and its peak concentration in the blood. The precise amount of daily protein that will interfere with levodopa absorption is not clear. Current opinion is that, in those with advanced Parkinson's disease, a daily protein intake in excess of the recommended daily allowance of 0.8 g per kilogram of body weight would diminish the response to levodopa. Furthermore, the closer the high-protein meal is to the time of taking the tablets, the greater the interference caused with the absorption of levodopa.

It is safe to take levodopa with most other medications. The exception is that antidepressants of the monoamine oxidase inhibitor-A type (MAOI-A) such as phenelzine (Nardil) and tranylcypromine (Parnate) should be discontinued for at least three weeks before starting levodopa. Large quantities of vitamin B6 (pyridoxine) can accelerate the conversion of dopamine in such a way that little reaches the brain, although this is no problem with the combined pills containing a peripheral decarboxylase inhibitor. The major tranquilizers used to treat psychotic symptoms such as hallucinations and delusions act by blocking dopamine and consequently produce parkinsonism. These medications should not be taken concurrently with levodopa.

The Immediate and Short-Term Side Effects of Levodopa Therapy

Although levodopa therapy is very effective in controlling the symptoms of Parkinson's disease, most people experience a number of undesirable side effects immediately or shortly after starting the treatment. These side effects differ in terms of how serious or bothersome they are and include the following:

❖ Nausea and vomiting can occur and are due to dopamine stimulating the vomiting center in the brainstem. With prolonged treatment, the vomiting center usually becomes habituated to the presence of dopamine and no longer responds to it. Because the stimulation of the vomiting center is most likely to occur when the amount of levodopa in the blood increases rapidly, one solution is to take your levodopa dose after a meal so that its absorption is slowed down. Another solution is to increase the dose of decarboxylase inhibitor, thus preventing the peripheral synthesis of dopamine. Alternatively, you might have to take additional medicine such as domperidone, to overcome the nausea. (Domperidone is not available in the United States; it can be ordered from Canadian pharmacies. However, Merck provides free carbidopa (Lodosyn) on order by physician.)

❖ Levodopa therapy can affect the sympathetic nervous system, which controls the heart and blood vessels. As a result, postural hypotension—that is, a drop in blood pressure when you stand up—can develop. In fact, blood pressure could fall so low that you might feel dizzy and faint. These problems can be partly overcome by taking salt tablets or wearing elastic stockings to constrict the blood vessels of the legs.

❖ Psychotic symptoms such as hallucinations, delusions, and confusion are experienced by about 20 percent of people taking levodopa.

Psychotic symptoms occur more frequently in older people with a later onset of the disease. Other possible mental effects include restlessness during sleep, vivid dreams, and nightmares. Depression may be made worse by levodopa therapy. These problems can be partly overcome by reducing the total dosage and by taking the last dose before going to bed.

❖ Sleep disturbance is a side effect of levodopa therapy that can be troublesome both to the person with the illness and to his or her spouse or partner. Sleep problems, which tend to increase with the length of treatment, are mainly caused by the alerting effect of levodopa. Insomnia, a common complaint, can be partly overcome by not taking any medication after the evening meal and by regular daily exercise to facilitate sleep. Another common side effect is sleep fragmentation, with many brief awakenings throughout the night. As well as more vivid dreaming, jerky movements during sleep can be a problem.

❖ Another side effect of levodopa treatment is the discoloration of urine and sweat. Before the kidneys eliminate the levodopa absorbed in the intestine, it is broken down into dopamine and then into a series of inert substances, one of which is melanin, a pigment that varies in color from orange to red to brown. When melanin is discharged into the urine, it gives it a reddish color that can leave stains on underwear—but this should not cause alarm. Similarly, when a small amount of levodopa is secreted through the sweat glands, the sweat too can occasionally be of a dark color and discolor clothes.

The Long-Term Complications of Levodopa Therapy

Levodopa has proved not to be quite the miracle drug it promised to be. With long-term use adverse reactions develop. After three to five years of levodopa therapy, the majority of people with Parkinson's disease experience some loss of benefit as well as medication-induced complications. These complications, which affect 90 percent of those treated for ten or more years, include unwanted involuntary movements, or *dyskinesias*, and *response fluctuations*. Response fluctuations include the "wearing-off" effect, a gradual loss of benefit at the end of the dose, and "on–off fluctuations," which are more abrupt episodes of loss of benefit. We discuss these long-term side effects at some length, as they influence the patient's quality of life later on in the illness and become a main focus of medical management.

Dyskinesias   The dyskinesias, or involuntary movements, induced by levodopa are commonly *chorea* (dancelike writhing movements) and *dystonia* (involuntary muscle contractions or spasms producing abnormal postures). They can also take the form of jerks or muscle twitches, and may affect a variety of muscle groups in the face, neck, trunk, and limbs, and sometimes the chest or diaphragm. Dyskinesias occur either at the peak of benefits or at the end of the dose. In his book, Ivan Vaughan graphically describes his experience:

My body is possessed of two demons. Off the drugs, with too little dopamine in the system, I suffer the three classic symptoms of Parkinson's disease: trembling, rigidity and slowness of movement. . . . With surplus drugs swilling around in my bloodstream, another demon takes over and my body begins to writhe to a different tune. My arms seem double-jointed as they snake up to my face, the hands bending grotesquely at right-angles. . . . Of the two demons, I prefer the drugless rather than the drugged.

Sidney Dorros, who described his experiences of the illness in his book *Parkinson's Disease: A Patient's View*, also gives a vivid description of dyskinesias—in contrast to Vaughan, he states a preference for the "overdosed, dyskinetic" state:

At times, though, the dyskinesia was so extreme that I felt as if I was spinning in a centrifuge. My arms and legs seemed to be pulling from their sockets, my inner organs seemed to be pressing to get outside my body or to turn themselves inside out. My muscles, particularly in my arms and around my shoulders, developed very sharp pains and cramps. The dyskinesia could be almost entirely eliminated by reducing the dosage of medication to the point of slight underdose, but underdosage was so disabling, depressing, and frightening that I preferred to be slightly overdosed even at the cost of involuntary movements.

Dyskinesias may develop as a result of dopamine receptors becoming supersensitive over time. Once these involuntary movements have developed, they can be induced by even very small doses of levodopa—clear evidence of intolerance and receptor-supersensitivity. It is not clear what determines when the dyskinesias develop, but there is some evidence that both the likelihood of developing them and their severity increase with higher dosages and the length of the therapy.

Gradual "wearing-off" effect, or end-of-dose deterioration   After some years of levodopa therapy, a proportion of patients become aware of the effect of individual doses: that is, they know when the medication has "taken" and is working and when it is not. After six years of the therapy, about two-thirds of people with Parkinson's disease develop "end-of-dose akinesia," or the "wearing-off" effect. The individual complains that the beneficial effect of the drug wears off two or three hours after the last dose. And with continued treatment, the degree of benefit from each dose lasts for a yet shorter period. While initially the benefits of a dose would last from six to eight hours, later on they may disappear after half an hour. The individual experiences this as a gradual slowing down. An analogy has been drawn with a clock or a mechanical toy that requires winding up. It is not known what precisely it is that causes this wearing-off effect, but it may be related to a reduced capacity of the remaining neurons in the substantia nigra to synthesize, take up, and store dopamine.

Rapid on–off fluctuations   With long-term levodopa therapy, periods of slowness, immobility, stiffness, or tremor, sometimes combined with depression, may occur. These "off" episodes alternate with "on" periods when the medication is working effectively and the individual is mobile, relatively symptom-free, alert, and able to work. The "off" periods occur mainly in the afternoon and evening and last several hours, and once these fluctuations start the duration of benefit from each dose may be reduced to two or three hours. In addition, during the "on" periods involuntary movements, or dyskinesias, may develop. The term *on–off fluctuations* to describe these rapid and sudden swings in efficacy of levodopa therapy during the day was first used by a patient of Dr. Roger C. Duvoisin, who compared the alerting and mobilizing effect of the drug to the switching-on of a light and the sudden return of the parkinsonian symptoms to the light going off. Such fluctuations in the psychomotor state of the individual with Parkinson's disease first appear two to five years after starting levodopa therapy and occur several times a day. Each swing in mobility and mood lasts from one to three hours. Initially the fluctuations may be relatively regular and predictable, but later they may occur relatively randomly so that planning work-related, social, and leisure activities becomes impossible.

In his book *A Shadow over My Brain: My Struggle with Parkinson's Disease*, child psychiatrist Cecil Todes describes his experience of on–off fluctuations:

> *How often did I find myself in my dinner suit, all primed for a party, sitting in the car or driving about outside, waiting for the drug to come through. Life with Parkinson's disease was a continual personal battle of trying to gain stability on drugs. The precarious balance between being Off and being On and moving into dyskinesia (grimaces) was very difficult to achieve.*

The exact mechanisms of these long-term complications are not fully understood, but three main factors may play a role in their development.

1. It is possible that these side effects are related to the by-products of breaking down dopamine. Long-term dopamine replacement therapy may contribute to the pathogenesis of the disorder, as it increases the production of toxic free radicals resulting from the breakdown of dopamine. These substances could speed up the degeneration of dopamine-producing neurons in the substantia nigra. Research suggests that the incidence and development time of these levodopa-induced complications correlates with the duration of levodopa therapy and the cumulative dosage taken by the patient over many years.

2. However, levodopa therapy cannot be the only factor responsible for the development of fluctuations, because before it was introduced as a symptomatic treatment for Parkinson's disease, fluctuations in motor function were already noted. In other words, the variability in motor function occurs with the progression of the illness, with or

without levodopa therapy. Progression itself, then, is another important factor that results in the loss of dopaminergic neurons and terminals. The loss of dopaminergic terminals in the striatum means that the storage and regulation of the activity of dopamine in this area are also impaired. As the illness progresses, levodopa can no longer compensate for the dopamine deficiency in the striatum because there are too few neurons remaining in the substantia nigra to synthesize enough dopamine to stimulate the dopamine receptors in the striatum.

3. Most importantly, perhaps, the reduced levodopa benefit after long-term therapy may partly result from a change in the brain's sensitivity to dopamine, whereby a process of "downregulation," or subsensitivity, of striatal dopamine receptors develops.

The Management of the Long-Term Complications of Levodopa Therapy

As already noted, after ten years of treatment 90 percent of people with Parkinson's disease who are on levodopa are affected by response fluctuations, and these fluctuations constitute one of the major therapeutic challenges facing doctors in the management of the illness. A number of strategies, already mentioned, are used to prevent or delay the development of the response fluctuations. The overall aim is to minimize the cumulative amount of levodopa that people take over the course of their illness:

❖ delaying the start of levodopa therapy until it is indicated by moderate to severe disability in daily activities

❖ using the lowest dose of levodopa that will control the symptoms

❖ combining levodopa therapy with a dopamine agonist that will permit the use of a smaller dose of levodopa.

To minimize these fluctuations and dyskinesias once they have developed, a number of strategies, some of them already mentioned, are employed:

❖ The dosage of levodopa is fractionated, so that smaller doses are taken more frequently during the day.

❖ A dopamine agonist such as bromocriptine or pergolide is added to levodopa—again, to permit the levodopa dosage to be reduced.

❖ A low-protein diet is recommended, or protein intake is rescheduled, so that amino acids in the diet do not interfere with levodopa absorption and entry to the brain.

❖ Brief "drug holidays" for a day or so are considered to allow the resetting of dopamine receptors that have been overworked during levodopa therapy. This *must* be done in the hospital.

❖ Methods of continuous dopaminergic stimulation are introduced to prevent the rises and falls of the levodopa level in the blood, which are partly responsible for the fluctuations in mobility and the dyskinesias.

Several methods for continuous dopaminergic stimulation have been developed and used.

❖ The standard Sinemet and Madopar tablets are absorbed in about 30 minutes. Sinemet CR (controlled-release) and Madopar LS or CR are special preparations that allow the gradual and controlled release of levodopa into the stomach over four to five hours, thereby maintaining adequate drug levels in the blood for about eight hours. In effect, instead of a sharp rise and fall, the CR tablets allow a steadier level of levodopa in the bloodstream over a longer period. As a result, the CR preparations produce longer "on" and shorter "off" periods, smooth the wearing-off response, and reduce the number of tablets that have to be taken each day; in fact, they can effectively control on–off fluctuations in a proportion of cases. They are more effective in those who have had the disease for a shorter time and who have also been on levodopa therapy for a shorter time. The tablets must be swallowed whole with a glass of water or broken *only* in half, never crushed.

❖ A small battery-operated mobile pump system, which includes a needle for insertion into the side of the abdomen, is used for continuous subcutaneous delivery of dopamine agonists. The pump itself can be carried in a pocket or attached to a belt. Subcutaneous delivery of lisuride controls motor fluctuations in many people, but it can also produce psychiatric side effects. Continuous subcutaneous injection of apomorphine, another dopamine agonist, has been more successful. The only drawback with this method is that many people find the pump too difficult to cope with. An easier alternative is the Penject system, which provides a single-shot subcutaneous injection of apomorphine.

❖ Continuous delivery of levodopa into the duodenum (a part of the small intestine) has been used to overcome the possibility that irregular emptying of the stomach may be partly responsible for unpredictable absorption of levodopa into the bloodstream. At the moment, the procedure is too complicated to be generally applicable.

❖ Intravenous injections are another way of reducing fluctuations, but this is not a particularly practical method.

When Should Levodopa Therapy Be Started?

Because of the disabling nature of the long-term complications associated with levodopa therapy, medical opinion is divided about when it should be started. Those who believe that the optimal period of therapy lasts for about two to five years recommend withholding treatment until it is absolutely necessary and then using as small a dose as possible for as long as possible. Others believe that the development of levodopa response complications is a function of the progression of the disease and disease severity rather than of treatment duration. They therefore consider that to withhold levodopa therapy is inappropriate.

There is also evidence that, by delaying the complications of immobility, treatment with levodopa increases life expectancy. As already noted, therapy has not altered the rate of progression of the underlying disease pathology, but the symptomatic deterioration has been slowed down. Before the levodopa era, within five years of onset 28 percent of people with Parkinson's disease were severely disabled (as measured on the Hoehn and Yahr scale, stages 4 or 5) or had died. In the post-levodopa era, only 9 percent of people treated with the drug reach the stage of severe disability within the first five years. Before the introduction of levodopa, mean life expectancy was ten years after onset, and slightly higher with a younger age of onset. Since the use of levodopa, 60 percent of people with the illness live to the age of 75, compared with 25 percent previously.

These various considerations should be weighed against each other when deciding when to start levodopa therapy. Since the circumstances and needs of each person are unique, a doctor can only inform the individual and the family concerned of the available options and their likely benefits and side effects, then in light of his or her expertise make specific recommendations. This advice depends on the age of the person as well as on his or her personal circumstances. For example, for someone with young-onset Parkinson's disease, who will have to live and cope with the disease for 30 to 40 years, consideration of the present quality of life needs to be balanced against long-term future prospects. Here it might be best to postpone levodopa medication for as long as possible. In contrast, for a 75-year-old with Parkinson's disease, the quality of life in the short term should be made a priority, and levodopa should be introduced when disability first appears.

Ultimately, doctors can only inform and offer expert recommendations. The decision about whether or not to take levodopa medication and when to start it should always be made by the patient. Ivan Vaughan states his personal preference clearly:

Of the two demons, I prefer the drugless rather than the drugged. . . . Yet there can be massive pressure from doctors (who should know better) and people around me to take as many drugs as are necessary to mask the symptoms of Parkinson's disease—but these people do not fully admit the consequences and discomfort of L-dopa's side effects. You can manage more easily on the drugs; you are less of a burden on those around you; but the social consequences of the writhing side effects can be as daunting to the sufferer as the symptoms they "cure." . . . I am not saying that being on the drug, even with side effects of dyskinesia, is worse or that people are daft for taking the drugs. But, given my personality, I prefer the non-drug state. In a strange way I feel more in control, even though I have less control in a motor sense.

Dopamine Agonists

Dopamine agonists are another class of medication used in the symptomatic treatment of Parkinson's disease. As described in Chapter 1, neurotransmitters are chemical messengers of the brain that allow the transmission of information between neurons, which are separated from each other by clefts called synapses. One neuron releases its neurotransmitter, which then acts on receptors on the next neuron, and so on. The information is transmitted across the synapse by a neurotransmitter stimulating the postsynaptic receptors—that is, the receptors of the second neuron on the other side of the synapse. In the brain each neurotransmitter—such as dopamine, acetylcholine, or noradrenaline—has special receptor cells that selectively respond only to neurotransmitters of its own kind. The lock-and-key analogy is often used here—each neurotransmitter is like a key that opens only the door to its own lock, or receptor.

Besides the naturally occurring neurotransmitters, synthetic substances called *receptor agonists* are similar enough in their chemical structure to fool the receptors into accepting and responding to them. The several types of dopamine receptors that exist in the brain are known as D1, D2, D3, D4, and D5 receptors. Dopamine itself can act on all of these receptors; stimulation of D2 receptors is most important for the relief of the symptoms of Parkinson's disease.

Bromocriptine (Parlodel), pergolide (Permax), pramipexole (Mirapex), ropinirole (Requip), and apomorphine are synthetic dopamine receptor agonists (Table 3-3). Each drug operates by directly stimulating postsynaptic dopamine receptors. Apomorphine is currently given by injection using a small battery-operated pump or by means of the Penject system. When tremor is severe, the patient may need help in operating either of these.

Although generally less effective than levodopa, dopamine agonists have several advantages. Unlike levodopa, these substances do not have to be converted to dopamine in order to be effective, and the absence of a conversion process alleviates some of the side effects of levodopa. In addition, by directly stimulating dopamine receptors, dopamine agonists lower the rate of dopamine turnover in the brain and thereby reduce the toxic by-products of breaking down and metabolizing dopamine. Because of this they may do less damage to dopaminergic neurons. Moreover, they do not compete with other amino acids for absorption, so neither the amount of proteins in the diet nor the time of eating proteins affects dopamine agonist medication.

It was originally hoped that dopamine agonists would replace levodopa, and thus eliminate or reduce its associated complications as well. But long-term experience has shown that their efficacy is limited. This is partly because whereas there are several types of dopamine receptors in the brain, the currently available agonists mainly stimulate D2 receptors, and it may be that the stimulation of additional types of dopamine receptors is necessary for maximum effect. Furthermore, although for the first few months of treatment dopamine agonists such as bromocriptine can be as effective as levodopa, in the long term they are not.

The short-term side effects of dopamine agonists are similar to those produced by levodopa, but more noticeable and distressing. They include nausea and vomiting, loss of weight, hypotension, sleep disturbance, depression and agitation, confusion, hallucination, dyskinesias, cardiac arrhythmias, nasal stuffiness, dry mouth, and headache.

Each of the various types of dopamine agonist that are currently available alleviates the symptoms of Parkinson's disease to a similar extent. But particular individuals may respond better to a particular one. Absence of effect or intolerance of one dopamine agonist does not mean that others will not be effective; sometimes when one loses its efficacy, its replacement by another dopamine agonist restores the benefit. Dopamine agonists are mainly used in conjunction with levodopa therapy. To reduce or postpone the long-term complications of levodopa therapy it is recommended that pharmacotherapy is initially started with a combination of levodopa and dopamine agonists.

Anticholinergics

As long ago as 1869, extracts of the plants *Hyoscyamus niger* and belladonna, which have anticholinergic effects, were used by the French neurologist Jean-Martin Charcot in the treatment of Parkinson's disease patients. As is evident from their name, anticholinergics are a class of drugs that operate by blocking the action of the neurotransmitter acetylcholine in the brain. This blocking action has beneficial effects on the symptoms of Parkinson's disease, but also produces side effects.

Benzhexol/trihexyphenidyl (Artane), orphenadrine (Disipal), benztropine (Cogentin), and procyclidine (Kemadrin) are some of the anticholinergics used in the treatment of early and mild Parkinson's disease (Table 3-3), mainly to postpone the introduction of levodopa therapy. As these drugs have a period of action of four to six hours, doses are taken three or four times daily. The main benefit of anticholinergics is in reducing tremor, excessive salivation, and dysphagia. They also alleviate rigidity, or muscle stiffness. Bradykinesia and balance and walking problems are not so well alleviated. Anticholinergics, also called cholinergic antagonists, are not as effective as levodopa.

Besides the concern inherent in giving cholinergic antagonists to people with Parkinson's disease, a disorder with some cortical cholinergic deficit, there is the problem of the side effects. These include blurred vision, constipation, dry mouth, urinary retention, reduced sweating, and a number of mental and cognitive side effects. Particularly problematic in the elderly person with Parkinson's disease may be forgetfulness and memory loss, depression, confusion, and hallucinations. The older patient with signs of dementia is especially at risk to the negative effects of anticholinergics. Treatment with these drugs is not advisable if the patient has glaucoma or prostate problems.

Anticholinergics should be withdrawn gradually—sudden withdrawal can result in the return of the symptoms and produce anxiety.

Amantadine

Amantadine (Symmetrel) was initially introduced as an antiviral agent. By chance it was found to have some antiparkinsonian effect. A 58-year-old woman with Parkinson's disease, under the care of the American neurologist Dr. Robert S. Schwab, was taking amantadine as a prevention against the flu when she noticed that her rigidity, akinesia, and tremor were unexpectedly alleviated. This beneficial effect was later replicated in wider-scale clinical studies. The precise mechanism of action of amantadine is not known, but it seems to have some anticholinergic properties as well as enhancing dopaminergic transmission by increasing the release of dopamine or blocking dopamine re-uptake. It may have some NMDA receptor antagonism.

Amantadine alleviates slowness of movements, particularly fine movements, and improves posture and facial mobility. It also has some beneficial effects on akinesia and rigidity, but tremor is not much relieved. The improvements are noticeable approximately two weeks after first starting the drug. A daily dose of 200–300 mg is usual and is well tolerated by younger people with Parkinson's disease. Its benefit usually wears off after three to four months, but after stopping it, the drug can usually be reinstated with concomitant benefits. The side effects of amantadine are blurred vision, dry mouth, constipation, confusion, hallucinations, an unusual rash on the lower limbs called livedo reticularis, and edema (accumulation of fluid in spaces between cells), all of which disappear when the drug is discontinued.

When directly compared with other antiparkinsonian medication, amantadine is less effective than levodopa but better than anticholinergics. It is primarily used as the sole medication for short-term therapy (6 to 12 months) in people with mild to moderately severe symptoms. It helps to postpone levodopa therapy.

Selegiline

Monoamine oxidase (MAO) is the enzyme that breaks down dopamine, and it exists in two forms, A and B. MAO type A is found in the adrenal glands, heart, liver, and other body organs; MAO type B is present in the brain. Substances that inhibit the action of MAO type A prevent the breakdown of dopamine as well as of adrenaline and of noradrenaline. MAO-A inhibitors are used as antidepressants. They should not be taken with food containing the amino acid tyramine, such as cheese, red wine, and pickled herrings, as they result in the so-called "cheese effect"—that is, fluctuations in blood pressure and hypertensive crises.

Selegiline (Deprenyl, Eldepryl) is an MAO type B inhibitor, which has the unique feature of selectively blocking the action of MAO-B, thereby preventing the breakdown of dopamine in the brain, while allowing the normal degradation of other monoamines such as noradrenaline, adrenaline, and serotonin. With selegiline no dietary restriction is required. Its mode of action is different from that of other medication.

The recommended daily dose of selegiline is between 5 and 10 mg. As it may cause insomnia if taken at night, it is usually taken in the morning. There are two reasons why the daily dose of selegiline is kept low. First, 5 mg inhibits MAO-B, the enzyme that breaks down dopamine in the brain, by 90 percent. Second, with a daily dose higher than 20 mg the selective action of selegiline on MAO-B is lost, and it also inhibits MAO-A so that the "cheese effect" is more likely to occur.

Selegiline was first used as a symptomatic treatment for Parkinson's disease by Dr. Walther Birkmayer and his colleagues in Vienna in the early 1980s. Subsequently, the demonstration that in laboratory animals the effects of MPTP, the toxin that selectively destroys neurons in the substantia nigra, could be prevented by prior administration of selegiline further confirmed the potential value of selegiline. Clinical trials were restarted, in which Drs. James Tetrud and J. William Langston demonstrated that for patients on selegiline the symptoms worsened at a rate that required the introduction of levodopa after 548 days. In contrast, for those on a placebo (not a drug, but an inert substance) the introduction of levodopa was required after 312 days. In other words, treatment with selegiline delayed the need to start levodopa therapy by about eight months. The larger multicenter DATATOP (Deprenyl and Tocopherol Antioxidant Therapy of Parkinsonism) study, in which the long-term effects of treatment with selegiline were examined, obtained similar results, showing that deprenyl (Eldepryl) delayed the need for the introduction of levodopa by an average of 13 months. However, when people with Parkinson's disease who took part in the DATATOP study were followed up, the results suggested that the benefits of selegiline were short-lived. Another large-scale study by the Parkinson's Disease Research Group in the United Kingdom suggested that, in the long term, levodopa in combination with selegiline seemed to produce no clinical benefits over levodopa alone. The results of this study also suggested that the long-term mortality rates were higher for those taking levodopa with selegiline than for those taking levodopa alone. This is clearly an issue that requires further investigation.

For patients whose Parkinson's disease starts in their sixties, in whom short-term symptomatic control and enhanced quality of life may be a priority, the combined use of selegiline and levodopa may be appropriate. When taken with levodopa, selegiline increases the duration of action of levodopa and prolongs the benefit from each dose. But at the same time the side effects of levodopa may be accentuated, and it may become necessary to reduce the levodopa dosage. Selegiline may also be useful for people with Parkinson's disease who have developed on–off fluctuations after long-term levodopa therapy.

In the short term selegiline has no major side effects of its own except occasional insomnia and nausea. The side effects that patients experience are mainly those associated with levodopa. Selegiline is not recommended for people with peptic ulcer. It may have an antidepressant effect that can be helpful for those who have become depressed. An occasional side effect of long-term levodopa therapy, or when selegiline is added, is hypomania—a sense of well-being, mild euphoria, enhanced ambition, increased talkativeness, increased sexual desire, and excessive motor activity and agitation. The dose may have to be reduced to prevent hypomania.

Other Medications

Besides the major classes of medication used in the symptomatic treatment of Parkinson's disease, which are summarized in Table 3-3, other drugs are used to deal with specific problems.

When tremor is the main problem, it may not respond very well to levodopa therapy or to anticholinergics in small doses. Propranolol, a drug normally used to treat high blood pressure or an irregular pulse, often proves effective in suppressing tremor; it has no effect on the other symptoms of Parkinson's disease. Alternatively, low doses of the minor tranquilizer diazepam (Valium) may be used to control tremor. Painful rigidity of the muscles is treated with muscle relaxants.

Occasionally, minor tranquilizers such as diazepam (Valium), lorazepam (Ativan), and oxazepam (Serax) are used to overcome the restlessness or insomnia that can sometimes accompany Parkinson's disease. The problem with the use of these drugs is that in Parkinson's disease they can produce drowsiness, dizziness, and sometimes increased slowness. Also, with prolonged use physical and psychological dependence may develop, such that their withdrawal will result in agitation and nervousness.

When it is severe, depression in Parkinson's disease needs to be treated directly with antidepressant medication. The tricyclic class of antidepressants is often used; these also have a mild anticholinergic action that can be beneficial in Parkinson's disease, and a mild sedative effect that can help with insomnia.

Constipation in Parkinson's disease is due to the reduced motility of the muscles of the bowel, and it is worsened by some types of antiparkinsonian medication. It is best treated by exercise and increasing the intake of water and dietary fiber, but if these are not effective, it may become necessary to use laxatives or enemas. Diuretics can be useful in relieving the swelling of the legs and feet that can occur in Parkinson's disease as a result of bradykinesia and the reduced muscular activity and mobility of the limbs. As mentioned earlier, akinesia results in reduced mobility and lubrication of the eyes, and soreness, redness, and scaliness of the eyelids. Artificial tears that mimic the liquid and salt composition of natural tears can help to increase the eyes' lubrication. Seborrhea, scaliness, and oiliness of the skin and hair, can be reduced by levodopa treatment; frequent washing of the face with special oil-controlling soaps and the hair with dandruff-controlling shampoos can also help to deal with the problem.

Drug Holidays

At times it may become necessary to stop taking antiparkinsonian medication for a number of days, or even weeks. For instance, it may have to be stopped for a few days for surgery that involves a general anesthetic, and for a few weeks before trying a new type of medication. Sometimes stopping medication for a few weeks can make the drugs more effective when they are restarted. This frequently occurs with Symmetrel.

This period of being off all medication is called a "drug holiday." Withdrawal of medication can make the symptoms much worse and the patient immobile. For these reasons drug holidays can be dangerous, and should always be medically supervised and carried out during hospitalization. The patient should never stop his or her medication without consultation. When surgery or treatment for other medical complaints is to be undertaken, it is important to inform the surgeon or other doctors concerned about the Parkinson's disease and the medication used.

SURGERY

Surgical treatment of Parkinson's disease has a history that goes back to the early 1900s. Those early surgical procedures involved *lesioning*—that is, cutting or destroying small areas of the brain that control movement. Complications were common, and success was highly variable. A much safer technique, using *stereotaxic surgery*, was first developed in the United States in 1947 by Drs. Spiegel and Wycis. It was applied to the treatment of Parkinson's disease in the 1950s by, among others, Professor Hirotaro Narabayashi in Tokyo and Dr. Irving S. Cooper in the United States. In stereotaxic surgery a special frame is fixed to the skull, then a hole is made in the skull and a needle-like electrical probe is inserted into the brain to produce a small focal lesion. The direction and depth of the probe insertion is determined with X-rays or scans, which are used to create a map of the various parts of the brain. This map then guides the surgeon during the operation. The procedure is carried out under local anesthetic and sedation, so that the individual is alert and can cooperate in the placement of the probe.

Between 1957 and 1972 stereotaxic surgery, mainly thalamotomies and pallidotomies (see below), was used relatively frequently to treat the symptoms of Parkinson's disease in various centers across the world. Since the mid-1970s, the therapeutic management of the disorder has been dominated by levodopa therapy, but more recently the long-term complications of that therapy have regenerated the interest in surgical management. Technologic advances in brain scanning have improved the precision of both stereotaxic probe insertion and the focusing of the lesion in the target area of the brain. This in turn has enhanced the success and safety of surgery. Current surgical approaches to Parkinson's disease are thalamotomy and pallidotomy, thalamic, pallidal and subthalamic nucleus stimulation, and brain implantation.

Thalamotomy

The thalamus consists of a group of neurons that connect the basal ganglia to the frontal lobes (the front part of the brain). The thalamus acts as a relay station between these areas. Thalamotomy involves placing a stereotaxic lesion in a specific part of the thalamus, usually the ventrolateral nucleus. In the late 1950s and 1960s, before the introduction of levodopa therapy, many thalamotomies were carried out on people with Parkinson's disease. They were effective for controlling tremor and to some extent rigidity, but they were less effective with bradykinesia and akinesia. The mortality associated with the procedure was 1 percent. The major complication following bilateral thalamotomy was dysarthria, or slurring of speech. Partial paralysis of one arm and/or leg, together with memory disturbance and impairment of judgment, were other short-term complications of the procedure in a minority of cases. Now thalamotomies are recommended in special cases only—those with severe, intractable, unilateral tremor.

In his book *Parkinson's Disease: A Patient's View*, Sidney Dorros gives a detailed minute-by-minute description of his thalamotomy operation, from the fitting of the frame to his head, through the drilling of a small hole in his skull, to the insertion of a surgical probe to "freeze" the target neurons. In his case, the unilateral thalamotomy, undertaken before levodopa therapy became available, was successful in that it resulted in complete elimination of tremor and rigidity on the left side of his body. However, this was accompanied by increased tremor and stiffness on his previously "normal" right side. With hindsight, he states:

> *People often ask me if I would have chosen to have the operation . . . knowing what I do now. The answer is, "Of course not!" But neither I nor anyone else knew at the time how soon a new drug treatment would be available that for me would be more effective and safer than surgery. One can only act on the best information available at the time of decision. On that basis, I believe my wife and I made the right decision.*

Thalamic Stimulation

This procedure allows long-term electrical stimulation of the same area of the thalamus that is lesioned in a thalamotomy, and is also most suitable for controlling severe tremor. It involves the surgical insertion of high-frequency electrodes into the ventralis intermedialis nucleus of the thalamus. The electrodes are connected to a programmable stimulator surgically placed under the skin, with which the electrical stimulation of the thalamus can be turned on or off and the intensity of stimulation controlled. During stimulation, tremor in the arms is controlled, tremor in the trunk and legs may be reduced, and balance may be improved. This procedure is less risky than is thalamotomy and may be preferable to it, especially when bilateral intervention is required.

Pallidotomy

Pallidotomy—the placing of a lesion in the globus pallidus, the output gateway of the basal ganglia—is one of the older surgical procedures used to treat Parkinson's disease patients. When this operation was performed in the 1950s and 1960s, the lesion was placed in the anterior and dorsal parts of the globus pallidus (the procedure known as anterodorsal pallidotomy). This relieved rigidity, but not the other symptoms of the disease, and it was modified in the 1950s by a Swedish neurosurgeon, Lars Leksell. This modification, which involved placing lesions in more posterior and ventral sections of the globus pallidus (known as posteroventral pallidotomy), seemed more effective and resulted in alleviation of tremor and akinesia as well as of rigidity.

Leksell's modified pallidotomy procedure has recently been refined and carried out stereotaxically. The stereotaxic map guides the surgeon, who places the needle-like probe into the appropriate part of the globus pallidus, after which a brief current is passed through the needle to create a small lesion.

Since 1985 a large number of people with Parkinson's disease have had Leksell's pallidotomy, carried out in Sweden by Professor Lauri S. Laitinen and his colleagues. The operation was reportedly of great benefit, allowing medication to be reduced by 50 percent to 75 percent. In particular, levodopa-induced dyskinesias were considerably reduced on the opposite side of the body to which the surgery was carried out. Many more patients have now had this operation, including Anne Marshall, whose experiences are described in an issue of the British publication *YAPmag* (the magazine of the Young Alert Parkinson's Partners and Relatives group). A made-to-measure frame was built to hold her head in position during surgery, which was conducted under local anesthetic. She was awake during the operation, which produced no pain, and was asked to describe her experiences while the surgery was actually being performed. Immediately after the operation the tremor in her right limbs was much less, and she could move them more freely. Her medication, Madopar, worked much more effectively and she no longer needed apomorphine.

The new pallidotomy procedure has now been carried out world-wide, and many people with Parkinson's disease have had the operation in the United States and United Kingdom. It has been successful in relieving levodopa-induced dyskinesias as well as rigidity and akinesia.

Pallidal and Subthalamic Nucleus Stimulation

These procedures are similar to thalamic stimulation, except that a different site is selected for the stimulating electrodes. The fine electrodes are inserted into the internal segment of the globus pallidus—this is for pallidal stimulation—or into the subthalamic nucleus (for STN, or subthalamic nucleus stimulation), which is another relay station between the striatum and the frontal cortex. The electrodes are then connected to a programmable stimulator surgically placed under the skin. Both high-frequency pallidal and STN stimulation have been shown to be effective in reducing bradykinesia, rigidity, tremor, and dyskinesias. Compared with pallidotomy these procedures have the advantage of not destroying the target brain areas, and of being reversible.

Brain Implantation

As already explained, in classic Parkinson's disease the symptoms arise from the loss of dopamine-producing neurons in a relatively small area of the brain, the substantia nigra, which results in dopamine deficiency in the striatum. Because of the relatively confined nature of its pathophysiology, classic Parkinson's disease has been at the forefront of the research into *brain implantation*—used here to refer to the implantation of dopamine-producing cells into the brains of people with Parkinson's disease. The rationale is this: if the implanted cells can survive, release the deficient neurotransmitter dopamine, and establish connections with the nonfunctioning neurons, then partial or complete reversal of the symptoms of the disorder may be possible.

Since the 1980s, after years of experimentation on animals, it has been possible to implant into the striatum of the patient, dopamine-producing cells from his or her adrenal glands—these are situated above the kidneys and have their own dopamine-producing cells—or from tissue obtained from aborted fetuses. The first implant of adrenal tissue into the brains of four people with Parkinson's disease were carried out at the Karolinska Institute in Stockholm in the early 1980s. Adrenal autografts—that is, tissue taken from the adrenal glands of the patient—were used, in order to reduce the risk of rejection of the grafted tissue. The benefits obtained were not impressive, and it was concluded that the procedure held little promise, and this technique is no longer being used. But at about the same time in Mexico, Dr. Ignazio Madrazo performed the same procedure and claimed better results. Over three hundred such operations have now been carried out, mainly in the United States.

From a review of the outcome of the surgery in these cases, a number of conclusions are possible:

❖ The benefits were usually minimal. People with Parkinson's disease who have undergone the adrenal autograft procedure continue to require levodopa therapy, although the duration of action of the drugs may be longer and the degree of disability during "off" periods may be smaller after the implants.

❖ Both the abdominal surgery to remove adrenal tissue and the neurosurgery carry the risk of complications, which occur in about 10 percent to 20 percent of those operated on.

❖ PET scans in live and postmortem studies have shown that the transplanted adrenal tissue did not survive. Therefore, the benefits obtained may have been due to the release of growth factors produced by the procedure itself, which stimulates the regeneration and growth of the surviving nigrostriatal nerve terminals in the damaged striatum.

❖ A number of symptoms, including disruption of the sleep-wake cycle, hallucinations, delusions, confusion, and mood changes, may be experienced by some people after the operation, the majority of which disappear in a few months. In a few cases, depression and sleep problems may be longer-lasting.

The general consensus is that the modest benefits of these autografts of adrenal tissue do not justify the risks of the procedure.

Subsequent experimentation on laboratory animals proceeded by using tissue obtained from animal fetuses. On the basis of the better results produced by these experiments, the implant work of the Swedish team was resumed in the late 1980s using neurons from the substantia nigras of aborted human fetuses. The technique was refined by using a stereotaxic procedure and a smaller needle to inject the implant tissue into the striatum. PET scans have demonstrated that the implanted tissue survives, and can develop a blood supply and new nerve connections in the receptor site. In general, implants of fetal nigral tissue have produced better results than have adrenal autografts, and several hundred people with Parkinson's disease have had them. The benefits differ from person to person, but have mainly been to do with a longer duration of "on" time, or response to levodopa. Rigidity and slowness are most alleviated, tremor least. However, truly impressive benefits, such as complete reversal of symptoms, have not been obtained in a single case, and only one person has been able to stop all antiparkinsonian medication after implantation.

Dr. Cecil Todes was the fourth person with Parkinson's disease to undergo brain implantation of fetal tissue in the United Kingdom. He obtained relatively little benefit from the procedure, and describes his reactions and feelings about it in his book *A Shadow over My Brain*: he felt "disappointment in the realization that the operation [had] been of no benefit . . . I felt that having the operation when I did was premature and an ill-considered risk."

Brain implantation as a treatment for Parkinson's disease is still experimental, and many procedural questions and ethical issues remain to be addressed. Besides the moral objections of a minority, the ethical issue of using 8–12-week-old fetal tissue has been raised, and guidelines have been drawn up. The main concern has been that, to meet the demand for transplants, a black market may develop and fetuses may be conceived and aborted for the sole purpose of providing tissue for the transplants. However, these problems may be averted by the novel methods for producing implantable tissues that are currently exploring the use of cultured cells, or tissues that have been genetically engineered, to produce the desired neurotransmitter.

Long-term suppression of the patient's immune system with appropriate medication may be necessary, in order to avoid rejection of the implanted fetal tissue by his or her brain. How long this immunosuppression should be continued, and the potential risks, are not known. There is also the possibility that the implant may eventually be subject to the same degenerative process that produced the disease in the first place. Furthermore, the efficacy of the procedure may be limited by the fact that dopamine is not the only neurotransmitter system affected in Parkinson's disease, and that other affected neurotransmitters are *not* replaced by the implanted tissue. Other procedural questions that remain to be addressed are the age span and the amount of the human fetal nigral tissue necessary for a viable implant, and the best implantation site in the striatum. Much work remains to be done before brain implantation is firmly established as a treatment for Parkinson's disease patients.

Who Should Have Surgery for Parkinson's Disease?

Surgery does not aim to cure the illness. As with drug therapy, the aim of surgery is to control the symptoms and to prevent or reduce disability. The other similarity with medication is that, although surgery may successfully control the symptoms for a while, with progression of the illness the old symptoms may become severe enough to reemerge or new symptoms may develop. Most people with Parkinson's disease who have undergone one or other of the possible surgical interventions still need to take some medication afterwards, but perhaps at reduced doses.

The decision to undergo surgical treatment is usually taken after discussion with a neurologist and/or a neurosurgeon, who provide full information about the likely benefits, side effects, and risks. These surgical procedures are now recommended for a minority of people with Parkinson's disease—those with unilateral symptoms, those with a predominance of tremor and rigidity but relatively little akinesia and bradykinesia, younger people, and those who have developed severe levodopa-induced dyskinesias.

Undergoing surgery is a major decision that should only be taken after finding out all the relevant facts. Once the decision is made, in addition to acquiring information about the likely outcome, the patient usually finds it reassuring to find out more about the practical aspects of surgery:

the procedures of admission and information about the ward, what to expect on the day of surgery, how long the operation is likely to take, what sensations and experiences to expect during stereotaxic surgery, and the process of postsurgical recovery. To be well informed helps to alleviate anxiety and fear.

KEY FACTS 3

Is there a cure?

No, unfortunately there is no cure for Parkinson's disease yet.

How can Parkinson's disease be treated?

It can be symptomatically treated with medication or with surgery. Compared with other neurologic illnesses, many effective forms of medical treatment are available for Parkinson's disease.

What are the main types of medication used?

Various kinds. Levodopa therapy (Sinemet or Madopar), dopamine agonists (bromocriptine, lisuride, pergolide, apomorphine), anticholinergics (benzhexol, benztropine, orphenadrine, procyclidine), amantadine, and selegiline are the main types of medication used in the various stages of the illness.

When does drug therapy start, and for how long do I have to continue taking medication?

The decision as to when to start drug therapy is dictated by the symptoms and the associated disability of each individual, together with his or her age and life circumstances. Once treatment is started, the patient needs to remain on medication for the foreseeable future. To achieve maximum benefit, the type and level of medication may occasionally have to be altered.

What are the main types of surgery?

Thalamotomy (cutting a specific section of the thalamus) and pallidotomy (cutting a specific section of the globus pallidus) are surgical procedures that have been used to treat Parkinson's disease symptoms since the 1950s. Thalamic stimulation through surgical insertion of electrodes, and thalamotomy, are methods of treating cases of severe tremor. Pallidotomy, and pallidal and subthalamic nucleus stimulation, are used for the treatment of cases with severe levodopa-induced dyskinesias and rigidity. Also current is the implantation of dopamine-producing cells from the adrenal glands of the patient or from the nigral tissue of aborted fetuses into the patient's brain.

What are the pros and cons of each treatment?

Levodopa therapy is the most effective treatment for Parkinson's disease patients, particularly for the first five years after starting it. The short-term side effects include vomiting and nausea, low blood pressure and postural hypotension, psychotic experiences, and sleep disturbance. The major drawback of levodopa therapy is that after three to five years most people develop medication-related complications such as dyskinesias, wearing-off phenomena, and on–off fluctuations. The advantage of dopamine agonists, used in the treatment of Parkinson's disease either in the early phases when the symptoms are mild or after levodopa-related complications emerge, is that they produce fewer of the medication-related complications associated with levodopa.

In the early phases when symptoms are mild, anticholinergics may be prescribed. These mainly alleviate tremor and are not as effective as levodopa. Blurring of vision, constipation, dryness of mouth, urinary retention, and memory problems are among their side effects. To control stiffness or slowness in the early phases of the illness, amantadine is occasionally added to anticholinergics.

The advantages of the available surgical procedures are listed above. In addition, tremor and slowness can be alleviated by pallidotomy. Partial paralysis and slurring of speech are complications that can occur with thalamotomy.

The implantation of fetal nigral tissue into the striatum has produced some beneficial effects on motor function, but brain implantation is still in the early phases of development and only time will tell whether it is a viable treatment. Unfortunately, even in the hands of the most expert surgeons all forms of surgery carry the risk of irreversible damage to the brain, or even death.

PART II

Living with Parkinson's Disease

4

Chronic Illness

Marjan Jahanshahi
Brigid MacCarthy

This chapter gives you background information about the general as well as the more specific ways in which a chronic illness such as Parkinson's disease can affect the lives of the person affected and of his or her family. Stress, and its effect on mental and physical well-being, has been a topic of intensive research. This research has increased our understanding of how people react to and cope with stressful life events, and of the factors that are important in determining good or poor coping. The onset of a chronic, progressive, and disabling illness such as Parkinson's disease is undoubtedly a major life event.

We believe that knowing about the variety of reactions to stress and loss, and finding out which environmental and personal factors influence an individual's ability to face the challenge of stressful life events, can be helpful in several ways.

- ❖ It will prepare the person with Parkinson's disease, and his or her carer and family, for what to expect.
- ❖ It shows that a large proportion of those who experience stressful life events cope remarkably well.
- ❖ It gives insight into the personal and environmental resources that people need in order to arm themselves against the impact of stressful life events.

STRESS, APPRAISAL, SOCIAL SUPPORT, AND COPING

To most of us, the concept of stress is a familiar one. The term entered common usage in the 1960s, and ever since then the public has been aware of stress as something to be avoided. From a commonsense understanding of stress we tend to assume that its effects are simple and obvious: that when something unpleasant or difficult to handle happens to them, people feel bad, either physically or mentally. However, most readers will recognize from their own experience that this straightforward equation—stressful event leads to adverse reaction—fails to describe the complex process of adjustment when they are "under stress." Research evidence has also clearly demonstrated that individuals show enormous variation in how they respond to basically similar stresses. This has led scientists to develop more subtle, complex descriptions, or "models," of how people cope with stress.

Stress is difficult to define. In current thinking on stress and coping, it is defined, in deliberately general terms, as changes in the relationship between a person and his or her environment. When some major change happens, whether pleasant or unpleasant, the individual has to make some effort to adjust to the new circumstances. This adjustment will draw on personal resources—physical, mental, and social. A "change" becomes a "stress" when there is a marked imbalance between the effort required to adjust and the personal resources available.

Psychologists have studied the degree to which major life events such as the death of a loved one, marriage, divorce, the onset of a disabling illness, the birth of a child, the loss of one's job, moving house, children moving away from home are perceived and experienced as stressful. Two main findings of this research are of interest:

1. There is general consensus about what life events are perceived and experienced as more or less stressful. For most people the death of a loved one such as a spouse or a child is the most stressful of all. In general, events that are unexpected and over which the individual has less control, such as death and illness, create most stress.

2. Apparently positive life events such as marriage, the birth of a child, or promotion at work are also stressful. So it is obvious that stress is created by any change, whether positive or negative, that outstrips the individual's ability to cope.

The harmful effects of stress on physical and mental health are produced by various means. First, stress creates a biologic and physiologic
imbalance in the body. Second, under stress people are more likely to
engage in potentially harmful behaviors such as smoking or excessive
alcohol or food consumption. Harmful effects can be measured in terms
of subjective feelings of well-being and physical health. However, these
effects are never static. While individuals try to adjust to and cope with
stressful life events, these coping efforts, in turn, influence and redefine
the nature of the stressful event. So instead of coping with stress being a
question of a few simple reactions, an adequate understanding of how
individuals deal with it requires consideration of three sets of factors—
what we might call antecedents, mediating factors, and outcomes.

Antecedents

The first set of factors to consider, present before the stressful event
happens, can be summarized as *environmental conditions* and *personal
characteristics*. By "environmental conditions" we mean the social and
economic resources and constraints to which everyone is subject. These
include the amount and quality of *social support* available—that is, people
in the individual's environment on whom he or she can rely, to whom he
or she can turn for practical support, emotional ventilation, sympathy, and
understanding. At times of stress or crisis, social support may be provided
by family, friends, or colleagues. Emotional support takes the form of gestures of understanding, caring, comfort, and sympathy, which help people
to feel less isolated under stress.

When an individual is facing major changes, access to both kinds of
support, practical and emotional, has been shown to contribute much to
his or her eventual sense of well-being. To function as an effective buffer
against stress, the quantity and quality of the social support provided must
match the individual's needs. In the context of chronic disease, high levels
of uncalled-for social support may at times constitute a threat to autonomy
and independence, and in effect reduce his or her sense of self-worth. Ultimately, it is for the individual to perceive the amount and quality of social
support available as satisfactory and matching his or her needs. For some
people, a few intimate relationships are adequate, whereas others require
a network of support from friends and family.

Financial security can also cushion the impact of many different kinds of stress. In the personal accounts given by people encountering stress there are many instances of households being better able to cope by having ready access to goods and services that can be bought.

Personal characteristics include individual motives and beliefs about the self and the world. Self-esteem, or the beliefs, attitudes, and feelings that each of us has about our worth as a person, is a strong determinant of reactions to and coping with stress. Motives are shaped by the goals to which we have made a commitment, and by our value system. Personal goals and values tend to be formed in young adulthood and change little during adult life. They set our priorities for action and shape our emotional and practical responses when we are faced with stress. Beliefs concerning the degree to which events are perceived as personally controllable or due to chance affect our approaches to coping with those events. In the case of a physical disorder, the degree to which symptoms are objectively controllable, the rate of progression of the disorder, and our beliefs about whether our health is under our own personal control or under external control by powerful others such as doctors, or chance factors, are all likely to be important in the choices of the strategies we use to cope with illness. These personal characteristics contribute to our perceptions of events in our lives and determine the ways in which we eventually cope.

Mediating Factors

As we said before, the relationship between stress and coping is not direct or simple. In fact, it can be tracked along a number of complex routes. The impact of stress on the individual is influenced or moderated by a number of mediating factors, the most important of which are personal appraisal and coping strategies.

It has been said that, like beauty, stress is in the eye of the beholder. Events are not inherently stressful—they are interpreted as being so. To experience an event as stressful, a person has first to appraise or label it as such. The process of *appraisal*, which begins when an individual notices the onset of a stressful change, involves an evaluation of that change as either beneficial or harmful. The outcome of this judgment will depend on the external circumstances and personal beliefs and values described earlier, and will in turn determine how the individual chooses to cope. The concept of appraisal is central to the argument that personal perception and interpretation play a significant role in determining eventual well-being under stress. An event that fills one person with dread may strike another as an interesting challenge, an opportunity for personal development or the pursuit of important goals. Such nonthreatening appraisals of potentially stressful life events can substantially diminish their negative impact on the individual. The importance of appraisal in determining the outcome of stressful events shows that we all have access to psychological mechanisms within ourselves that can help us combat stress.

The concept of *coping* is equally difficult to define. Coping is considered to refer to all the various ways in which an individual faced with a stress-inducing situation, or *stressor*, tries to deal with or overcome his or her problems. These include his or her practical efforts, as well as the mental and emotional strategies he or she uses to come to terms with or reduce the emotional impact of the stressor. In general, people try to cope in two main ways: either by actively trying to change some aspect of their environment or of events—referred to as problem-focused coping, or by controlling the negative emotions they experience as a result of the stressful change—referred to as emotion-focused coping. Health-related examples of problem-focused strategies include seeking information about alternative therapies, participating in a medical treatment, or finding a new job that minimizes the impact of disability. The individual may also focus his or her coping efforts on changing the way that he or she interprets a specific stress in order to change its emotional meaning. These efforts are not passive, but involve an active process of restructuring of goals and values in line with the limitations imposed by the event. Examples of such emotion-focused strategies are finding new interests, discovering new faith or a different philosophy of life, and changing priorities.

When faced with the stress of illness, besides using strategies for controlling the symptoms, most people look for social support and resort to emotion-focused coping. Research has shown that when people seek to combat the demands of chronic physical illness, certain sorts of coping strategy—such as information-seeking or action-taking—lead to positive well-being. In contrast, strategies involving avoidance, denial, and blame are related to distress and a poorer overall adjustment to the illness. So coping strategies differ in terms of their effect on the individual's short-term or long-term adjustment, and can be either adaptive or maladaptive. Any coping strategies that improve people's adjustment to their new situation and enhance their sense of well-being are considered adaptive. Coping strategies that interfere with acceptance and adjustment are labeled maladaptive.

Clearly, not all coping strategies are equally effective, although research findings indicate that it is important to keep an open mind about what particular strategies are likely to be effective in particular circumstances. Misusing alcohol and drugs and unnecessary risk-taking are two prevalent strategies that rarely seem to have a positive effect. Denial and emotional distancing are less clearly maladaptive. In some circumstances—again, depending on the exact relationship between external circumstances and personal resources—they may be the only viable option.

Of course, no one relies exclusively on either problem-focused or emotion-focused efforts to cope. People who use a range of specific coping strategies have more positive outcomes, but it also seems that those who systematically use a limited number of ways of coping do better than those who randomly grab at a large number of strategies. Efforts focused on changing emotions and personal interpretations are likely to be more effective in situations where the source of stress is relatively intractable, while problem-focused efforts have more impact when there is considerable scope for manipulating external circumstances. In Western societies, stoicism, bearing it all with a smile, the "stiff upper lip," being in control—however it may be described—is a highly valued coping style. In practice, this idealistic but rather superficial means of coping can be kept up for only a short while, and usually at great emotional cost. More effective and realistic coping should incorporate and allow emotional expression, as well as more problem-focused ways of adjusting to illness.

Outcomes

Finally, and most importantly, it is worth taking a fresh look at the outcomes of coping. What do we mean by saying that an individual coped well with a stressful event? As we noted before, good and poor outcomes are defined in terms of the individual's adjustment to his or her circumstances and physical and psychological well-being. Satisfactory outcomes are associated with improved adjustment and physical and psychological well-being. Deterioration in adjustment and in physical and mental health are features of unsatisfactory outcomes. In the case of a chronic illness, we might also examine the effect of the patient's emotional state on his or her longer-term physical well-being. The significance of this latter factor has been harder to demonstrate clearly, perhaps because of the inevitable deterioration that is a feature of most chronic illnesses.

Many factors contribute to the way in which stressful events, such as the onset of a chronic illness, affect people. There is some evidence that the longer-term effects of stress are more closely related to an individual's expectations and aspirations than to external circumstances. Coping efforts bent on either meeting or changing personal agendas are likely, therefore, to be more successful. Indeed, personal accounts of coping with stress make it very clear that people are capable of infinitely flexible and courageous adaptations to very difficult circumstances.

In writing about his experiences of living with Parkinson's disease, Ivan Vaughan likens the stress of the illness to standing in front of a dam that is starting to leak. As a coping mechanism, he at first resorted to minimizing the significance of the diagnosis:

I felt as though I were standing in front of a dam. The walls were springing leaks in different places one after another. I raced round frantically trying to patch them up, but with my eyes closed in case I caught sight of the flood of water that threatened to engulf me. I could not acknowledge the seriousness of the illness because if I did so fear and panic would undermine the self-confidence I was still able to generate. Can't you see, Jan? [his wife]—it's a race between my developing ways of coping and people finding out about the illness. I accept that I've got the illness, honest, but I've got to pretend that it is not too serious, otherwise I'll be too intimidated to deal with it.

THE OBJECTIVE BURDEN AND THE SUBJECTIVE BURDEN

Adapting to any major crisis requires an effort to cope. But the consequences of an event, however traumatic, cannot be predicted simply by examining its basic features. As already suggested, individuals show an enormous range of reactions to essentially similar events, and vary as much in their ability to cope constructively. Also, as people *respond* to the threat or challenge that the stressful event poses, the nature of that event changes. They may manage practical consequences well or badly, so that the original event's impact is altered. Or they may alter the way they view it, so that it is perceived as more or less threatening. As we said before, the individual's appraisal of the stressful event and the particular coping strategies that he or she employs play a fundamental role in determining its physical and emotional impact.

Burden is a term that professionals use to help people think about the impact of a chronic disorder on the patient and his or her family. Distinctions are drawn between the visible difficulties and deficits to which a household with a chronically disabled member is prey—the so-called *objective burdens*—and the degree of distress *subjectively experienced* by the household members as a result of the objective burdens they face. With a chronic illness, the potential objective burdens, for patient and family members alike, may include the physical and social consequences of providing physical care, economic hardships, dwindling social networks, and loss of autonomy. The subjective burden represents not only the degree to which specific objective burdens are experienced as distressing, but also the overall impact on mental health and well-being of coping with a chronic disease.

Studies of people coping with different disorders have confirmed that objective and subjective burdens do not always closely coincide. These findings emphasize the importance of appraisal, personal perceptions, and interpretations in determining how stressful any one individual will find a particular set of circumstances. The levels of subjective burden, determined by personal agendas, expectations, and aspirations, can exaggerate or reduce the impact of any single objective burden. This being so, helping people arrive at more realistic appraisals of stressful events can, to an extent, diminish their distress and their subjective burden. Personal perception and appraisal act like a filter that modulates the relationship between the objective and subjective burdens, either enhancing or diminishing the anxiety, distress, and even depression experienced by the individual exposed to a stressful life event.

ACUTE AND CHRONIC ILLNESS

The image that most people have of being ill is modeled on episodes of acute illness such as appendicitis. Injury or pain and suffering descend suddenly. There is a crisis; doctors are called or consulted; hospitals, nurses, maybe operations, are all part of the picture. For a short while everyone may feel extremely worried about the patient's chances of survival. But after the crisis is past the patient recovers and life eventually returns to normal. The essential priorities in the management of *acute illness* are getting medical attention and treatment quickly, speedy cure, and survival.

The picture with a *chronic illness* is quite different. The onset of most chronic illnesses is not marked by a sudden crisis, but more characteristically by a gradual decline in physical well-being. Sometimes the onset, as with Parkinson's disease, is so slow and unremarkable that the symptoms may be mistaken for several other, minor disorders before a correct diagnosis is reached. Even after diagnosis, the person with Parkinson's disease will usually have only occasional involvement with hospitals and doctors. Survival is not at issue in the early stages of most chronic illnesses, so people are spared that intense acute anxiety. But the lack of a definitive focus for concern, the absence of an immediate crisis that everyone can recognize, bring their own difficulties. Of most importance, the patient, the family, and everyone else concerned have to come to terms with the fact that life will *not* shortly return to a familiar version of normality and that their expectations of the future must subtly change to accommodate a lifelong illness. The priorities for managing a chronic illness are very different: to delay deterioration, to limit discomfort, and to maintain the best possible "quality of life" whatever stage the disease has reached. These apparently modest aims are immensely challenging.

An episode of *acute illness* has a marked effect on the social status of its victim. For a limited time, the need for the patient to seek refuge in the role of sick person is fully recognized. This "sick role" gives him or her time off from normal responsibilities and grants him or her the right to be looked after, to be more dependent or helpless than at any time since young childhood. It also gives the patient the space to concentrate on fighting the illness and recovering. Although many adults feel intensely frustrated by the temporary loss of personal autonomy that goes with being cast in the sick role, they recognize the advantages of complying, of being a "good patient." There is no lasting stigma attached to this temporary status—after recovery, the previously sick person resumes all his or her old social roles, as spouse or partner, parent, colleague, friend.

But the effect on the personal status of a person with a *chronic disease* is significantly different—being cast in the sick role does *not* provide a welcome refuge that will facilitate a rapid recovery. Instead, it can be experienced as debilitating, threatening the individual's will to combat the disabling aspects of the disease, and ultimately promoting handicap. Loss of autonomy is an important issue for most people with chronic disorders, and successfully minimizing that loss at every stage is a key factor in maintaining a reasonable quality of life. Adjusting to the consequences of the disease may entail either immediate or gradual surrender of some social roles—for example, the work role—and subtle changes in the responsibilities inherent in others, such as those of spouse or partner, father or mother. In addition, most Western societies, with the high value they attach to autonomy and free choice, have difficulty in responding positively to the diminished social participation of chronically ill people.

Future aspirations, expectations of oneself, of employment, of interaction with spouse or partner, with children, family, and friends, are all altered by chronic illness. And the disability-associated loss of familiar social roles, activities, and interactions in turn results in a sense of psychological and emotional loss and diminished self-esteem.

We experience similar reactions to loss of any sort, whether the death of a loved one or the loss of normal function and familiar roles brought on by chronic illness. All loss is associated with grieving, a process that often has four phases.

1. shock, disbelief, and denial
2. anger
3. mourning and depression
4. acceptance and adjustment.

Different people pass through these four stages at different speeds. One individual may pass from the initial phase of shock to the fourth stage of acceptance and adjustment in a matter of months or even weeks. In contrast, progressing through the four phases may take another person years. The fact is that despite the overall similarities in people's reactions to loss, the processes of *grieving, acceptance,* and *adjustment* are very individual. In a sense, each person has to bear his or her own cross and come to terms with the loss in his or her own unique way.

Another characteristic of coping with loss is that the process is continuous and ongoing. Particularly with an illness such as Parkinson's disease, the nature and extent of the associated problems wax and wane over the years and people may find that they occasionally revert, emotionally, to an earlier phase, feeling angry, depressed, or unable to accept the reality of the disease. This may happen, for example, when there is a sudden deterioration of symptoms after a period of relative stability both of the symptoms and of the associated disability.

THE "PHASES" OF CHRONIC ILLNESS

One important determinant of how well people cope with a chronic progressive illness such as Parkinson's disease is, of course, the rate at which it progresses. For some luckier individuals, this will be a very slow process. For others, the symptoms will become worse very quickly. Four broad phases can be distinguished.

1. *Prediagnosis and immediate postdiagnosis phase*   Symptoms develop gradually and become clinically manifest over time. This first phase is often marked by feelings of uncertainty and shock.

2. *Early phase*   The period when the signs and symptoms are so mild that no treatment is yet required, or when changes are well controlled with treatment. Impairment and disability are either nonexistent or mild.

3. *Middle phase*   Usually the longest. As the disease progresses, impairment and disability will become greater. Treatment will still

effectively control the symptoms, but they will show variations in severity during the day, with the wearing-off effects and on–off changes already described. Medication-related dyskinesias including dystonia may cause additional problems.

4. *Late phase*   By now the disease is producing severe symptoms. Medical treatment produces little relief, and the medication-related fluctuations and side effects lead to marked disability.

Besides the variations in symptom severity and in disability, these four phases also differ in terms of the physical challenges that they present for both patient and carer, and in terms of the emotional challenges—the feelings of loss, depression, and anxiety that may be associated with each phase. And although Parkinson's disease affects the life of each individual in a unique way, for the majority the early phase is probably the least stressful, while the other three may be times of intense upheaval, anxiety, and depression.

The Prediagnosis Phase

As described earlier, the symptoms of the illness develop gradually over many years, and the length of the prediagnosis phase differs widely from person to person. For some time before the formal diagnosis, the individual will have been aware that something is wrong, without knowing exactly what, or its true significance. Even after the symptoms become clinically manifest, there may be a period of "diagnostic uncertainty," when doctors are not sure how to label the illness. One patient wrote:

It took about nine months from the first appearance of symptoms before I was diagnosed, and nobody seemed to know what was wrong.

This is also a period during which the symptoms may be noticed by the person concerned, but hidden from everyone else. This secrecy partly results from uncertainty about the meaning of the symptoms and partly from an unwillingness to be seen as complaining unnecessarily. One person with Parkinson's disease revealed:

It took me almost six months to tell my friends and family.

So the prediagnosis phase is likely to be characterized by uncertainty and confusion, while the individual and those close to him or her struggle to make sense of rather vague or subtle changes in his or her physical and mental well-being. Typically in this phase, people search for ways of understanding any emerging disability, and may settle for explanations that are inaccurate or unhelpful.

The Immediate Postdiagnosis Phase

Once given the diagnosis, people vary widely in their immediate reaction to being told that they have Parkinson's disease. Diagnosis may be associated with shock, confusion, anger, apprehension, resistance, and denial; or acceptance, and relief that finally the symptoms that have been slowly becoming evident have been labeled and are not of psychological origin or due to a tumor, but caused by a recognized disorder. In his book *The Spaces in Between* the graphic designer John Harris recalls:

The shock had been profound, as much to the family as to me, and that should not be underestimated. The very name had conjured up images of some doddery old geriatric, dribbling at the mouth, shaking and staring into space. Was this going to be me in ten years' time?

This sense of shock is expressed by others.

I was shattered, as I thought that they would not be able to do anything for me.
I felt angry and sorry for myself.

Two main reactions. Fear, because it is a progressive and incurable condition, but also relief that somebody had finally put a name to it and confirmed that it was not "all in my mind."

I was shaken up, and it took me five weeks before I told my wife and later some friends that I had developed Parkinson's disease. I was scared of being disabled. Working in the hospital I knew the sequelae of Parkinson's disease.

I was filled with disbelief for a few seconds, as during a career as a nurse I had met only elderly people with Parkinson's disease. I was only 43! Then the enormity of having Parkinson's disease hit me and I was devastated. All I could think of was that it was a life, if not a death, sentence. . . . My husband and I cried for two days, as did my daughter, aged 17 at that time.

When the child psychiatrist Dr. Cecil Todes was told by his internist that he probably had Parkinson's disease, his reaction was, by contrast, one of relief. *In A Shadow over My Brain,* he writes:

I was so relieved at not having a terminal brain tumor that anything less was welcome, especially as, in time and space, the end point seemed so far removed for the newly diagnosed sufferer.

The sense of relief following the diagnosis was expressed by another patient, too:

I was very afraid of what the diagnosis might prove to be. At one stage I guessed it was Parkinson's and was relieved when that was confirmed. I had imagined far worse scenarios, such as a brain tumor.

Just as in the prediagnostic phase, another early reaction to the diagnosis may be the desire to keep the illness a secret. Ivan Vaughan recalls:

I was absolutely determined to conceal from friends and colleagues that I was ill and, when I could no longer keep it secret, to minimize the seriousness of the illness. . . . I tried to avoid meeting people. I hid from friends I met in town and pretended I was not in when friends came round. Jan and I refused invitations to dinner parties or to visit friends. If I could not avoid seeing people, I would refrain from telling them what was wrong. I always preferred to be thought of as odd rather than as someone who was seriously ill.

The Early Phase

During the early phase, which may be quite prolonged for some people, disability may be minimal. Nevertheless, people with a chronic disease have to make a major psychological transition at this point. Both their self-image and their perception of their social status must adjust to the knowledge that they are no longer perfectly healthy, and never will be again. For some, this will entail little effort. If the individual is relatively elderly and perhaps does not place a high value on physical vigor, or if the level of disability progresses slowly enough to allow gradual adaptation, this transitional phase may have little emotional impact. But old and young alike are confronted with the reality of coming to terms with the knowledge that they have Parkinson's disease. Feelings of loss are very common during this phase, when people recognize that they have permanently lost their sense of physical invulnerability, and that some of their plans for the future may have to be altered. There are likely to be numerous practical issues to sort out, some of which will have to do with employment and future finance.

The Middle Phase

In the middle phase, which is usually the longest, levels of disability are moderate but the impact of the disease will be extremely variable. When it progresses slowly, adaptations can be made to new impairments, and this will in turn reduce the degree of disability or handicap resulting from each deterioration. At this point, the main challenge for both patients and family members is to strike the right balance between health and illness. A major concern is to obtain the maximum relief from medication. Levodopa may remain effective for some, but for others a decrease in its effectiveness will mean that other medications will be tried. As a result, contact with health professionals may become more frequent.

Psychologists have identified a style of coping with this stage of Parkinson's disease that they characterize as "sanguine and engaged."

This is exemplified by patients actively trying to cope with altered circumstances and enjoying the challenge of managing the practical and emotional consequences of the disease. In this phase, those whose disabilities increase too fast, or for whom medication loses its efficacy too quickly to allow this continual process of minor adjustment, are most vulnerable to serious depression. People in this situation tend to feel they are engaged in an unsuccessful struggle, and they often become very worried about the future.

The Late Phase

By now the disease is giving rise to severe symptoms that are no longer responsive to medication. Medication-related fluctuations and side effects are distressing in their own right. Now that disability has become severe, depression is much more common. Both patients and caregivers lose much of their ability to influence the course of events—the disease is more clearly in charge now, and a sense of helplessness may prevail. Physical demands become pressing. The patient gives up his or her active participation in a number of personal, family, and social roles, and the loss of independent functioning in turn entails a loss of privacy and dignity, which places high demands on mutual trust between patient and caregiver. As the scope for practical action is severely curtailed, coping efforts at this stage tend to focus more on emotional responses.

From what we have said, it will be clear that adapting to a serious chronic illness is not a simple process, completed at or soon after the point of diagnosis. It involves a continual series of adjustments, the timing and outcome of which are determined both by aspects of the disease process and by the psychological and social resources on which the individual can draw. The relationship between the severity of the illness and the psychological well-being of individual patients is not as simple and direct as one might expect—people who are more disabled are not necessarily more unhappy than less disabled people. What seems to happen is that psychological well-being ebbs and flows as the disease progresses, and this ebb and flow reflects the outcome of people's efforts to cope. Strategies that worked well at an earlier stage will not necessarily be adequate to deal with new challenges posed by a further deterioration, or a new combination of disabilities. While searching for new coping strategies the individual is likely to feel anxious or unhappy, but once ways are found to manage the practical and emotional implications, he or she will regain a psychological equilibrium.

IMPAIRMENT, DISABILITY, AND HANDICAP

In these last few sections dealing with the effects of stress on health and well-being, we have largely ignored the *symptoms* of Parkinson's disease. No one would minimize the importance of tremor, akinesia, bradykinesia, and rigidity—after all, the impact of a chronic illness on an individual's life is a consequence of the symptoms. But how do they translate into everyday life? A useful way of thinking about the consequences of the symptoms of Parkinson's disease is to use the distinction suggested by the World Health Organization (WHO) between *impairment, disability,* and *handicap.* We tend to use these terms interchangeably in everyday language, but let's clarify how they differ and why such a distinction may be helpful in understanding the effects of Parkinson's disease.

Impairment is most closely linked to the physical symptoms of the disorder. In a sense, impairment is the net result of the combined effects of the symptoms of tremor, rigidity, akinesia, and so on. The term refers to deficits or the changes from normal function that occur as a result of the symptoms. In Parkinson's disease the most significant impairment is in motor function—in other words, the impairment relates to how the person starts and carries out all forms of movement, from the simplest to the most complex. This motor impairment is not limited to particular movements or to specific parts of the body. It affects all movements and all parts of the body to different extents. Movements of the hands and arms appear to be most severely impaired.

Disability is the way in which impairment affects daily activities or restricts the individual's behavior. So in Parkinson's disease the motor impairment, when it becomes severe enough, leads to problems in getting dressed, drinking from a cup, using a knife and fork, writing, speech and nonverbal communication, walking, driving, and so forth. These are all forms of disability.

Handicap refers to the impact of the disease in its widest personal and social sense. The handicapping effects of illness are considered in relation to broad areas of life: mobility, work, social and leisure activities, relationships with others (colleagues, friends and family), physical independence, and economic self-sufficiency. While impairment and disability are measured against some general notion of normality, handicap can be judged only in relation to each individual's life, his or her immediate social context and future expectations—that is, in terms of how he or she functioned, worked, and played before the onset of the illness, or in terms of the life he or she would have been expected to be leading if the illness had not occurred. Loss of a job, marital breakdown and divorce, or the inability to play the piano after the onset of the illness are handicaps for people who were working or married or who derived great pleasure from playing the piano. These enjoyments would not be at stake for those who are single or have never worked, or who have never played the piano. For this reason, the WHO definition of handicap is "a disadvantage for a given individual, resulting from an impairment or disability, that limits or prevents fulfillment of a role that is normal (depending on age, sex, and cultural factors) for that individual."

Social prejudice, legal restrictions and regulations, and environmental obstacles can magnify, or even cause, handicap. Most public places do not adequately cater to people with disability. Public transport, and most theaters and restaurants, are inaccessible to people with a motor impairment who are confined to a wheelchair, and fire regulations may restrict their use of public premises. Social attitudes can play a major role in creating handicap. Ignorance, fear, and discomfort in the presence of disabled individuals lead people to treat them differently, to exclude them from ordinary social participation. Furthermore, the person with the illness may sometimes share some of these biases. For example, a sense of embarrassment or not wanting to be seen as different can lead people to give up certain social roles or to restrict their social participation. Also, the degree of handicap depends on the individual's coping mechanisms and on how he or she adapts his or her lifestyle to accommodate the illness and the associated impairment and disability.

The WHO has summarized the relationship between impairment, disability, and handicap in the following way:

$$\text{Impairment} \rightarrow \text{Disability} \rightarrow \text{Handicap}$$

When looking at this simple equation it is important to remember that the link between impairment, disability, and handicap is not always direct, or one-to-one. Not all impairments lead to disability, and not all disabilities are handicapping. Some people may be disabled with relatively little impairment, while others, despite having severe disabilities, may not be handicapped at all.

The degree of impairment and disability is undoubtedly important, but handicap depends on many other things as well. The life circumstances of the individual (age, marital status, job, financial security), the physical and social setting in which he or she lives (house or apartment, with or without elevator or facilities for wheelchair; whether or not he or she lives alone; whether there is a social support network available), his or her personal characteristics (self-esteem, beliefs, goals, motives, appraisal of the illness, and so on)—all play a part in preventing or producing handicap.

We have suggested in the preceding pages many intervening, or mediating, variables that determine the nature and severity of the disability and handicap experienced as the result of a given level of impairment. This complexity has an advantage—namely, that impairment and disability do not inevitably lead to handicap. Instead, individuals have the opportunity to make the most of their personal and social resources in order to prevent impairment and disability from producing handicap.

QUALITY OF LIFE

As we mentioned earlier, the traditional medical model of disease is primarily concerned with acute illness. Within this model, the individual falls ill, is treated, then recovers quickly, and contact with the medical profession ceases. Although this conventional picture does not fit well with chronic illness, here too medical management is often solely aimed at treatment of the symptoms, mainly through medication. The WHO considers this traditional approach to be inappropriate for chronic illness, in which the primary concern should be with "quality of life."

"Quality of life" is difficult to define, as it has many meanings. Under normal circumstances, a person's quality of life is related to how he or she functions and feels; it includes his or her physical and mental health, social activities and relationships, and economic, work, and environmental circumstances. When an individual falls ill, "quality of life" embraces the total effect of the illness, and its subsequent treatment, on physical, psychological, social, and occupational function, as perceived by that individual. In relation to the chronically ill, "quality of life" refers also to the personal and emotional reactions of individuals to the differences they perceive between their actual life and their desired life.

Quality of life is influenced by three sets of factors:

1. the wishes and expectations of the individual and of his or her family
2. the limitations imposed by the illness on the individual's ability to fulfill his or her wishes and expectations
3. the individual's reactions to these limitations, which include both emotional reactions and behavioral changes, such as changing jobs or finding new hobbies.

Like handicap, quality of life is extremely individual, and this is why there are many factors determining how chronic illness impacts it. Beliefs, desires, and expectations, habits and living circumstances, culture and social environment, are all important determining factors. Of course, limitations are also largely dictated by the nature of the symptoms and the associated impairment, disability, and handicap. The WHO recommends that in cases of chronic illness, instead of concentrating solely on medical treatment of the symptoms, doctors and health professionals should shift the emphasis to managing disability and handicap. The primary concern should be with promoting and maintaining a good quality of life for the ill person and his or her caregiver and family.

KEY FACTS 4

What is stress?

Any change, whether positive or negative, that creates an imbalance in a person's life and outstrips his or her ability to cope, becomes stressful. The most stressful life events are those that are unexpected and over which the individual has less control, such as the death of a loved one or the onset of an illness.

What factors determine the effects of stress on an individual?

People differ in their reactions to stress and in terms of how well they cope with it. The *outcome* of stress can be either an improvement or a worsening of adjustment and physical and emotional well-being. The effects of stress on the individual are not direct but, rather, are influenced by antecedent and mediating factors. *Antecedent factors* are present before the stressful encounter; they include the personal characteristics of the individual (such as his or her sense of self-esteem, motives, beliefs about personal control), and the environment in which he or she lives (which includes financial circumstances and the availability of social support). The features of the stressful event that he or she has to face (rate of progression and controllability of symptoms in chronic illness) are also important. *Social support*— that is, the availability of people on whom the individual can rely for sympathy, understanding, emotional and practical help—has been shown to protect individuals against the negative impact of stress. *Mediating factors* such as the individual's personal appraisal of the situation and his or her coping abilities moderate the effect of the stress—that is, either magnify or reduce its impact. *Appraisal*, or personal perception and interpretation of the stressful event as negative or positive, is a major determinant of reactions to it. The *coping strategies*—that is, the behavioral, practical, and emotional methods used by the individual—can help him or her to come to terms with the change and reduce its impact on his or her life. So the effects of stress are not straightforward, but can be modified in many complex ways.

What are objective and subjective burdens?

The term *burden* signifies here the impact of chronic illness on the individual and on his or her family. *Objective burdens* are all the demands and restrictions imposed on the family's resources by chronic illness, such as the physical strain of caregiving, the shrinking of social networks, economic hardship, loss of independence or autonomy. *Subjective burden* is the distress experienced by the ill person, the caregiver and other family members as a result of the objective burdens. Objective and subjective burdens do not have a one-to-one relationship. Some experience very little subjective burden even when exposed to major objective burdens, while others feel greater subjective burden despite facing smaller objective ones. The distinction between objective and subjective burdens highlights the importance of personal appraisal, of the individual's perception of the stressful event and his or her circumstances, in determining the way in which he or she copes.

How do acute and chronic illness differ?

An acute illness such as appendicitis is associated with sudden pain and suffering followed by medical intervention and restoration to full health. During the usually short while that the person is ill, there may be anxiety, survival may be at stake, and he or she can adopt the "sick role" and be exempt from normal responsibilities. Once cured, the individual resumes previous roles and returns to normal function. The onset of chronic illness is often much more gradual; usually there is no event clearly marking the transition from health to illness, other than diagnosis of the symptoms by a doctor. When chronic illness is progressive, the symptoms become worse over time; daily activities, and social and occupational functioning, will show a gradual decline. The chronically ill person gives up familiar roles at work, at home, and socially. In the later phases, loss of autonomy and increasing dependence may occur. In chronic illness, survival is not an immediate issue. The focus is on delaying deterioration, limiting discomfort and distress, and ensuring the best "quality of life" possible.

How does chronic illness create a sense of loss, and what are the related psychological stages?

The symptoms of chronic illness result in loss of normal function with disability in daily activities. The relinquishing, over time, of familiar personal, occupational, and social roles, alterations in habitual ways of living and interacting, pose a threat to self-esteem. Future expectations and aspirations are fundamentally changed. All of this can create a sense of emotional loss in the chronically ill person. Reactions to loss, whether of a loved one through death or of normal function and roles through chronic illness, are similar. Loss, like grieving, has four phases: (1) shock, disbelief, and denial, (2) anger, (3) mourning and depression, (4) acceptance and adjustment. The pace of psychological transition through these phases varies from person to person—a few months or many years. Also, as the nature and severity of problems posed by Parkinson's disease change over time, people may occasionally revert temporarily to an earlier phase of emotional reaction—for example, when new or more severe symptoms develop.

How do the demands and challenges posed by chronic illness change with the "phase?"

Coping with a chronic illness is not a "one-time" challenge, but a continuous and ongoing process with many ups and downs. The rate of progression plays a major part in determining the demands and challenges faced by the ill person, the caregiver, and the family. In Parkinson's disease, four "phases" can be distinguished:

1. *Pre-diagnosis phase*   Often marked by uncertainty and confusion; followed by the immediate post-diagnosis phase, which may be associated with shock, anger, resistance, and denial, as well as relief that the symptoms finally have a recognizable label.

2. *Early phase*   Symptoms are very mild, disability is nonexistent or equally mild. Patients must now modify their self-image and future expectations to adjust to the knowledge that they have a progressive illness. Practical arrangements may be instigated to prepare for future unemployment, loss of earnings, and disability.

3. *Middle phase* (usually the longest)   Moderately severe symptoms and disability. Medication is more or less effective in controlling the symptoms. Social and occupational roles may be relinquished. Much effort may center on obtaining a combination of medications to produce maximal control of symptoms. Depression may ensue when a sudden or severe worsening of symptoms occurs.

4. *Late phase*   The illness is producing severe symptoms, no longer controlled by medication. Medication-related complications such as on–off fluctuations, wearing-off, and dyskinesias add to the disability. Feelings of helplessness may set in, as the disease may seem to take over and physical dependence increases.

What are the differences between impairment, disability, and handicap?

These terms differ in the extent to which they relate either more closely to the symptoms of the illness or to the individual's characteristics and circumstances. *Impairment* relates most closely to the symptoms. In Parkinson's disease, motor impairment results from the combined effects of tremor, rigidity, bradykinesia, akinesia, and postural instability. This gives rise to *disability* in daily activities. When impairment becomes severe, the individual has difficulty with daily activities such as dressing, bathing, shaving, cooking, eating with a knife and fork, drinking from a cup. *Handicap*, which has been defined as "a disadvantage for a given individual, resulting from an impairment or disability that limits or prevents fulfillment of a role that is normal (depending on age, sex, and cultural factors) for that individual," relates more closely to the individual and his or her social circumstances than to the symptoms. Chronic illness can create restrictions with mobility, work, social and leisure activities, relations with others, physical independence, and economic self-sufficiency. The association between impairment, disability, and handicap is not direct: not all impairments lead to disability, not all disabilities are handicapping. Some people may be severely disabled despite only mild impairment; others may not be handicapped at all by severe impairment and disability. Social prejudice, legal restrictions, environmental obstacles, can all help create handicap. The individual's psychological makeup, appraisal of the situation, and the coping strategies he or she uses are important in determining handicap. The complex route to handicap allows people ways of using their personal and social resources to prevent impairment and disability from creating handicap.

5

From the Perspective of the Person with Parkinson's Disease

Richard Brown

This chapter considers the broader aspects of Parkinson's disease as seen from the patients' perspective, and the impact of the symptoms on their lives. As Chapter 4 has outlined, depending on their circumstances and their outlook on life, people react very differently to the problems and limitations imposed by chronic disease; some of these reactions can be positive and others negative.

I had two major problems in setting out to write this chapter. First, I do not have Parkinson's disease. I can only suppose, from my experience as a clinical psychologist and the knowledge I have acquired through talking to many people who have, what their lives must be like. I realize that I will be wide of the mark at times. Second, my experience has taught me that Parkinson's will not affect any two people in exactly the same way. Indeed, the main message of this chapter is that you cannot separate the disease from the person, and that you cannot separate the person from the world in which he or she lives. Even if I did have the illness, my experiences and thoughts about it would be very different from those of others—what might be true or appropriate for me might have very little relevance for another person with Parkinson's.

For these reasons, I have tried to deal with the broad issues of living with Parkinson's disease. Where I can, I illustrate these issues with examples. Some of you may recognize yourself and your life in these descriptions, while others may find little that seems familiar. I hope, though, that you will all find something of value here, even if it is just an alternative way of looking at your situation.

First, I'll consider the impact of Parkinson's disease on various aspects of an individual's life. The categories that I have used—daily activities, mobility, leisure, and so on—are in some ways artificial. Obviously there is often a close relationship between them. Factors that affect one area will also influence others; strategies for dealing with one aspect of handicap can be applied to others. However, there are also some important differences between them, which I will highlight as they arise.

DAILY ACTIVITIES AND SELF-CARE

Once we leave infancy behind us, we take responsibility for a number of key areas of our lives—we wash and toilet, dress, and feed ourselves. These activities probably represent the most basic level of independence. They are accomplishments that we take for granted for most of our childhood, not just as adults. But there is obviously more to independence than this. It may also include, for instance, being able to do your own shopping, cooking, and housework; turning on the television when you choose; reading a book; or using the telephone. We all have a core of activities that form our lives as individuals, that constitute an important part of our sense of personal identity.

As described in Chapter 4, all of us at some time or other go through periods when we have to suspend these activities for a short time—for example, if we are taken ill, admitted to the hospital for an operation, or break a limb. In such cases it is relatively easy to cope with the lack of independence, because we know that soon it will be regained. But in Parkinson's disease, the decrease in independence happens gradually. This has both positive and negative implications. On the positive side, it is possible to make gradual adjustments, both practical and emotional, as the changes occur. There is no sudden, overnight loss of independence with which you and others have to cope. On the negative side, everyone with Parkinson's is aware of the progressive nature of the disorder. Although they will hope for a dramatic new treatment or even a miracle cure, most will be aware that the future probably holds the prospect of increased dependence on others.

Unlike some other aspects of handicap, problems with the *activities of daily living* (ADLs) show a relatively predictable increase as the disease progresses from the early to middle and late phases. This is because these activities are among the most closely related to the physical symptoms of the disease.

In the earliest phase of Parkinson's, daily activities are largely unaffected. You may be slightly slower at carrying out some tasks, but they can still be done independently. To some degree, the amount of difficulty experienced will depend on the pattern of the symptoms. For example, Parkinson's disease usually starts on one side of the body before progressing to the other. If the disorder starts on the right side rather than on the left, a right-handed person may have more early problems with simple tasks. The sort of difficulty that occurs in the earliest stage tends to be with fast repetitive hand movements. For instance, you may notice that brushing your teeth or polishing shoes requires a bit more effort and takes longer. Handwriting may be noticeably slower. It is sometimes this type of difficulty that is the first sign that an individual has Parkinson's disease. But although possibly annoying, such difficulties will have little impact on his or her ability to look after him- or herself.

As the disease progresses, problems with the activities of daily living become more marked, although the vast majority of everyday tasks are still achievable. They simply take a bit more time and effort. Previous difficulties may be more noticeable, and new problems may develop. For instance, slowness or tremor may make getting dressed a chore, particularly where buttons and other fasteners are concerned. Some of the problems will be associated with a general decrease in mobility (discussed in the next section). For example, it may become more difficult to take a shower if getting in and out is a problem; extra care may be needed to minimize the risk in potentially dangerous actions such as lifting a saucepan of boiling water.

However, although such everyday tasks are more difficult, or require extra attention in order to avoid accidents, it is still rare for independence to be seriously affected at this stage. This is mainly because there are many opportunities to work around any problems, such as:

❖ changing the time when you attempt a particular activity, so as to make the optimal use of your best time of day

❖ replacing old ways of doing things with new ways that are less problematic, such as showering rather than having a bath, or using zippers or Velcro rather than buttons.

❖ using any of the many simple aids and tools that are available, such as a button-hook, or a handrail in the tub.

Of course, how helpful these strategies are depends on how willing the individual is to change and adapt. The person who rigidly tries to do the same tasks, in precisely the same way, at precisely the same time, will have many more problems than the person who is always ready to try out new ways of doing things. The subject of *strategies* for coping with some of the problems of living with Parkinson's disease is dealt with more fully in Chapter 9.

In the late stage of Parkinson's disease, the physical symptoms have progressed so that many of the everyday tasks may be difficult or even impossible without help from someone else. For some, the early and middle stages of Parkinson's disease will last for seven or eight years, while others may continue to take care of themselves without major difficulty for twenty years or more. Indeed, a few people never seem to progress to the late stage. However, those who do, sooner or later, reach this stage may find themselves dependent on others for some activities. This will be particularly true when general mobility is severely affected and the individual requires a wheelchair. He or she will often need help when moving from bed to wheelchair, or from wheelchair to toilet.

Other problems that severely limit self-care are severe tremor and abnormal involuntary movements. These may make *tasks requiring fine control,* such as shaving or eating, virtually impossible. However, there are still things that can be done. There will still be times of day when the individual has some mobility or when the symptoms are relatively mild. Making best use of these times will enable him or her to maintain some independence. Even when the symptoms are at their worst, there will always be something that the individual can do, whether alone or with someone else's help. These little acts, however insignificant they may seem at the time, are very important in maintaining self-esteem—as the following case illustrates:

John's Parkinson's disease had started 15 years earlier. Although still mobile about the house, he had problems with severe abnormal invol-

untary movements which made it difficult for him to do simple tasks such as making himself a cup of coffee or shaving. He either had to leave these things undone or call for help from his wife, both of which he found frustrating and sometimes demoralizing. However, he enjoyed the challenge of thinking of ways around his problems, and attempted to treat it as a bit of a game. So he started making his coffee when he was in a good phase and storing it in a thermos flask with a straw; he switched from a safety razor to an electric one, and bought a telephone with large buttons and a storing facility for frequently used numbers. He valued the opportunity to demonstrate his continued independence about the home, and the ability to use his brain in his battle with the "dreaded movements."

MOBILITY

Together with daily activities and self-care, mobility is probably the most significant aspect of life affected by Parkinson's disease. The ability to move around independently, in our homes or outside, is critical to us all. It enables us to carry out the many activities to do with work, leisure, and day-to-day tasks that define much of our lives. Where mobility is reduced, the resultant handicap can be widespread. It is for this reason that so much of the clinical management of Parkinson's is concerned with maintaining mobility.

While walking is the most obvious aspect of mobility, there are many other actions and behaviors involved in moving our bodies from place to place. "Mobility" includes climbing stairs, bending down, getting up from a chair, and turning over in bed, as well as our ability to travel longer distances on bicycles, in wheelchairs, in cars, and on public transport.

Moving Your Body

First, how is your ability to move your body "under your own steam" affected when you have Parkinson's disease? In the early phase there will be little impact. You may notice some physical changes—your stride may be shorter and you may walk a little more slowly—but there is little hand-icap. Getting up out of a chair and turning over in bed will present no sig-nificant problems. In other words, you will still be able to do all the things you could do before, if sometimes a little more slowly. Any handicap will be slight.

Walking: A Complex Problem

As the disease progresses, problems with mobility begin to arise. In par-ticular, difficulty with walking may become more obvious; this is due to a number of factors, which may develop at different rates and emerge at dif-ferent stages:

❖ decreasing stride length
❖ increasing fatigue
❖ flexed posture
❖ problems with balance
❖ "freezing"

Stride length will continue to shorten, and walking may become more tiring. The person with Parkinson's may be able to walk only short dis-tances before he or she needs to take a short rest. In addition, another set of symptoms starts to emerge—problems with *posture* and *balance*. The body starts to become flexed, with the knees bent and the head forward. There is an increasing tendency to walk with the weight forward, on the balls of the feet or on the toes, and with the heels off the ground. This posture is less stable, and the individual may feel uncomfortable and slightly off balance when walking. Unfortunately, the normal reflexes that we use to maintain balance cease to function properly in Parkinson's disease. An extra problem that develops later on in some people is "freezing," as described in Chapter 1. When walking, taking the first step may be a problem—the feet may seem to be stuck to the ground. At other times, such as when going through a doorway, the feet may suddenly stop. In both cases, getting started again may take some time and effort.

Falls

One major problem when you have Parkinson's disease is falling. This is a result of the many factors described previously—the change in stride pattern and posture, the loss of normal balance reflexes, and freezing. While problems with walking may be inconvenient and restrict your actions, falls present a real danger, with the risk of severe bruising or broken bones. The loss of postural reflexes tends to mean that when an individual falls, he or she falls more heavily than usual. So while anyone else may stumble and reach out a hand to steady him- or herself, the person with Parkinson's will fall like a felled tree.

Falls may occur by tripping over small obstacles, when attempting to stop suddenly, when changing direction, when trying to walk too fast, or through suddenly "freezing" when on the move. Stepping backward—for example, when opening a door—is also a problem in Parkinson's disease and may lead to a fall.

While falls can be dangerous in themselves, they can also have a wider impact. Some people, although unsteady, may never fall but may be afraid of doing so. Others may fall once or twice and become fearful. Such individuals may avoid walking, or stay within their own homes where they feel more confident. As a result, they suffer a severe loss of mobility. Clearly, this handicap is caused more by fear and loss of confidence than by the physical symptoms of Parkinson's disease.

Other Mobility Problems

As mentioned earlier, other actions such as rising from a chair or getting out of the bath may present problems as the disease progresses.

Penny had moderate Parkinson's disease, which had started about eight years earlier. Although quite capable of moving about the house on her own, and looking after herself, she found that she was always getting stuck in chairs, particularly the comfortable armchair that she most enjoyed sitting in. She would try to lean forward and push with her arms, but would be unable to shift herself more than a few inches before falling backwards. She would either have to call for help, or gradually shuffle forward to the edge before struggling to her feet.

Why should simple actions suddenly become so difficult? One reason is that they are not really so simple. They seem so because we have been practicing them since early childhood, but in fact they require the precisely timed and coordinated movement of many different muscles. Parkinson's disease seems to interfere with carrying out such *automatic* actions. People who have it often report having to think about the individual components of an action, then having to carry out each one deliberately and consciously. Unfortunately, because we have never had to think about these actions before, it is not always obvious what we have to do to achieve them. As in the preceding example, it is common to see someone with Parkinson's disease struggling to get out of an armchair—pushing up with the arms and legs but unable to rise successfully to his or her feet. In fact, it is only by watching someone *without* Parkinson's that you can see how it should be done. First, he or she brings the feet in, as close as possible to the chair, or even slightly underneath it. Second, the upper body leans forward. These two actions serve to move the center of gravity of the body over, and slightly in front of, the feet. Only then, with the upper body still moving forward, does the person push up, using arms and legs together. However, ask him or her how it's done, and he or she will probably be unable to tell you.

Cars and Driving

Of all forms of transport, as a society we have grown to depend most upon the car. For many people with Parkinson's, the question of driving is a critical issue. Should they be driving? When should they stop? How will they manage if they do stop? And the emotional impact of giving up driving is likely to be as important as the practical consequences. For many, this signals the point at which the disorder is starting to have a real impact on their life. Depression is a common reaction.

Each state has its own laws regarding when an individual is considered unsafe to drive. You should check with your state's Department of Motor Vehicles to determine whether your medical status puts your legal right to drive in jeopardy. Obviously, you should also exert common sense in this area—you should not drive in any circumstances in which you cannot safely manage driving, and your family members or friends may be better judges of your abilities than you are yourself.

Slowness of movement initiation and execution, rigidity, and dyskinesias are the symptoms that most affect driving. When the symptoms are mild, such as when the individual is slightly slower than before or has a slight tremor, he or she can continue to drive. But when disability becomes moderate or severe, it is safer to stop driving. Some people with Parkinson's give up driving before they need to, perhaps through lack of confidence. Others time their car trips to coincide with their best "on" periods and continue to drive safely for short distances for a number of years. If you do decide to give up driving, it is important to look at all the alternatives that are available, preferably before stopping, including having your caregiver able to drive. (This is dealt with more fully in Chapter 10.) Depending on where you live, there will probably be a whole range of options, from public transport, taxis, car services, and paratransit, to getting lifts from friends and members of local voluntary groups. Making full use of these options is critical if stopping driving is not to mean that you feel housebound.

However, although alternative means of transport are available, they bring with them some new problems. There may be a long walk to a bus stop, for example, and stairs or escalators to deal with. You may have to cope with crowds pushing on and off buses and trains, and the often unpredictable starts, stops, and turns, which can be difficult when you are standing or walking toward the exit. All of these can be dealt with, though, and some suggestions are offered in Chapter 9.

WORK AND LEISURE

Why is mobility important? The main reason is that it allows us to get from A to B, either in the home or outside of it, and the reason for getting to B is usually in order to *do something*. Mobility, therefore, is a means to an end, not merely an end in itself. Besides self-care activities such as washing, dressing, and going to the toilet, we spend most of our time resting, working—either at a formal job or doing household chores—or at some form of leisure or social activity. Occupying our time in a purposeful, productive, and enjoyable manner is crucial to maintaining both our mental well-being and our physical well-being.

Work

Parkinson's disease may appear after a person has finished his or her normal working life and has retired. For such people, the main impact of the disease will be on their ability to engage in their usual leisure and social activities. For younger people, however, the impact of the illness on their career is an important concern. Apart from the obvious financial implications, a person's job often forms such an important part of his or her sense of personal identity that giving up work can leave a gap that is difficult to fill. Most people, therefore, will want to continue working for as long as they can.

However, the obvious question—"Will Parkinson's disease affect my ability to work?"—is an almost impossible one to answer in general terms. Fortunately, the immediate answer for most people is that there is no reason why they should not be able to continue working as effectively as before. In the early stage, when the symptoms are mild and well controlled by medication, it should be business as usual. With time, and progression of the disease, though, that business may change. But even then no two people's situations will be the same. As we have already seen, individuals vary enormously in the rate of progression, their particular pattern of symptoms, and their response to medication. People vary just as much, of course, in the kind of work they do. For those with active, physically demanding jobs, mobility may be a limiting factor in their ability to work. As noted in Chapter 1, writing is a major problem for many people with Parkinson's disease. Tremor and dyskinesias can make even the neatest handwriting illegible. Even when tremor and involuntary movements are not a problem, the legibility may still be reduced, particularly if the handwriting size decreases—so-called *micrographia*. Writing is not the only form of communication that may be affected: some people with Parkinson's find speech a problem *(dysphonia)*. The voice may be softer and more monotonous—at worst it may be virtually inaudible.

When it comes to the influence of the disorder on an individual's ability to perform his or her job, what is critical is how the job and the disease "fit" together. With luck, the person's job and his or her own "personal" Parkinson's disease will be compatible, allowing him or her to continue working for many years, perhaps to normal retirement age. If the individual is unlucky, the symptoms will make it impossible for his or her usual work to be carried out, even early on. The choices may then be early retirement, a progressive reduction of working hours, or, if possible, changing the nature of the job. These are reflected in the following varied experiences of three people with Parkinson's disease.

Dorothy worked in her local bureau of vital statistics. An important aspect of her job was entering details into the official registers of births, marriages, and deaths. She had always taken pride in her handwriting. One of the first signs of her Parkinson's disease, even before it was diagnosed, was a gradual deterioration in the size and clarity of her writing. Things improved once she started taking levodopa, but soon started to deteriorate again. Although her other symptoms were still mild, and her hand-writing was still legible and adequate by most people's standards, it was not good enough for her to continue her work. She chose to retire a few years early and make the most of the time when her Parkinson's disease was still mild.

Tom worked from home as a freelance book editor. His job involved reading manuscripts, copyediting—that is, correcting typescripts before the publishers sent them for typesetting, and proofreading. After 16 years, his Parkinson's disease had made him largely housebound, and dependent on his wife for much of his day-to-day care. However, he was still able to sit at his desk and read, and his handwriting, although slow, was still legible. He was not able to carry on for more than an hour or two without getting tired, but working from home, he could take a rest whenever he needed to. Although he knew that he might have to reduce his workload at some point in the future, he saw no reason why he should not continue working indefinitely.

Dave had been a taxi driver for 20 years before his Parkinson's disease was diagnosed. He continued working for five another years, but found it increasingly difficult. He was uncomfortable sitting for long periods without being able to stretch his legs, and an increasing need to go to the toilet proved inconvenient. However, he was reluctant to give up work completely. His employers were sympathetic, and found him a position in the control room, taking calls and assigning fares to the other drivers. He was able to maintain links with long-standing friends and colleagues, continue to use his local knowledge, and keep a salary coming in before he reached retirement age.

Early retirement or changing the nature of their work is perfectly acceptable to many people. For others, however, making such decisions is seen as a defeat. Rather than adapting their working life around the limitations of the disease, they try to carry on as before despite increasing difficulty.

Fatigue plays a central role in limiting people's ability to continue to work, as was noted in most accounts in John Williams's *Parkinson's Disease and Employment*. Fatigue is a fact of life for many people, and one for which they are not always prepared. Perhaps because even everyday tasks require more effort, they are liable to tire more easily and require breaks to "recharge their batteries." Unfortunately, medication does not necessarily relieve this feature of the disease. As with symptoms such as tremor and freezing, rushing, or working under pressure—which, sadly, are features of many people's jobs—is likely to make it worse.

Fatigue is not simply physical. Many people with Parkinson's disease report that they find it difficult to concentrate for long periods without a break. Depending on the nature of the job, this mental fatigue may be the main limiting factor. One of the people who figured in Williams's booklet, a pharmacist, found that he had to concentrate so hard on manipulating the equipment and pouring medicines from one bottle to another that he was afraid of making a mistake in the prescriptions. In his case, lapses in concentration could have had serious consequences. At home, of course, it is possible to take things easy for a while, or schedule physically or mentally demanding tasks for the "best" times of the day. At work this may be more difficult to arrange, and will depend on the nature of the job and whether employer and colleagues are willing to make accommodations. It is important to remember that you are protected in the workplace by law. The Americans with Disabilities Act (ADA) provides strict guidelines for the employment of people with disabilities. We refer you to Mark Stolman's *A Guide to Legal Rights for People with Disabilities* (New York: Demos, 1994).

Another common theme in the accounts that Williams gives is the importance at work of other people—employers, colleagues, employees. This is dealt with more fully in Chapter 10, but it is important to introduce it here because it raises a crucial issue about living with Parkinson's disease—the willingness to be open and honest with others. Within the workplace it is commonly feared that *telling other people* about the illness will lead to the individual concerned being treated differently, and to his or her disadvantage. The person with a disabling condition tends to expect people to feel sorry for him or her, to underestimate his or her capabilities, or to feel embarrassed and steer clear. There may even be the fear that he or she will be fired once employers know about the illness.

Bob worked as a salesman for a farm equipment manufacturer. He had always enjoyed his job, and had taken pride in the fact that his name was always near the top in the monthly sales figures. His job involved long hours and a lot of driving about the countryside. When he was 53 he discovered that he had Parkinson's. Although the disease was still mild and well controlled by medication, he was extremely worried about the impact that it would have on his work, and on his employer's attitude. Because the farm equipment market was sluggish at that time, and his work was judged on results, he was afraid that his employer would dismiss him and take on a younger salesperson. At his age, he was worried about his ability to find another job. As a result, he told no one about his Parkinson's disease. He kept his visits to the office to a minimum, and avoided meeting colleagues socially in case they noticed any of the symptoms.

In contrast to Bob's feeling that it was essential to maintain secrecy, the overwhelming message coming from the writings of those with Parkinson's disease is the exact opposite—they were amazed at how helpful and supportive everyone at work was once they knew. Many, such as Dave, the taxi driver mentioned previously, were able to continue working because of the support of others (despite the ADA, it is still possible for people to be made so uncomfortable in the workplace that they quit even if it is legally unnecessary). It is encouraging to hear that people's fears about telling others are seldom realized.

Eventually Bob found that the pressure of work and the stress of keeping his Parkinson's disease a secret were too much. He went to his manager and told him that he wished to resign. Explaining about his illness, he was surprised to discover that his manager had suspected the truth for some time, as his own mother had it. He was also unwilling to accept Bob's resignation, saying that his experience and long-term contacts with clients were too valuable for the company to lose. He asked him to continue, adding that the company would be willing to make some allowances if he found things too difficult, perhaps by reducing the size of his sales territory. Bob accepted and continued working productively for several years before choosing to take early retirement.

Leisure and Social Activities

Leisure and social activities form an important part of our lives. For the person who is working, they provide the opportunity to switch off the stress of work and to relax. Depending on the activities concerned, they may provide either physical or mental exercise—which are important for everyone, but particularly for someone with an illness such as Parkinson's. For retired people, such activities constitute a major way of occupying their time.

If anything, people's *hobbies* and other leisure pursuits are even more varied than the types of work they do, so it is difficult to generalize about how much of a problem in this area Parkinson's disease will be. Individual symptoms may interfere or not, depending on the nature of the activity, although factors such as fatigue may have a more general impact. Fortunately, we have far more flexibility in organizing our leisure pursuits than we do our work. We have the freedom to choose what we do and when we do it. The danger, as will be discussed below, is that with Parkinson's disease the individual may take this freedom to an extreme and choose to do nothing for much of the time.

Hobbies and other leisure activities can be broken down into two broad areas—activities that we do in our own homes and those that we do outside. Often, our home activities will be solitary, while those outside will involve other people. With Parkinson's disease, it is the latter, social, activities that are most at risk.

There are many reasons why people with Parkinson's may cut back on *social activities* outside the home. Often these relate to problems of mobility: individuals may be unable to walk as far as they used to; they may have given up driving; public transportation may be expensive, unreliable, or inconvenient. All of these may make getting out more difficult. Fatigue may also play a role—the effort of getting to their destination may leave people with Parkinson's disease too tired to enjoy themselves once they get there. The result may be that, more and more, they spend time at home.

But psychological factors may be even more responsible for this reduction in social activities. Someone who is subject to falls, "freezing," or unpredictable on–off fluctuations may lack the confidence to venture far from home. These, and many of the more visible signs of the illness such as tremor and dyskinesia, may be a source of embarrassment. Many of the accounts written by people with Parkinson's describe accidents or other incidents in public situations. This is from Sidney Dorros's book— *Parkinson's Disease: A Patient's View*:

Suddenly, as I got close to a crowd, I froze in my tracks. I could not take a single step more, and had I not been supported by my wife and friend, I would have slipped to the floor. They practically carried me to a nearby couch and stretched me out on it. I had to rest there for over an hour before I could move.

Eating and drinking in public, whether in restaurants or at the homes of friends, is another important social activity that is often avoided, even in the early stages. Tremor or dyskinesia may make eating and drinking difficult or messy. Cutting food may be a problem, as may swallowing. Dorros describes a typical scene:

I remember how this "on–off" effect affected me when my wife and I and another couple had dined at a fashionable restaurant in a hotel near our home. During dinner I was so dyskinetic I tipped over my water glass and scattered food off my plate in all directions.

Another example is provided by Dr. F., an internist, in another booklet compiled by John Williams, *Parkinson's Disease: Doctors as Patients: Eleven Autobiographical Accounts*:

My table manners have deteriorated and I sometimes need help with cutting up meat. Involuntary movements of my legs sometimes cause trauma to those of adjacent guests. I try to avoid cocktail parties: I spill my drinks if standing up and if sitting tend to be treated as an ashtray or a social leper with whom the occasional guest will spend five minutes before "circulating on."

The social embarrassment associated with the symptoms and avoidance of social situations is also described by Dr. J.:

One of my biggest handicaps and fears is in being invited out to tea or any social gathering. I am fine for perhaps 20 minutes, then tremor takes over and I feel lost and miserable. I know I can avoid such gatherings, I don't go very often, but then one becomes a recluse and that is not good either.

It is easy to see how people may want to avoid such situations, perhaps from an early stage. From childhood, we are taught about the importance of "behaving properly" in public. Society tends to dictate rules and standards that we expect of ourselves and of others. But it is those very rules and standards that make "disabled" or "handicapped" people withdraw, often voluntarily, from participating in a full and active social life.

Resting

While much of our time is spent working, looking after ourselves or our families, socializing, and taking part in leisure activities, we all need time to unwind. "Rest" includes sleeping, sitting in a chair and looking out at the garden, reading a book, watching television. All involve little or no physical activity and allow us to "switch off." Indeed, it is these very features that make resting so vital to people with Parkinson's disease, as a way of countering fatigue and "recharging their batteries" before carrying on with more energetic activities.

However, these passive ways of passing the time are a double-edged sword. Although resting is good, there is a real danger that it can become the main way in which those with Parkinson's spend their days. Because activities are more difficult and more tiring, passive pastimes seem increasingly attractive. When combined with giving up work, a decreasing tendency to travel outside, and a shrinking social network, the individual may find him- or herself spending more and more time indoors doing nothing in particular.

Even people who previously led remarkably full and active lives may fall prey to the temptation to do nothing. The eminent historian A. J. P. Taylor, who had Parkinson's disease, confessed:

Gradually I get more reluctant to go out more than a few hundred yards. I can see that soon I shall be quite content to sit in the open air of my back yard or patio. I lose interest in what is happening further afield.

And again in an account by J.K., a psychotherapist, in John Williams's booklet *Parkinson's Disease and Employment: The Experiences of Forty-three Patients:*

At such times I doubt my skills as a therapist and would like to contract out. How much easier to potter around in the garden. This tendency to avoid challenge is real and pervasive. I would like to avoid any social or professional encounter at which I may be viewed as less well than formerly.

Most people slow down, socially as well as physically, as they age. This process of cutting down on previous activities and on our social lives is sometimes referred to as "disengagement." But research has shown that it tends to happen at a younger age and to a greater degree in people with Parkinson's. In a recent study by Dr. Singer, he noted:

[people with Parkinson's disease] are less likely to engage in household tasks, or to have a close circle of friends; at the same time, they are more likely to engage in such solitary leisure activities as watching television and reading, and much more likely to report ways of spending time which are not "activities" at all—namely, napping and idleness.

There is nothing abnormal in this pattern of behavior. However, when comparing Parkinson's patients with different age groups in the general population, it was found that people under the age of 65 who had the disease were leading the lifestyle of others aged 80 or more. This led Singer to suggest that Parkinson's disease can lead to *premature social aging*. Obviously, it is important to guard against this pattern setting in—suggestions for ways to keep active, physically, socially, and mentally, are given in Chapter 10.

FINANCIAL INDEPENDENCE

All of us have a standard of living to which we have grown accustomed. When something threatens our financial security and independence, it can have a profound effect on many aspects of our lives and on our self-respect. Parkinson's disease can affect our financial status in two ways—if he or she has to give up work or accept a job with less pay, and through the extra costs of living incurred by having the illness. On the plus side, there are benefits that he or she may be able to obtain; these are described in Chapter 9.

As with employment itself, the impact of the illness on their finances is going to affect younger and older individuals differently. Those who have already reached retirement age and stopped working will suffer no change in their income—they will already have made the necessary adjustments to their lifestyle in order to accommodate any reduction in income associated with normal retirement. Such individuals will have their Social Security pension and, ideally, a private pension and savings as well. The major impact of Parkinson's disease will be on those younger people who are still of employment age; their particular financial problems are discussed in Chapter 8. Where the person with Parkinson's has been the sole or the main breadwinner, some couples choose for the other partner to start working, or to work more hours, to bring in extra income. This has obvious practical advantages for the finances, although the radical change in roles may have a wider impact on the relationship (see below).

Loss of financial independence can be a major source of stress for those who are unprepared, and who have not made the necessary adjustments. It should be remembered that people often retire or work shorter hours so as to reduce stress, but there is little point in this if work stress is replaced by financial stress. As discussed in Chapter 9, careful financial planning is important to lessen the impact of any income loss.

RELATIONSHIPS

We human beings are social animals. The people around us often play central roles in our lives, be it at work or at home. They are vitally important to us, and the nature and quality of our interactions with them contribute to our sense of satisfaction and happiness.

We can think of our lives as the layers of an onion, with ourselves in the middle. Surrounding this core are our family, friends, and work colleagues, then health professionals and others whom we may come across occasionally, and finally strangers. These various groups differ for us in both the amounts of time that we spend in contact with them and the intimacy of that contact—the extent to which we share our lives and our feelings with them. We can also think of this "onion" in terms of the places or situations where we meet these various individuals—at home, at work or in social settings, in medical situations, in stores, and in all the other places out there in the world. In each of these places and for each of these groups we can think of ourselves as having different roles. At home we may be husbands or wives, and parents; at work we are colleagues, while in a social setting we are friends. In the hospital we are patients, while in stores we are customers. Even though the person inside is the same, we are viewed as different in each context and, to a degree, we act differently as we play our different roles.

Because of these multiple roles that we each have, and the many different kinds of people with whom we make daily contact, it is not possible to describe here every situation and every kind of encounter. What we *can* do is consider in a more general way the different groups of people in turn, and how Parkinson's disease may affect the nature of our relationships with them.

The Immediate Family

There is no such thing as an "average" family. For some, there may be a vast extended family of children, grandchildren, and relatives of all kinds, who provide the main focus of their lives. For others there may be just a few people, some of whom they rarely see. For most people, the immediate family of spouse or partner and children provides the most important and most intimate set of relationships. It is these people who will share, most closely, many of the ups and downs of Parkinson's disease.

For those with a spouse or partner, telling them about the illness is rarely a choice. Almost always, they will be fully involved in the processes leading up to and including the diagnosis. However, relationships will vary in the amount of openness and communication that is, or seems to be, appropriate.

One of the major stresses on a relationship is the effect that Parkinson's disease can have on established roles and patterns of behavior. In any relationship, there is usually a division of labor and responsibility, built up over the years. One partner may be the main breadwinner and the other the main housekeeper. Care of children may be shared equally or may be the main responsibility of one of the partners. One may take more initiative in organizing and maintaining social contacts and recreation for the two of them, and so on. In the early stage of Parkinson's disease there are unlikely to be any changes to these established patterns. But in the middle stage, as symptoms become more evident and difficulties in various aspects of life may start to emerge, there is a tendency for previous roles to change or even to be reversed. If you are the one with the illness, and you have been the main breadwinner, your partner may choose, or need, to start bringing in more money. You may suddenly find yourself having to take on unaccustomed roles about the house so as to relieve the burden on your partner. Later on, if you become less capable of functioning independently, such flexibility may not be possible. This can bring with it another change—the role of partner becomes that of a caretaker, perhaps full-time.

All of these changes can have their effect on a relationship. There may be dissatisfaction, at times, caused by the loss of a previously valued role, or by the need to take on additional unwanted or unfamiliar roles. Also, certain roles may be psychologically incompatible—it may be difficult, for example, for a woman who has been in the caregiver role all day, and has just helped her partner to wash, undress, and get into bed, to suddenly switch to the role of lover. The following case illustrates this:

Len had his Parkinson's disease diagnosed at the age of 48, and gave up his work as a car mechanic six years later. He had worked all his life, and found it difficult to adjust to the idea that he was no longer the main provider for the family. He continued to work on friends' cars for some of the time, but spent most of his day indoors at home doing nothing in particular. His wife, who had always taken care of all the household matters, found his presence an increasing irritation. To help with the finances she took on a part-time job. But Len was unwilling to do any of the day-to-day jobs such as shopping or cleaning. If he did do them, after persuasion, his half-hearted efforts tended to cause more arguments. After a time, his wife was offered a full-time job which she decided to accept, and she derived considerable satisfaction from the challenges and stimulation of her new career. Len, of necessity now, took on many of the household jobs. To his surprise he learned that he enjoyed cooking, and took particular pride in devising special surprises for dinner when his wife returned from work. She, in turn, lowered some of her high standards and worried less if the carpets were not vacuumed every day.

A common problem is not knowing how much to do for the person who has the disease. Where is the line to be drawn between helping that person but not depriving him or her of independence? Pat talks here about her husband:

> *He is incredibly kind, but he seems to think that he has to do every-thing for me. If he sees me trying to get up from a chair he rushes over to help me up. If I even move towards the kitchen he tells me to sit down and asks me what I want. I know I shouldn't, but sometimes I want to scream: "I may have Parkinson's disease but I'm not totally useless!" I really wish he would find some other interest and give me a bit of space, but I don't know how to tell him—he would be so upset. I really am very lucky, but sometimes I want to hit him I feel so frustrated.*

And Ed, about his wife:

> *She is marvelous the way she copes with the Parkinson's disease—I wouldn't be able to be as brave as she is. After all these years, I feel that it's the least I can do to look after her, she deserves it. I can't say that it isn't a strain, physically and mentally. She doesn't demand help but I know that's just her—she has never asked for things, but I know she would be upset if I didn't offer. I must confess that there are times when I would just like to go out to with my friends like I used to, but I couldn't leave her on her own—it wouldn't be fair.*

These examples illustrate the importance of striking the right balance between helping the patient and not taking away his or her autonomy and independence by being there at all times. This balance can only be established by honest communication of needs, and by flexibility to the changing demands of the illness.

The Sexual Relationship

One aspect of a couple's relationship that may be affected by Parkinson's disease is their sex life. Whatever their ages, an active sex life can form an important part of the relationship, even if they make love less frequently and the physical passion diminishes over the years. Unfortunately, sexual problems are common when one partner has Parkinson's.

What sort of problems can occur? Sexual problems are often classified as problems of arousal—men find it difficult to achieve or maintain an erection (impotence), while women fail to lubricate, making penetration uncomfortable, or may suffer an involuntary contraction of the vagina making penetration impossible or painful (vaginismus). Many people, however, become aroused normally but have problems with orgasm. Men may ejaculate too soon (premature ejaculation) or are unable to do so (retarded ejaculation). Women too may have difficulty in achieving orgasm (anorgasmia). As important as these physical signs of sex is the question of satisfaction. Some people find that they enjoy sexual relations less, and therefore want it less often, even if the physical "machinery" is still working.

All of these problems are found in couples in which one partner has Parkinson's disease. In a recent study of younger couples, about 80 percent reported that they were having sexual relations less often. In terms of the nature of the sexual problem, about 60 percent of men reported erectile dysfunction or impotence, and 65 percent had a problem with premature ejaculation. Among women with Parkinson's, 55 percent reported lack of sexual arousal. Of course, the difficulties were not restricted to the person with the illness: partners, too, reported the same types of problems. This study revealed important differences between couples when the patient was the man, and those in whom it was the woman. Many more problems were reported by both partners where the man was the one with Parkinson's. This gender difference probably reflects the fact that, traditionally, men play the active role in the sexual relationship.

Exactly how may Parkinson's disease affect the sexual relationship? First, there are the physical symptoms. Unfortunately, many of these, such as fatigue, difficulty in sustaining repetitive movements, freezing, tremor, and abnormal movements, can potentially interfere with the act of sex itself. And increased physical tiredness may also be a problem for the partner. Sidney Dorros, in *Parkinson's Disease: A Patient's View*, describes his, and his wife's, problem:

Sexual relations presented the greatest challenge to timing. My peak period of mobility was so short that if I started to get amorous towards the end of the drug cycle, I would run out of energy at a most crucial point in the love-making cycle. It didn't increase Debbie's libido for me to say, "Excuse me, I've got to take my pills now," and then wait half an hour before continuing. She would usually fall asleep before the half-hour was up.

Obviously, the more physically active the individual's normal role in sexual relations, the more handicapped he or she is likely to be by the physical symptoms of the disorder. And while the physical limitations of Parkinson's may be important, the *psychological* aspects are probably even more significant, involving both the individual *and* his or her partner. Unfortunately, particularly in the later stage, physical attractiveness may be diminished by some of the symptoms. These may include the involuntary movements, uncontrolled salivation, and sweating experienced by some, and there is the added possibility that limited facial expression and a monotonous voice may make it more difficult to effectively communicate interest or excitement. Furthermore, as noted previously, some partners may find it difficult to switch from the role of caretaker to that of lover. Perhaps most damaging to a couple's sex life, though, is stress. Anyone's interest in sex, and his or her capacity to perform, can be seriously affected by stress and worry, whether deriving from outside or from within the home. If there is a general tension in the relationship, it is unlikely that the couple's sex life will escape unaffected. If either partner has worries about work, finances, or the future in general, this too will have an adverse effect.

Unfortunately, if problems start, sex itself can become a source of stress, and a vicious circle may develop.

Mark's Parkinson's disease started nine years ago when he was 47. Both he and his wife worked, although he had recently started working part-time. Financially, they were finding things more difficult. Although Mark had always played an active role in the home, he was recently finding it more difficult to make a full contribution, placing more responsibility on his wife. This was a subject of concern for him. The marriage had been a happy one, and both he and his wife had always enjoyed their sex life. Gradually, however, they were having sex less and less often, and when they did it was not always as satisfying as before. For Mark, this was a particular worry, because he felt that his illness was removing an important aspect of his relationship with his wife. He attempted to initiate sex more often, but she was frequently too tired. When they did have sex, Mark worried that he was forcing her to do something that she would rather not be doing. On occasion he was unable to obtain a full erection—which added even more to his worry. His erection problems became worse, so that both of them suffered increasing disappointment and frustration. The worry was there not just during sex, but beforehand, too. Would they be able to have sex tonight, or would there be another "failure?" Despite persevering for some time, their attempts became less and less frequent, until sex essentially stopped altogether.

As in this account, problems with sex, if permitted to continue, can lead to a situation where it is avoided altogether—it is either too stressful or it requires too much effort, and both partners eventually give up trying. Before this point is reached, there may be an extended period when the couple continue to struggle to maintain some level of sexual relationship. Most difficult is when there is a difference in the two partners' desire for sex—in the amount that they want, for instance. Although it happens rarely, a few people experience an enhanced desire for sex as a result of taking levodopa. More commonly, the imbalance will be caused by one of the partners losing interest. Whatever the cause, one may feel that he or she is giving in to pressure from the other, while the other may feel guilty for asking him or her to do something for which he or she has no enthusiasm. Emotions such as guilt and resentment are a poor foundation for a sexual relationship, and there is always a danger that the effects may spill over into other aspects of the couple's life. Even when their sexual life has stopped, there may still be lingering negative emotions, particularly if it has ceased by neglect rather than by a spoken agreement between the two of them.

Many of these difficulties can be dealt with through honest and open discussion or, perhaps, with the help of an experienced therapist. The subject of how to deal with problems in the sexual relationship and how to seek professional help is covered in some detail in Chapter 8.

Other Family Members and Friends

Besides your spouse or partner, other family members may be involved in your life—children, grandchildren, brothers and sisters, and so on. Most important are probably any children who still live at home with you, but family members and friends too may be affected to some degree by your illness, whether you live in the same house or just meet them socially.

It is a common fear for people to think, when told that they have Parkinson's disease, that others will avoid or reject them if they know the truth. As already noted, this leads to the decision to make it the *Big Secret*—the assumption is that, if no one knows about it, life can go on as before. And, of course, this may work to some degree in the early stages when the signs are mild; but, clearly, it will not work forever. Some people worry in particular about telling their children for fear of frightening or worrying them. Unfortunately, this approach can have the opposite effect of that intended. All children, whatever their ages, are observant and they have fertile imaginations. If not kept informed it is likely that they will develop their own ideas about what is going on, and these versions may be far more frightening than the reality.

Louise had her Parkinson's disease diagnosed when she was only 45. She and her husband had three children, two teenage daughters and one son aged seven. The diagnosis came as a severe blow to Louise. She decided that she wanted to carry on as before, and she was particularly concerned that the children should not know until it was absolutely necessary. Her daughters were studying for their SATs, and she was afraid that the news could be too upsetting for them. Her son, she thought, was too young to understand and would be frightened.

However, it was increasingly difficult to maintain this situation. Her symptoms, although mild, were noticeable. Tablets had to be hidden and taken in secret, and one excuse after another had to be given for medical appointments. Eventually, Louise's son asked her when she was going to die. He had seen the tablets and heard about the appointments, as well as overhearing vague "coded" adult talk about the illness, and had come to his own conclusions. Louise and her husband decided immediately to tell their children the truth. Not surprisingly, their daughters too had noticed that something was wrong, but because their parents clearly wanted it to be a secret they had felt unable to raise the subject. They too had formed their own conclusions. Talking together, and with friends, they had been through all possibilities from multiple sclerosis to cancer.

There are also risks in not telling children who have left home, or other relatives. The Big Secret approach, although rarely successful in hiding the truth from anyone for long, can lead to reduced contact. You may avoid seeing them, particularly in social situations, and they may feel embarrassed or awkward coming to see you. Familiarity and knowledge demystify illness and turn it into an everyday fact of life. Your family should be informed so that they know as much as you do about Parkinson's disease, what its symptoms are, and what you can and cannot do.

The same advice applies to friends. As already discussed, there is a real tendency for many people with Parkinson's disease, and their partners, to withdraw from social contact and avoid social situations. The importance of maintaining a network of friends and a social life cannot be overemphasized, particularly if other aspects of your life such as work or hobbies have been restricted by the disorder. Trying to keep the Big Secret will almost certainly lead to turning down invitations. Eventually the excuses will wear thin, and the invitations are likely to stop coming; contact, once lost, is almost impossible to reestablish. Even if maintaining the same level of social life as in the past may be neither physically nor financially possible, it is important to keep up the contacts. Keeping in touch with long-established friends will inevitably involve letting them know that you have Parkinson's disease and explaining the symptoms and its treatment. Friends, just as much as strangers or work colleagues, can misinterpret some of the signs and symptoms.

Peter had decided not to tell his work colleagues about his Parkinson's disease. But despite his efforts to act normally, he was aware that others were treating him differently. In one-to-one situations, they seemed somehow less chatty and friendly than before. Eventually he asked a friend what was wrong. His friend was unable to be specific, but told

Peter that he seemed more reserved; he laughed and smiled less, and seemed to be a bit depressed. Although Peter was not depressed, he realized that his facial expressiveness had subtly changed, and had taken on more of the mask-like expression characteristic of Parkinson's disease. His friends had been picking up these signals and interpreting them as boredom or depression.

It is possible that some old friends *will* be unable to cope with the reality, or with their perceptions of Parkinson's disease. Some people, for reasons of their own, feel acutely awkward or embarrassed around people with physical disorders. In such cases, no amount of information will help, and contact *may* be lost. While regrettable, this will emphasize the importance of those friends who remain close. Finally, there is no reason why the person with Parkinson's should not make new friends—indeed, the illness may bring about a broadening of social life rather than a restriction. If the individual has given up work, the extra time may allow him or her to meet new people and develop new interests better suited to his or her current situation. New friends will come to accept the whole person—Parkinson's disease and all.

MOOD

I have left this section until last because it is so intimately bound up with what has been discussed so far. Up to now we have been considering the impact of Parkinson's disease on specific aspects of life. Most of our discussion has been in terms of practical constraints or the effects on relationships with other people. In addition, of course, Parkinson's disease can have a profound impact on a person's general outlook on life, on mood, and on sense of well-being. Our opinions about ourselves, both good and bad, are very important when it comes to how we view the world and how we interpret things that happen to us. This sense of personal identity and "self-concept" is partly a function of the many facets that make up our life—work and family, hobbies and interests, relationships with friends and colleagues. It follows that when an important aspect of our life is threatened, or is taken away, it can have a marked effect on our sense of personal identity. For example, people who have worked all of their adult life will almost inevitably feel diminished if they have to stop working through illness.

Perhaps the first challenge that Parkinson's disease offers to the individual's sense of identity is the very knowledge of having it. You may feel that you have stopped being a "person" and started being a "patient"; that you have changed from being "normal" to being "disabled." Later there may come times when you are unable to do something that you particularly value, such as participating in a sport or other leisure activity, or driving your car. For some people this can threaten, if only temporarily, their sense of self-worth. Potentially most threatening is becoming dependent upon other people for help in basic self-care. People will react in very different ways to these challenges to their sense of identity. Some seem able to keep a core sense of themselves as a person, as separate from the things that they can and cannot do. Others may become angry with themselves and with those around them, while yet others may become withdrawn. In any event, a large number will show signs of depression, some for a short period, some for many years.

Depression: A Broad Spectrum

Mood problems are common in people with Parkinson's disease. Perhaps as many as one-third may experience some degree of depression at any one time. What is meant by the term "depression?" For many it's simply "feeling blue" or "down in the dumps." Hearing a particularly good joke or doing something enjoyable may enable these individuals to "snap out of it." In other cases, the mood change may be more fundamental and long-lasting. There may be a general sense of sadness and pessimism that is more difficult to shake off. The individual may be tearful and derive less enjoyment from things going on around. He or she will tend to be passive and unmotivated, as well as worried, tense, or irritable. Severe depression involves more than just sadness and mood change. Individuals become preoccupied with depressive thoughts. Everything they see and hear will tend to be viewed negatively—the world, their situation, and the future. They may feel guilt or self-blame, or feel that they are being punished. This negative outlook on everything may even lead the individual to attempt suicide. Other symptoms of depression are sleep disturbance, loss of appetite and weight, a sense of lethargy, and lack of interest in anything at all.

Where, along this broad spectrum, is the person with Parkinson's disease likely to lie? In principle, he or she may experience depression from its mildest to its severest form, but the evidence suggests that depression in Parkinson's disease has some particular characteristics. Most typically, it shows itself as *depressed mood*. The person feels sad and tearful and may be pessimistic about the future, and these feelings may be prolonged and difficult to shake off. However, other features of depression appear to be far less common. For instance, very few people with the illness who are depressed express thoughts of self-blame or guilt, or feel that they are being punished. While they may think about death and even wish, at times, that they were dead, suicide and attempted suicide are very rare.

Why Is Depression Common in Parkinson's Disease?

There are two contrasting views on this matter. One is that depression in Parkinson's disease is a direct result of the biological changes in the brain—many of the brain chemicals affected by the illness are also implicated in mood change and depression. This can be termed the *biological approach*. The alternative view, which may be called the *psychological approach*, is that depression in Parkinson's disease is a reaction to the disabling and handicapping nature of the disorder; that it is the loss of important roles, the restriction of activities, and the increased dependence on others that are the key factors in causing the depression.

Which is likely to be correct—the biological or the psychological view? The answer is probably both. Both are likely to play a role, although from one individual to the next the relative importance of one or the other will vary. It is my view, though, that biological factors account for only a small proportion of the depressive symptoms of Parkinson's disease and are significant in only a minority of cases. I believe that in most people psychological factors are the most important cause.

Are Some Individuals Vulnerable to Depression?

Although depressed mood is common in Parkinson's disease, it is by no means certain that everyone with the illness will become depressed, nor that the individual who becomes depressed will stay depressed. Some people with severe Parkinson's disease will remain cheerful and optimistic, while others, who have only the mildest of symptoms, may become severely depressed. This begs the question, "Why do some people with Parkinson's disease get depressed and not others?"

A related question is "Who is vulnerable to depression?" Although anyone can become depressed, it does seem that some are more prone than others. One important predictor is whether they had periods of depression before the onset of their illness. A previous history of depression seems to greatly increase the chance that an individual will become depressed at some time during the course of his or her Parkinson's disease. Reasons for this increased risk are probably complex. The individual may have some biological predisposition to depression, or he or she may be the type of person who reacts to any stressful event or loss by becoming depressed.

Taking the psychological approach, we can suggest that depression will be more likely, the more the illness interferes with the individual's life. As we have seen, Parkinson's disease *can* (but need not) affect a person's ability to carry out everyday activities—to participate in hobbies and other forms of recreation and social life, to work and to maintain financial independence, to engage in relationships with other people. As discussed in Chapter 4, it is the interaction between the disease symptoms, the individual, and his or her normal lifestyle that defines handicap, not the symptoms alone. So someone who suffers handicap, or the threat of handicap, will be more vulnerable to depression than another individual with the same symptoms who experiences little change in his or her normal pattern of life.

Perhaps the group under the greatest threat of handicap are the young. In the context of Parkinson's disease, by "young" I mean those between the ages of 40 and 60–65. It is known from research studies that this group is also the most likely to become depressed. People in this age group are likely to be still working, any children they may have are growing up or already adult, and they are passing through the stage of their lives when their peers may be enjoying the period of greatest financial and personal freedom. People in this age range may find themselves with spare money and time to enjoy themselves for the first time in many years. Parkinson's disease may directly challenge this freedom, and the threat of losing it may be difficult for some people to cope with.

Barbara was diagnosed as having Parkinson's disease when she was in her early fifties. Despite coping well for a while, she developed severe on–off fluctuations, and her husband eventually gave up work to care for her. Their children had left home, and together they had been planning a long trip, touring India in a camper. This adventure had been an ambition of theirs for years, throughout the time when their children had been growing up. They now realized that they would never be able to make this journey. This, perhaps more than the Parkinson's disease itself, was a source of great regret.

In contrast, when Parkinson's disease starts later in life, particularly after normal retirement age, the individual may feel that his or her chances of living a full life have been more or less fulfilled. Furthermore, as noted earlier, many of the necessary adjustments for retirement may have already been made. Older people probably have fewer financial commitments and have already learned to get by on less money. Also, it is usual for older people to have less active social lives and to enjoy more leisurely and less physically demanding pastimes. For all these reasons, Parkinson's disease has less opportunity to cause severe handicap in them than in younger individuals. I am not suggesting that older people do not suffer handicap or depression—they do—but that younger individuals, or those with more active lifestyles, are going to have the greatest relative handicap and to be most at risk of becoming depressed.

When Are the Vulnerable Times for Developing Depression?

Why do people get depressed at some times yet remain cheerful at others? A simple account might suggest that you are more likely to become depressed as the disease progresses. In fact, depression seems to show two peaks, one in the early stage and one in the late stage. One critical period is the time immediately after diagnosis. As suggested earlier, for some people, being told that they have Parkinson's disease comes as a relief, particularly if they have feared something worse; reassurance and information from their doctor, combined with prompt and effective treatment, may allay fears and prevent any emotional reaction. However, for others the news can be devastating, particularly if they have a distorted view of the illness, such as distant memories of an aunt or grandparent in the late stages. Although such individuals may be perfectly able to carry on as before, fear of the future and the threat of having to let go of important aspects of their lives can cause depression. In cases like these, the depression can sometimes become more of a handicap than the disease itself.

Most people will eventually come to terms with their illness, particularly once they realize it need not stop them from working or enjoying themselves. However, as the disease progresses and begins to have more of an impact, there may be times when an individual again becomes depressed. When new symptoms start to emerge or the medication ceases to be as effective, he or she may be required to make new adjustments, both practical and emotional. Some particularly stressful change or life event may happen, leading to a long-term loss of some valued role or opportunity. Major events such as giving up work or giving up driving can have wide-ranging consequences in people's lives, as well as threatening their self-esteem and sense of identity.

Except for such periods of change, depression is typically less of a problem in the middle stage of Parkinson's disease. It is only in the late stage, when the illness may have the greatest impact on the most basic abilities required for mobility and self-care, that depression becomes more common again. Again, it is independence and self-esteem that are being challenged.

Anxiety

Depression is not the only emotional problem experienced by those with Parkinson's disease. Although less common, anxiety may also be a feature. As with depression, anxiety ranges from the mild to the severe. Some may experience a general restlessness and sense of unease, accompanied by general worry about life and the future. At the other extreme, the anxiety may be quite disabling, taking the form of panic attacks in which the person feels acute fear, with breathing problems, rapid heartbeat, nausea, and even the fear that he or she is going to die.

To a degree, some anxiety may be a natural reaction to the challenges of living with Parkinson's disease. If the individual has had a fall, he or she may be anxious when walking for fear of falling again. He or she may have stopped work and have real worries about managing financially.

Although any anxiety is unwelcome, it can become a real problem when the individual starts to avoid the things that are causing the anxiety. The person who has fallen may avoid crowded places or public transportation. Someone who feels anxious in front of friends or family members because of symptoms that (to him or her) are embarrassing may start to steer clear of social contacts.

Teresa describes herself:

I have always been a "nervy" sort of person, but it never really affected my life. When I developed Parkinson's disease, however, I found myself worrying more and more about little things. When my balance began to be affected it really started to get worse. If I felt a bit wobbly I would immediately get anxious. Even though I had never fallen, I was afraid that I would fall and hurt myself. If anything, the anxiety made my unsteadiness worse. When at last I did fall it seemed to confirm my worst fears. I was in a supermarket. I tried to stop suddenly and crashed forward, bringing down a load of packets from a shelf. Although I wasn't badly hurt, I was terribly embarrassed. My Parkinson's was really bad for several hours afterwards, and I had to take some extra medication. A few days later I tried to go into the same shop, but I suddenly felt terrible. I was sweaty and shaky, and my heart was pounding in my throat. I sat down, but I still felt awful. After a while I had to go home. That was weeks ago, and I still haven't plucked up the courage to go back. Just thinking about it makes me feel sick. What is worse is that I am starting to feel nervous about going into any place where there are lots of people. If I am not careful, home will be the only place where I feel safe, which is silly. After all, I've only fallen once, but I can't stop worrying that I might fall again.

Anxiety, then, may serve to restrict a person's life, perhaps even more than the disease itself. The panic attacks experienced by some are the most severe form of anxiety. As we see here, even one attack in a particular location may lead to the individual avoiding the situation in the future. There is some suggestion that such panic attacks are somehow related to the disease itself, or to its treatment. A significant number of people feel a growing sense of panic during "off" periods, often fearing that they will stop breathing or die. Once they come "on" again, these fears disappear completely. One person with Parkinson's disease put it this way:

When I am "off," problems can often become mountainous. But when I come "on," these problems fade away and the tasks appear quite feasible.

Fortunately, depression and anxiety are not inevitable, and even if the individual *is* depressed or anxious there is plenty that can be done. Chapter 11 deals with ways of avoiding these problems and of coping with them if they do occur.

KEY FACTS 5

How will the symptoms of Parkinson's disease affect my life?

Parkinson's disease is much more than the sum of the symptoms. Because people lead such different lives, the impact of the illness can be very different from one person to the next, even if the symptoms seem similar.

Will there be changes in my ability to do everyday things?

As the disease progresses, there is usually a steady decline in the individual's capacity to carry out ordinary everyday activities as well, or as easily, as before. This is because many of these tasks are highly dependent on the aspects of movement directly influenced by the disease. Such changes, however, tend to take place relatively slowly, which permits the individual to adjust his or her life, to learn new skills, or to make use of special aids and equipment. However, just as important as the practical side of these activities is the psychological side. Being able to look after oneself is very important for self-esteem and a sense of personal identity. Maintaining as much independence as possible for as long as possible is probably the number one priority for all those with Parkinson's disease.

When an individual is largely dependent on another, even small acts of independence are vitally important.

What about mobility?

As it progresses, the illness may influence walking and balance. Difficulty in walking can have a dramatic effect on other aspects of our lives, both inside and outside of the home. One of the major problems is balance; falls can occur, particularly in the later stage of the disease. Other aspects of mobility affected include apparently simple tasks such as getting up from a chair or turning over in bed; in Parkinson's disease, these actions are no longer carried out automatically, but often require conscious thought. But although walking and other actions may prove difficult, physical therapy and special aids can be helpful, and there are many tricks and tips that can be learned. All of these can contribute substantially to maintaining mobility, allowing you to continue to lead an active life.

How are work, leisure, and social activities likely to be affected?

For those of us below retirement age, work is probably the most important way in which we occupy our time. Perhaps here more than in any other aspect of life, the impact that Parkinson's disease is going to have will depend on the "fit" between your symptoms and the nature of your work. Some people will be able to continue working until late into the disease, while others find it very difficult even in the early stages. As in other aspects of life, flexibility is important, as is your willingness to discuss your problems with those around you, particularly your employer. For those still working, leisure and social activities are important for relaxation, whereas for those who have retired, such activities may be their main way of spending time productively. Fortunately, people can be more flexible in choosing their leisure activities to suit their situation than they can be in choosing their work. Everyone, however severe his or her illness, can find relaxing, enjoyable, and rewarding pastimes. Although solitary activities are important, social contacts are vital for a sense of well-being. Unfortunately, there is a real tendency for those with Parkinson's disease to withdraw from social contact and to lose touch with friends and relatives. Avoiding this should be a major priority for all of those with the disease.

Will my financial independence be threatened?

Parkinson's disease can be expensive. The impact of the costs, however, will depend upon your previous circumstances. Obviously, retiring early can have a major impact on income, although this may be offset by savings such as giving up the use of your car and eligibility for benefits such as Social Security. One danger of decreased income is a reduction in "luxuries," which tend to include socializing and getting out and about.

How will my relationships with others be affected?

We all have people in our lives whom we see more or less often, in different settings. Family, close friends, and work colleagues are probably the most important. All of these will be affected in some way by your illness. Clearly, the closer the relationship, the greater the impact, and it is to be expected that any relationship will have to go through periods of adjustment and change as the disease progresses. For this reason, it is essential that others are involved as much as is necessary at all stages.

What about the psychological aspect?

The knowledge that you have Parkinson's disease can be a major blow, even before there are any problems. For some people, it may mean the loss of a particular role or activity that they greatly valued; sometimes even apparently small losses can take on major significance. It is perhaps not surprising that depression is common in Parkinson's disease. Although some of the problem may relate to the nature of the disease itself, most is probably related to the handicap that it brings with it. Minimizing handicap, therefore, is probably the best way of safeguarding against depression. Anxiety, too, can be a problem—worry can stop an individual from doing things that he or she is perfectly capable of doing.

6

From the Family's Perspective

Brigid MacCarthy

This chapter is about what it is like to live with someone who has Parkinson's disease—the challenges, the difficulties, and the rewards. The first assumption here is that most people with Parkinson's have one person who is involved in helping with daily activities, looking after him or her when the illness progresses and moderate to severe disability develops, and providing emotional support. Of course, this is not true of all individuals with the illness, some of whom live alone, without a full-time caregiver. Nevertheless, some of these probably have relatives or friends who to some extent have become involved in their care since the onset of the illness. The second assumption in much of this chapter is that, in the majority of cases, the spouse or partner is the primary caregiver. But although this seems to be borne out by statistics, we recognize that younger children, grown-up sons and daughters, sisters and brothers, and occasionally parents, friends, neighbors, and professionals may also fill this role.

Relatives often say that it is really difficult for them to understand what having and living with Parkinson's disease is like, as these comments reveal:

I often try to imagine what she feels like but I can't—it must be horrible.

We accepted from the start that there is nobody except the person who is ill who knows what it's like. Unless you've got it yourself you can't really appreciate it. I will look at it from a different point of view.

Just as relatives often feel that it's difficult to enter into the experience of the person they are caring for, so too they often feel that it's hard for outsiders to understand what it's like for caregivers—which is "living with Parkinson's disease" in another sense. This perceived lack of understanding and appreciation of the impact of the illness on the caregiver can sometimes add to his or her sense of burden and of being cut off from others. Hearing and reading about the experiences of other people coping with similar situations can help caregivers to feel rather less isolated, to realize that their efforts to cope are not so uncommon. If others have found different ways of dealing with the problems, maybe their tactics are worth a try. Also, the accounts of people who have found a way of coming to terms with their situation, however grave, show that there is hope even in the most distressing circumstances, and can be enormously encouraging.

In the course of our work with people with Parkinson's disease, we have talked to a large number of their relatives. We wanted to get their perspective on what was important to them in their efforts to cope with the illness. What follows summarizes the insights gained from those conversations and interviews. As far as possible we have used people's own words or summarized their stories, changing minor details only, so as to protect their confidentiality. Not all the experiences described here are positive or encouraging—that would be unrealistic. Instead, the different stages of adapting to living with the disease are described through the caregiver's eyes; the issues that arise in each phase are outlined, and the problems that have to be dealt with and the emotional cost those problems can bring are acknowledged.

The chapter is organized according to stage of illness.

BEFORE DIAGNOSIS

As you will have gathered from earlier chapters, the first signs of the disease often seem rather trivial. A barely noticeable tremor, for example, rarely leads people to guess that an individual may have Parkinson's disease. Usually, the first visit to the doctor is prompted by such relatively minor problems starting to interfere with work or leisure activities. For instance, one man whose job involved using a high-speed saw had to change the way he did his job after one arm became stiff. The need to find relief for such difficulties can speed up the process of diagnosis and put an end to a troubling period of uncertainty. But for many relatives, as for the patients, the time between the onset of these niggling problems and receiving the final diagnosis can be extremely stressful.

The changes can be hard to pin down, or difficult to understand, and do not necessarily announce themselves as a physical illness:

I found the way he spoke to me very upsetting, because I thought the tone of his voice was hostile to me, but in fact it was the illness and I didn't realize.

Often doctors, too, are puzzled or uncertain, or go along willingly with attempts to minimize symptoms:

It started with a slight tremor, and he put the words into the doctor's mouth, saying, "I suppose it's old age, one shakes."

Or, doctors may try to treat a completely different illness, so that when distressing symptoms are not alleviated by apparently appropriate treatment, both patient and relatives begin to feel helpless—not a strong position from which to hear a diagnosis that may at first be very upsetting.

She had very bad arthritis, then she had the hip operation done, and she was doing fine. Then all of a sudden, just like that, she couldn't walk. Their attitude was, "Well, the operation was perfect, we've done the legs," so they sent her to another specialist who diagnosed Parkinson's disease.

During this early phase, the person concerned may become less active and unable to find anything of interest in activities that were previously central to his or her pleasure in life. This may lead relatives and friends to misinterpret the first symptoms as signs that he or she is profoundly unhappy. Sometimes both relatives and professionals may perceive this as malingering—which may leave the individual feeling blamed at a time when he or she is feeling particularly helpless. In the absence of a correct diagnosis, these changes can be very destructive to vital relationships:

We all thought he was faking it, and that was a very difficult time for everybody. He sort of withdrew into himself completely.

Mutual trust and support, which will be so important in future years, can be severely eroded during the search for an appropriate explanation of the symptoms.

Alternatively, because of the apparent similarity of some of the early manifestations of Parkinson's disease to depression—for example, slowness, lethargy, changed tone of voice, and lack of facial expression—the individual's symptoms may be diagnosed and treated as depression. Then, a referral to a psychiatrist may lead to the kind of frustration that was experienced when the wrong physical diagnosis was given. Time and emotional energy are lost in attempting to accept the distressing idea that the patient has a psychological problem, only to discover that another wrong diagnosis has been made:

He went through all the tests of the psychiatrists and they found nothing at all wrong with him, and the next doctor we saw looked at his hand and said, "Well, it's only a slight tremor," and no treatment was suggested.

Sometimes family members suspect that the problem is Parkinson's disease, because they have known other people with the illness or because they have some relevant professional background. This can be particularly stressful if they remember people in the more severe stages of the disorder. But more difficult still is the situation in which the family try to keep their suspicions from the ill person, so that husbands, wives, or children feel that they have to deal with the implications of their worries alone. This means carrying uncertainty and anxiety without support, and with the additional strain of having to hide thoughts and feelings from the person with whom they are usually closest.

THE DIAGNOSIS

Occasionally, relatives are not present when the diagnosis is made, so they may hear it directly from the patient. Not many of the relatives we talked to recalled that it had been personally traumatic at the time. For some it legitimized unexplained symptoms, and usually it heralded a period—years, in many cases—when life returned to normal, with symptoms at last being alleviated by the right medication. Generally the diagnosis was easier to accept if the individual concerned was already elderly. Where both spouse and patient were already about retirement age or beyond and the impairments were still fairly mild, many families took the view that it was only an aspect of aging, and that they and their contemporaries should expect to experience ill health in some form.

Simply being given a name for puzzling changes can be enormously helpful for people with Parkinson's disease and their relatives. Once the problems they face have been identified, they can begin to adjust. They must now make choices about the balance they want to strike between making concessions to the illness and carrying on as normal. In these early stages, all concerned have to make practical and emotional decisions about how much in their lives has to change. Do jobs, houses, favorite activities have to be changed? Must household roles be modified? What about plans for the future? Is there bound to be a change in the quality of relationships? Will the family members be able to hold on to the same image of the person now under the spotlight as before the diagnosis? The relatives we talked to in the course of our work reacted with widely different ideas, attitudes, and coping strategies. Not all of these were helpful, but they were what they felt were called for at the time.

For many who had feared a more threatening diagnosis, knowing brought relief and a feeling of "Thank God, it could have been worse." This was particularly likely if the individual was not significantly disabled at the time and the illness was progressing only slowly. Others felt fearful, particularly if they had known someone in the final stages of the disease, before today's sophisticated drug regimens were in general use, or if they assumed that dementia was an inevitable part of its course. These relatives were enormously reassured by seeing the remarkable effects of appropriate medication, and discovering that dementia infrequently occurs in Parkinson's disease. Others were very concerned for their children—worrying that the illness might be hereditary.

Couples dealt with the acknowledgment of the diagnosis in a variety of ways. But what was universally clear was that the sooner they could arrive at a shared perspective and a way of dealing with the news that was comfortable for both, the better. Often one or another partner found it very hard to accept the news initially. The wife of one patient reported that she had been unable to go home and face her husband until she had visited a close friend to talk over her own feelings. Only then could she prepare herself to be supportive. Uncertainty before the diagnosis, and the perceived need for secrecy in the early post-diagnosis phase, can add an extra burden that makes the situation intolerable. With secrecy, barriers arise between individuals who are desperate for support and the very people who are their potential sources of that support. One wife describes how relieved she was when she finally let out the Big Secret.

It's much better now because our friends know and they make allowances. When you're trying to hide something, it's not actually that you're ashamed, but you don't want people to see it. I don't want sympathy, but now it doesn't matter because it's out.

Another woman spoke of being unable to reverse the feelings of isolation she suffered when her husband insisted that no one else should know his diagnosis:

I couldn't really face up to it. I couldn't cope with it, so I just sort of withdrew. When my husband first had it he didn't want me to tell anyone, and I found that very difficult. I would really have liked to tell someone, just to share the fact, and I think that's probably driven me too far within myself about it now.

THE PHASE OF MILD TO MODERATE DISABILITY

Once the diagnosis has been made and a treatment plan defined, the family and the patient have to arrive at a way of living with the associated disabilities. As already noted, usually there is a period, often several years long, during which the consequences of having the illness are barely noticeable. Once he or she has been stabilized on the appropriate medication, the individual may even be more mobile and feel in better health than for some time. The slow and gradual decline in physical ability experienced by most patients, with long periods of equilibrium in between, allows everyone concerned to make gradual adjustments to daily routines, so that the emotional impact of inevitable changes is minimized. Those individuals whose decline is more abrupt tend to find the necessary adjustments more upsetting and difficult to make.

At this point, although the picture varies enormously from one patient to the next, family members report little observable difference in their relative's ability to look after him- or herself and to cope with daily routines. In the very early stages, changes in self-care and in other activities, if they are apparent at all, are likely only to affect the time that ordinary chores take to complete. It is easy to misconstrue such changes in pace as laziness or lethargy. Relatives have described the difficulty they have had in adjusting the pace of their own schedules to match the patient's slowing down, particularly before they have realized that it was an inevitable aspect of the illness. Mild occasional clumsiness can also be a problem. One woman described her anxiety each evening when her husband wiped the dishes, a task he insisted on doing. She recognized his need to make a contribution to the running of the household, but couldn't ignore the frequent broken dishes.

Loss of balance or falling occurs relatively rarely at the stage of moderate disability, but its unpredictability and high public profile make it particularly difficult to adjust to. One woman reported that a couple of very public falls at the office had cost her husband his job long before he ceased being able to do the tasks the job required. Another felt she had to supervise her husband constantly at his favorite hobby, which was gardening, after he had been injured by becoming entangled with garden tools when he fell. Sometimes caregivers reported feeling irritated by the symptoms, but were reluctant to mention this to the individual concerned. Cognitive difficulties such as absentmindedness, when they were a feature of a person's illness, were difficult because they were unpredictable, and peculiarly disruptive to the quality of the relationship between spouses. More than any other disabling feature of the illness, cognitive problems seemed to lead to changes in the balance of dependency within relationships. A few family members whose relative had developed a blank face, having lost his or her full range of facial expressions, commented on how puzzling and distressing this symptom was. One thought her relative was feeling permanently hostile, while one wife had constantly to challenge her assumption that her husband was bored with what she was saying.

"On–off" periods also raised particular dilemmas. Unpredictability made the scheduling of activities difficult, and they experienced special difficulties in matching their own pace to the much more erratic one of the person with the illness:

When he comes on he gets super-energetic: it's as if he's missed something and he's trying to make up for it now. He even avoids sitting down. I think he's frightened in case he can't get up and get going again.

Relatives felt forced to go at the pace of the patient, so that leaving the house on time or trying to keep to a timetable became highly stressful. This in turn made some family members tend to abandon interests and activities of their own, to avoid the conflict or impatience triggered by thwarted efforts to keep some time for themselves.

In the phase of mild to moderate disability, it was not the physical or mental burdens of supporting someone through their daily routines that were the source of difficulty, but having to cope with subtle shifts in the balance of responsibility and initiative-taking. More specifically, concerns fell into three common categories: functional unpredictability, role reversal, and reduction of outside social contact.

Dealing with Functional Unpredictability and Erratic Performance

At this stage, many people with Parkinson's become rather erratic in the pattern of their activities. Lack of confidence and anxiety may often be greater obstacles in this respect than the individual's actual level of disability. This is partly caused by the "on–off" element of the disease, which undermines confidence and motivation. Relatives reported that they initially misread this loss of confidence and motivation as shirking, and had been impatient of it when it first appeared. The person with the illness can also miscalculate his or her ability to do familiar tasks; either underestimating or overestimating his or her disabilities can be peculiarly burdensome for others. One woman reported that her husband would regularly promise to go out and look for work in the morning, but by the afternoon felt incapable of helping with even the lightest domestic chores. She felt that her husband was equally unrealistic in the morning and in the afternoon, and she longed for him to settle for a realistic appraisal of his abilities, and stick to it. Spouses reported that they found themselves constantly checking up on what had been done—some found it distressing when household chores were unexpectedly left half-finished. Unpredictability seems to make even major burdens more complicated.

As with daily activities, at this stage changes in mobility are likely to be more a question of subtle, qualitative differences rather than marked decline. Slowness and hesitancy are characteristic, and are much easier to deal with if both patient and spouse are elderly, when rushing about is no longer the norm. Again, if the person with the illness is going out less at this stage, it is more likely to be due to loss of confidence than to physical limitations. The family members that we spoke to often described their impatience both at the slow or irregular pace they had to match and at the need to encourage the person to undertake seemingly ordinary outdoor expeditions. However, as one man remarked:

I just have to bite my tongue, no matter how desperate I am to get a move on. Rushing her makes her go to pieces completely.

The performance of apparently simple tasks may by now have become difficult for the patient, particularly those that involve the complex coordinated actions that are carried out rather automatically by most of us, such as walking. As explained earlier, it is because these skills are performed automatically, and without any apparent effort, that relatives find it very difficult to understand why the tasks that involve them are so hard for the patient to perform:

He looks just like a normal person when he walks down the stairs. Then he gets to the bottom and he can't walk along the hall.

There may be a big difference at this stage between the level of obvious impairment, which can be quite slight, and the degree to which people with Parkinson's disease feel they are handicapped. This discrepancy can test relatives' sympathy to its limits:

He says, "You ought to have it for just one day and then you'd realize what a struggle it is." He's right, but all I see is him wandering about.

Role Reversal

Spouses found they had to take on different practical and emotional roles within their relationship with the individual concerned. For wives this often meant assuming responsibility for managing family affairs, and making major decisions, sometimes for the first time. Husbands had to learn domestic skills—again, sometimes for the first time. Subtle changes in the relationship can occur in the effort to cope with the patient's emotional needs, as he or she struggles with loss of confidence and occasionally depression:

He was always the strong one, now I feel I have to be strong for both of us.

As discussed earlier, the point at which a person has to give up work depends on a complex combination of factors, such as the nature of his or her job and the supportiveness of employers. The consequences for a household of one of its members giving up paid employment are equally varied. Some couples or families reported that giving up work had been a welcome release; others saw it as a major step downward and postponed it for as long as possible:

I think once he stops work, it will be the end of him. I think it's because he fights to go to work every day that he keeps going.

Leaving a career affects not only the financial status of the household, but also the amount of time family members spend in each other's company and sometimes the allocation of status. One barrier to a spouse taking on full-time employment in order to make up the deficit in the household income is the uncertainty caused by the need to rush home to deal with emergencies. When the individual with the illness has been the main wage-earner, being reliant on his or her partner for money is a source of tension for some couples.

The wives to whom we spoke who worked full-time were sometimes annoyed to discover that no housework had been done by their husbands, who were unaccustomed to thinking of domestic chores as their responsibility and, possibly, lacked both the skills and the energy to contribute. A further source of irritation was dissatisfaction with how the task had been done, or being criticized for doing it differently. These problems cropped up during transitionary periods and tended to persist if not dealt with by open discussion. One husband reported having fallen victim to chronic nagging, which he now felt too demoralized to attempt to confront.

Withdrawal from Outside Contact

The unpredictability of the symptoms, which can be detrimental to self-confidence, seems to be an important factor in some individuals' gradual withdrawal from social contact, and even from old levels of intimacy within their family. Undoubtedly, reduced mobility also plays a vital role. We found that those families that were able to continue keeping a car were much more able to maintain outside contacts when the individual's disability increased. As he or she chose to make less and less contact with the outside world, some relationships were tested to breaking-point when partners were thrown together more than they ever had been before, with little or no option for spending time apart. For hard-pressed spouses coping with a full-time job and some degree of physical dependency, social life and non-essential leisure activities are likely to be seen as dispensable:

We do watch a lot of TV and nothing else, but I tend to ignore that, because I've worked all day and have to manage the house. I'm wrong really. But she never suggests we should do anything else and I just sort of let it happen.

Other Problems

While the *objective burdens* may be quite limited, the *subjective burdens* experienced by family members at this stage can be very variable indeed. The subtle shifts in the balance of the relationships described may be felt very strongly by individual spouses. Others experience the changes as fairly trivial or even welcome:

> *His illness, although it's had its bad effects, has also brought some good effects in that he is a nicer person—he is not so go-getting, he values our quality of life more.*

The burden was felt more acutely if the spouses were ill themselves, or emotionally vulnerable for reasons unrelated to the onset of the Parkinson's disease. Then difficulties were more likely to be experienced as an enormous strain. Additionally, spouses who were young and supporting someone who had contracted the disease relatively early seemed to have a harder time. Sometimes this was because there were children involved, who also had to be looked after by the spouse, so that their resources were stretched to breaking-point.

THE PHASE OF SEVERE DISABILITY

The exact symptoms associated with this stage of the disease are fully described in Part I. From the family member's point of view, they are now living with a person whose most basic abilities to care for him- or herself day by day are interfered with by the disease. For some patients, the most severely handicapping aspects will be intermittent during any given day, while others will have become almost totally dependent on other people's efforts to help them cope, with just a few precious opportunities to preserve mutuality in their relationships. As noted earlier, generally this stage is reached after a long period of slowly progressive illness, but in a few cases it arrives rapidly and abruptly, leaving everyone in the family with little opportunity to make the gradual adjustments that seem to aid adaptation over time. At this stage, the relatives that we spoke to tended to express much more resignation to their situation, and concern and sympathy for the plight of the patient.

Falling caused major anxieties, and efforts to be vigilant became very restrictive. Relatives felt they could not leave the individual alone in the house for more than a few minutes, and often preferred to keep him or her in sight even within the house. This obviously intensified the sense of being thrown together unavoidably, and made organizing practical tasks such as shopping or cooking very difficult. "Freezing," although less of a hazard, could place couples in awkward situations, particularly in public places. Some couples had worked out ways of "unfreezing" the patient—for instance, one man found that laying a stick in front of his wife's toes could help her move forward. Such ingenious, shared solutions were much appreciated by both. The involuntary movements were very disruptive and cut off the less resilient individuals and their spouses from important sources of interest and satisfaction, such as trips to movies and restaurants.

In addition to major practical problems, in the more severe phase of the illness the symptoms that relatives were most aware of, and felt most burdened by, were not necessarily the core symptoms. For instance, few focused specifically on difficulties arising directly from mobility, rigidity, or tremor. Usually by this stage they had developed adequate strategies to deal with their immediate effects and adopted a matter-of-fact attitude to them. Issues of greater concern were signs and symptoms that are perhaps less obviously part of the core problems and are less easily managed by medication. It was the *mental and cognitive problems* of the individual, when they were a part of the illness that were experienced as particularly distressing. Memory lapses and paranoid ideas were upsetting to all parties and often changed the quality of the relationship by undermining trust. *Sleep difficulties* also presented major problems—the individual's sleep was often restless and disturbed by nightmares, leaving spouses feeling anxious about his or her welfare round the clock, and sometimes guilty if they slept through the night themselves.

Practical Difficulties Related to Physical Dependence

Caregivers also reported a number of difficulties that were the consequences of the sheer severity of the disease. All sorts of practical problems arose from extreme physical dependence. When people become severely impaired they may have difficulty in performing independently the most basic self-care skills. Family members may become involved in helping with *toileting* and *feeding*, work that can be very demanding, both physically and psychologically. Having to be responsive to another person's biologic rhythms can be inordinately tiring, and the actual tasks may involve some heavy lifting and maneuvering. But caregivers commented more often on the emotional strain of being engulfed by the physical needs of another adult. Trying to do practical tasks in or out of the house accompanied by the ill person could be overwhelmingly difficult.

Transportation posed major dilemmas. By this stage, most people had stopped driving because of severe disability, and many were reluctant to use public transport. Lapses in concentration, uncertainty in making choices, and general loss of confidence added to the physical difficulties of getting on and off buses and trains. Caregivers who were able to drive found having a car a lifeline. However, maneuvering someone who is stiff or jerky in and out of a car can be a physically taxing chore. Some relatives spoke of the difficulty of pushing a heavy person in a wheelchair in public spaces, particularly if they had to cope with sudden and expansive involuntary movements. Also, who does the driving can be a loaded issue. Some spouses reported that their taking over the driving had caused subtle changes in the balance of relationships that needed tactful handling:

> *Everywhere we go I have to drive. That's something else I do now which I've never done before. I think he misses the fact that we haven't even got him on the insurance policy now, and he's driven all his adult life. It's been a real blow to his self-esteem.*

Caregivers also found it hard to tolerate the mess that occurred at mealtimes and complained about an enormous increase in disorder generally. This was particularly the case for the few people with Parkinson's disease who had problems with incontinence of the bowels. The main issue that spouses commented on was the change in the level of intimacy entailed by having to help an adult with toileting.

When the Caregiver Becomes Ill

Sometimes the patient or the caregiver contracts another major illness—for example, has a stroke or develops severe arthritis—whose consequences become completely unmanageable in combination with the problems of coping with severe Parkinson's disease. In *Parkinson's Disease: A Patient's View,* Sidney Dorros describes his increased dependence on his wife Debbie, and the necessity of role reversal brought on her by her developing breast cancer:

> *For over a dozen years I had been receiving a great amount of physical and emotional support from Debbie. By 1976, I had become very dependent on her to run our household, solve family problems, maintain social relationships, transport me around, and cope with the many problems of my illness. Then a sudden collapse of Debbie's health and strength reversed our roles within a few weeks: she became the patient and I the nurse. The small improvement in my mobility induced by bromocriptine coupled with a strong motivation to help Debbie enabled me to return a little of the aid and comfort she had given me for so long. First she developed severe back pain which confined her to bed for two weeks. But shortly after she resumed normal activities, a much greater tragedy struck—belated discovery of breast cancer.*

When the disability became severe, and individuals became dependent on their spouses for most of their needs, the physical demands of looking after an ill person could be difficult for the spouses, who were often elderly and disabled themselves. This is reflected in the remarks of some of the people with Parkinson's.

> *My husband is 62 and takes care of me. However, he has chronic diabetes and is at times quite sick himself. Things can be very hard, especially if we are both not well at the same time.*
>
> *My wife is my primary caregiver. She has osteoporosis of the spine, and also suffers from irritable bowel syndrome and hypertension.*

My husband is 73 but he is doing all the housework, assisting me to walk by helping me to keep my balance, dressing me and getting me in and out of the bathtub.

Some spouses we spoke to, who were severely ill themselves, were desperately concerned about what would happen to the person with Parkinson's if they themselves became too ill to cope.

Difficulties in the Relationship

At a time when good communication is essential, both speech difficulties and lack of facial expression are often obstacles to easy communication and shared understanding. Family members reported that they tended to give up trying to confide because it was difficult to gauge how the individual felt about what was being said. They also spoke of concealing their own worries because they recognized that worry of any kind increased the physical problems of their relative—who, on the other hand, often worried about the caregiver's well-being and quality of life.

Problems in relationships, which at earlier stages had reflected subtle shifts in the balance between partners, now developed into resigned tolerance of the status quo. Being thrown together for most of their waking hours imposed a severe strain on relationships that had never been based on shared interests. One man spoke with feeling of his and his wife's mutual frustration at having to go on shopping expeditions together—he simply hated shopping, and she felt inhibited in her enjoyment of looking around the stores, knowing his discomfort. This increase in daily contact was often imposed at a point when the possibility of reciprocity or meaningful communication was much reduced, which was an additional and severe burden.

I see the expressionless face and the slowness in responding as a kind of veil over her. Trying to push my way through this veil is frustrating, and I'm inclined to feel a bit angry.

At this point, spouses began to describe the person with Parkinson's as nothing like the person they first knew. Conversation can grow very limited, particularly if the household has few outside contacts. The caregiver's sense of isolation can be intensified when there is little mutual support available within the relationship. They often commented that they had learned not to expect any support in a crisis.

I can only describe it as having to have a complete sense of responsibility for him. If I am sick, he seems to need much more from me.

Personal Grief

The subjective difficulties that caregivers described, unlike in the earlier stages, arose more directly from the physical problems imposed by the disease. They spoke of how upsetting it was to have to stand by helplessly and watch suffering—for instance, during periods of prolonged stiffness or uncontrollable dyskinesias. Several spoke of feelings of sorrow, concern, and sympathy for the afflicted person. Spouses who were unable to help their partner, because the main difficulties seemed intractable, found their situation hard to bear—they reported feeling totally helpless.

I cry, but it's no use crying. My mind just goes blank. If I could help him, it would be much easier for me.

There were also many expressions of admiration for the patient's endurance. A few people who were severely disabled actively considered suicide, and all spouses faced with this problem found the distress and anxiety it caused insufferable. At this stage, also, caregivers have accepted not only that the joint future they had planned together has been lost, but also that their futures are significantly different. This alteration of expectations was also associated with the caregivers' sense of loss.

Mixed Feelings and a Sense of Isolation

Of the toll taken on themselves individually, caregivers reported feeling that their physical and emotional resources were stretched to the limit by

the length of time they had been struggling with a progressively deterio-
rating situation:

*They're only small things, but when you've dealt with them week after
week, year after year, it becomes difficult. Most days I'm all right, but I do
lose patience. I suppose it's because now I am old and not so well myself.*

It was more common for caregivers to speak of feeling irritable, and yet
very guilty about getting angry with someone so obviously helpless. Their
own opportunities for involvement with outside activities were severely
limited by the consequences of the disease, which seemed to contribute,
in turn, to the loss of alternative sources of informal support. Feelings of
extreme isolation were quite common:

*Neighbors are for emergencies only now. No one wants you when
someone is always sick.*

*I would say it's sheer misery. Half an hour is the most I go out for,
and yesterday it seemed like ten years since I had last been out.*

OTHER PEOPLE AS CAREGIVERS

This chapter has mainly reflected the experiences of those caregivers who
are spouses or partners and who share a household with the person with the
disease. Of course, other groups of relatives and friends become closely
involved in providing support, and most of the points made so far apply to
all caregivers. However, coping with Parkinson's does present each kind of
relationship with some unique issues. I shall now deal with specific problems confronted by parents, grown-up children, and more distant friends or
relatives who do not live with the patient; and finally, with the problems
encountered by those who do not have a primary caregiver.

Parents

When the well-being or life of a child is threatened, parents are faced with
peculiarly painful emotions. This is true even if the child has reached

adulthood. These emotional challenges are common to all severe disorders, and Parkinson's disease is no exception.

Primary threats to a child's well-being cannot but strike parents as untimely. It is just not part of the ordinary pattern of events for parents to survive their children or to be in better shape and healthier. Also, people who have contracted the disease in their parents' lifetime are likely to be younger than average at the age of onset. As was discussed earlier, those who are elderly when they become ill find the disabilities easier to accept, partly because they can be labeled as an ordinary part of old age. Parents seeing their adult children becoming disabled have to deal with this double issue of untimeliness plus the particular burden of grief about the loss of future hopes and expectations.

If parents are sharing a household with the ill person, roles and boundaries have to be renegotiated just as they do between spouses. Parents may find themselves resuming caring roles, with the grown child returning to a relationship of dependence long since outgrown. Negotiating these changes can be very stressful and may rekindle conflicts dating from adolescence if the adult child's need for independence is not carefully respected.

Parents may feel anxious about how their child will manage after their death—an issue of great concern for parents caring for children with lifelong disabilities. Support groups for caregivers, discussed in Chapter 9, are valuable sources of information and practical help. The majority of local support groups also have separate meetings and programs for caregivers. Parents coping with other sorts of disorders, too, find that looking carefully at available residential or sheltered accommodation and planning for an eventual move allays some of their worst anxieties. Similarly, establishing good working relationships with homecare or respite services also proves helpful in reducing future uncertainties.

Grown-up Children

Some adult children sharing a household with a parent who has Parkinson's find that he or she becomes much bossier, playing the role of authoritarian parent and insisting that the household conform to his or her preferred regimen.

She asks us to do something and if we don't do it right away, she gets super-irritable, because her life is revolving around her routine.

The problem seems much more common among this group of caregivers than among spouses or partners. In an effort to keep on top of their disease, some parent-patients fall back on old ways of relating to their children that are no longer appropriate, either to the age of the children or to the shift in dependency.

Adult children reported great concern for their own future, including fears that they would not be able to develop their own independent life. At the stage when young adults would normally be struggling to shake off old patterns of dependency, they are forced to recognize that they will be providing care and support for some indefinite period. This raises concerns about studying, housing, having a family of their own. One such caregiver put it this way:

I worry about the future more than the present. What if I were to get married—I couldn't move away and I would have to live in the same house.

Alternatively, when adult children have already moved away and have families of their own, caring for the parent with Parkinson's was sometimes an additional burden—although often willingly taken on:

My mom has now had Parkinson's disease for ten years, and I have been most involved in looking after her since my dad died. My brother lives too far away to help on a day-to-day basis, but she spends all holidays with his family. I come over most days after picking up my children from school. I do all her shopping and heavy cleaning. It is an added strain, but I see it as my duty as her daughter to do as much as I can to help.

Friends and More Distant Relatives

Many of the same issues arise—although usually with less urgency— for those who are closely involved in providing support for someone with

Parkinson's but who do not actually live with him or her. Although the burdens may be less pressing because fewer daily activities are shared, an alternative source of stress is the lack of control over certain aspects of living that can have an impact on the quality of life of a disabled person. Caregivers report finding it frustrating and additionally upsetting not to be on the spot for much of the time. The unpredictability that is a feature of the disease and that tends to make caregivers who do share a household overvigilant can be particularly difficult for caregivers who live separately. The solution in these circumstances is for caregivers to become effective *care-managers* rather than care-providers. Their main role then is to coordinate other people to provide the hands-on care that they themselves are unable to give. Sometimes feelings of guilt and uncertainty about where to draw the line as far as disrupting their own lives is concerned can make it difficult for relatives and friends to perform this function as efficiently as they might.

PEOPLE WITHOUT A CAREGIVER

In a study of Parkinson's disease in Aberdeen conducted by Dr. William Mutch and his colleagues, 19 percent of people with the illness lived alone. Clearly, this group of people inevitably have the same physical needs as those with caregivers close at hand, and having to function independently can often delay the disabling effects of the symptoms. However, this group has to find practical help eventually, and when they do they rely on formal, professional caregivers such as *home care attendants*, or on individuals with whom they may not have long-standing relationships. The expectations and obligations within such relationships are likely to be relatively clear-cut, and many people are more comfortable with that. Certainly, negotiating complex emotional issues such as balancing dependence and autonomy is easier and can be dealt with more concretely. The down side of this kind of arrangement, for more vulnerable people, can be a sense of being intruded upon or forced into a level of intimacy and dependence with a stranger that is quite unwelcome. It is vital that people in this position feel able to state their needs explicitly.

KEY FACTS 6

For people with Parkinson's disease, the primary caregiver is most often the spouse or partner, although other relatives such as adult children, siblings, or parents may also take on the role. Frequently, only one person acts as the primary caregiver, and he or she may have to combine this with other duties such as earning a living and running a household. Parkinson's disease in a close relative changes the life of the caregiver in fundamental ways; the adjustments involved change according to the phase of the illness.

Before diagnosis

Changes are slight or subtle, requiring little practical adjustment, but they can create tension and confusion while the diagnosis is still unknown. In some cases, the ill person may be blamed for behavioral changes over which he or she has no control. Particular strain is caused if anxieties and uncertainties are not discussed.

The diagnosis

Being given a label for puzzling changes can bring enormous relief. Reactions to hearing the diagnosis for the first time are determined by knowledge and by any previous experience of the disease; some see Parkinson's as part of normal aging, whereas others are influenced by memories of people in advanced stages of the illness, before effective drugs were available. Best outcomes occur when caregiver and patient arrive quickly at an open and shared perspective on the news.

The phase of mild to moderate disability

This period is characterized by gradual adjustment to living with disability. Abrupt deteriorations and rapid decline are more difficult to tolerate. People with Parkinson's have not lost their ability to function, but they may perform tasks significantly more slowly and their ability to carry out tasks varies unpredictably. Caregivers find that they struggle with a tendency to be impatient and need to be wary of taking over prematurely. Many couples report that shifts in responsibility and some role reversal occur at this phase. With increasing disability, social contact may be gradually reduced.

The phase of severe disability

Caregivers' attitudes tend by now to be characterized by resignation and/or sympathy. Usually the core symptoms are not the source of greatest distress, because strategies for dealing with the challenges they present have evolved gradually during the previous stages. Cognitive problems, if present, do cause distress. Falls make caregivers increasingly vigilant. This need for vigilance can create a sense of being thrown together too much, make organizing domestic routines difficult, and may encourage caregivers to impose unnecessary restrictions on themselves and on the other person. It also increases the sense of isolation, as the outside world becomes less and less accessible. Relationships can be radically changed by the patient's need for help with basic functions such as toileting and feeding. Caregivers' own ill-health may be an additional burden. Loss is a dominating theme—caregivers recognize they have lost their old relationship with the patient, as well as their vision of the future. A sense of personal grief may be associated with witnessing the increasing disability and dependence.

Caregivers other than spouse or partner

Despite the common ground of shared experiences, caregivers who are looking after not a husband or wife, but another relative or friend, do have specific issues to deal with. When *parents* are the caregivers, the main issue is the untimeliness of Parkinson's disease, normally held to be a disorder of old age, hitting a young adult. Parents may find it difficult to acknowledge their adult child's continuing need for independence when they have to return to their long-outgrown role of providing a high level of physical care. Parents also worry about the child's future after their own death; those who make detailed practical plans seem to find this issue easier to deal with. When *adult children* are the caregivers, there are often conflicts over the degree of separation the child can achieve, and parental attempts to reassert old power structures may prevent the child from developing as much autonomy as he or she might. When *friends or relatives* do not share the household but have a major caregiving role, there may be worries about their lack of control over the situation. Caregivers who are able to coordinate a network of formal and informal care have much to contribute, though some are hampered in this respect because they feel guilty about not performing the tasks themselves.

7

Parkinson's Disease and Dementia

Dementia is a progressive loss of intellectual abilities and impairment of memory to the degree that a person can no longer perform his or her usual social and occupational duties. Memory is impaired in a specific way; short-term memory—that is, memory for new events or items of information—is lost, but memory for events that occurred in the more distant past may be preserved. A person with dementia may not remember what he had for breakfast half an hour ago but may be able to recall childhood experiences. Other symptoms may include impaired judgment, inability to think or to learn, and changes in personality. The individual may be disoriented, not remembering the date or time or where he or she is, and engage in restless wandering. Simple tasks such as dressing and eating, cooking a meal, or finding the way to a local store become impossible. In the later stages of the illness, the person may not recognize even his or her closest relatives or friends.

In most people, Parkinson's disease is not associated with dementia. Dementia is believed to occur in approximately 15 percent to 20 percent of cases, although some studies show its incidence to be somewhat higher. The co-occurrence of dementia inevitably poses additional challenges for the person with Parkinson's disease and for his or her caregiver and family.

THE NATURE OF DEMENTIA IN PARKINSON'S DISEASE

Dementia affects all groups in society about equally and is not limited to a particular sex, socioeconomic group, ethnic group, or geographic location.

Dementia is primarily a disease of old age; although it occasionally occurs in middle age, the risk of it developing increases with age. Approximately 5 percent of people aged 60 or over develop dementia. Among those aged 90 or more, the rate rises to 30 percent. Alzheimer's disease is the most common type of dementia, and about half or two-thirds of people with dementia have Alzheimer's disease, which is named after Alois Alzheimer, the German neurologist who first described the disease in 1907.

The cause of Alzheimer's disease is not known. Its symptoms are associated with abnormalities in brain cells. At postmortem examination under the microscope, the brain of a person suffering from Alzheimer's disease has a number of characteristic features called "tangles," which are abnormal fibrous tissues in the brain cells, and "plaques," abnormal deposits of a protein called amyloid. In Alzheimer's disease, tangles prevent the transport of chemicals in the brain cells, and plaques interfere with the transmission of signals between them; in addition, *acetylcholine*, one of the major neurotransmitters of the brain that plays a fundamental role in memory and other cognitive functions, is in short supply.

Other forms of dementia exist besides Alzheimer's disease; for example, multi-infarct dementia accounts for about 25 percent of cases. As mentioned earlier, an infarct is a small area of dead tissue. In multi-infarct dementia, a blood vessel is burst or blocked by a blood clot, so that the blood supply to an area of the brain is cut off, the cells are deprived of oxygen and nutrients, and consequently die. With the death of a large number of brain cells, their functions are lost and dementia develops.

The risk of dementia in Parkinson's disease is 10 percent to 15 percent higher than in the general population of the same age. An outstanding question is whether dementia in Parkinson's is simply Alzheimer's disease co-occurring with Parkinson's, or whether there is a Parkinsonian dementia that is quite a separate disease. At least in the early stages, the picture of dementia in Parkinson's is somewhat different from the profound loss of memory and intellectual abilities seen in Alzheimer's disease. The Parkinson's dementia is marked by forgetfulness, slowness of thought processes, loss of "executive functions"—decision making, planning, reasoning, coping with novelty—and lethargy.

Some scientists propose that "cortical Lewy-body disease" may be the basis of dementia in Parkinson's. This condition is marked by the occurrence of abnormal deposits of a protein called *ubiquitin* that result in the appearance of Lewy bodies in the cerebral cortex and elsewhere. Some investigators have argued that the nature of dementia in Alzheimer's disease is qualitatively different from that in Parkinson's. Others believe that there is no justification for such a distinction, in terms either of the pathologic changes in the brain or of the nature of the cognitive deficits associated with them. These scientists consider Alzheimer's disease to be simply more severe than the dementia seen in Parkinson's. The debate, of both theoretic and practical interest, remains unsettled. The fact that cognitive function, particularly language and memory, is generally not as severely or as comprehensively impaired in the person with Parkinson's who has dementia as it is in someone with Alzheimer's disease, at least in the early stages, has implications for the management of the illness, in that caring for the person with Parkinson's and dementia may be less demanding in those early stages. Later on in the illness, the dementia may be as severe as that seen in Alzheimer's disease and require similar amounts of caring.

THE SPECIAL NEEDS OF THE PARKINSON'S DISEASE PATIENT WITH DEMENTIA

In the following sections, we suggest ways of dealing with some of the special needs of the person with Parkinson's disease and dementia. More thorough coverage of the special needs of people with dementia can be obtained from many other sources. In particular, we recommend R. T. Woods's *Alzheimer's Disease: Coping with a Living Death* as well as the information and self-help pamphlets available through the Alzheimer's Disease and Related Disorders Association (ADRDA).

Getting Help from Others

The primary care physician is usually the first person to be consulted when loss of memory and intellectual functions becomes severe enough for the person with Parkinson's or a relative to become concerned. She may refer the patient to a neurologist, or sometimes to a geriatrician or psychiatrist. After history-taking, followed by examination and referral for laboratory tests including a neuropsychological assessment, the doctor will diagnose—if the patient or caregiver is correct in his or her suspicions—the early signs of dementia. Change in the person's intellectual abilities and memory can be evaluated adequately if previous baseline assessments are available for comparison. This is one of the reasons why continuity of care from a single physician or specialist is advisable, since the medical record will contain all records of such assessments and reflect the changes that have occurred over time.

Once dementia has been diagnosed, unfortunately there is not much that can be done in the way of medical treatment of the condition, and contact with the neurologist, geriatrician, or psychiatrist may cease or become less frequent. The particular circumstances and needs of the person with dementia and his or her caregiver have now been determined, and other professionals such as clinical psychologists, social workers, occupational therapists, and home care nurses may become involved in the management of the case. The primary role of these professionals is to provide advice and emotional support. They can also arrange for practical help to be provided, such as help with the day-to-day care—bathing, dressing, feeding, day and night sitting services—as well as with tasks such as shopping, cleaning, and cooking. Unsurprisingly, the burden of caring for a person with dementia is more likely to lead to strain and trauma when borne alone by the caregiver than when shared with others. Sharing the care is not an admission of failure, rather an acceptance of the fact that it is impossible for a single person to deal with all the demands that caring for someone with dementia presents.

Medication

As already suggested, there is no cure for dementia, and no medication can slow down the process of mental deterioration. When dementia is present in

Parkinson's disease, the mental state of the person is often given priority over the physical state and mobility. *Neuroleptics*, or the "major tranquilizers," are the type of medication normally used to treat the disruptive behavior of dementia, but they are contraindicated in those with Parkinson's and dementia because they would worsen their motor symptoms. When neuroleptics are absolutely necessary, those that are least likely to exacerbate the symptoms of Parkinson's, such as clozapine, are used. When the person is agitated, minor tranquilizers such as lorazepam or oxazepam can be prescribed by the doctor. These drugs are addictive, and cause sedation, further confusion, and amnesia. Antidepressants such as trazodone (Molipaxin) and fluoxetine (Prozac) can have a general calming effect, improve sleep, and alleviate repetitive behavior, tearfulness, and depressed mood.

As far as the medication taken to control the symptoms of Parkinson's disease is concerned, dementia may limit the value of levodopa therapy. Side effects such as hallucinations and confusional states are more likely and will probably necessitate lowering the dosage of levodopa—the person may not be able to tolerate higher dosages. Some of the medications given for controlling the symptoms of Parkinson's, such as anticholinergics, may have to be discontinued, since forgetfulness and confusion, which also are side effects of these drugs, can exacerbate the problems of the person with dementia.

The presence of dementia affects not only the choice of medication to be used to treat the individual, but also his or her ability to take the medication without supervision. Because of memory impairment, he or she may not remember to take the medication, or may be unable to take the appropriate dose at the correct time. It may be necessary for the caregivers to supervise this or to set out the required number of pills in separate containers that are clearly marked with the time at which they are to be taken. Alternatively, the time of taking the medication can be linked to mealtimes, to make it easier to remember, or a timer can be set to go off when the dose is due.

A 60-year-old man who has had Parkinson's disease for 10 years recently developed some memory problems. Together with his wife, he has developed ways of reminding himself to take his medication on time:

Until recently I took responsibility for taking the pills myself and often forgot, so I got slowed down so much I was staying in bed all the time. I have a kitchen timer set at three-hour intervals which I carry around with me to remind me to take my medication. We have a white board in the kitchen set with medication times, which I tick off when I take my medication, so my wife can check that I haven't forgotten to set the timer or take the pills.

Difficulties in persuading the person with dementia to take his or her medication may also occur. Gentle persuasion, combined with strategies such as disguising soluble medicine in drinks or using smaller pills that can be more easily swallowed, may overcome this problem. To ensure safety, it is important to discard unused supplies and to keep current medication locked away.

Coping with Dementia-Associated Problems

The specific set of symptoms associated with dementia differs from person to person. This, together with the immense variability in the nature and severity of the symptoms of Parkinson's disease, means that no two people with Parkinson's *and* dementia pose the same problems in terms of their care and management. The major difficulties engendered by dementia result from the loss of memory and intellectual functions, which also affects people's ability to look after themselves, to communicate, and to socialize. Wandering, agitation and aggression, mood disorders and incontinence are other problems.

Forgetfulness

Forgetfulness is at the root of many of the other problems of the person with dementia. Certain aids can be used to supplement memory and improve orientation, such as a clock with large numbers and hands or a calendar clearly displaying the date each day, or a checklist of things to pick up (purse, money, keys) or make safe (gas, windows, doors) before leaving the house. Having prominent, set places by the door for keys and purses, or on a shelf in the living room for eyeglasses, can prevent mislaying and save hours of searching. The best memory aids are those that are familiar, with a simple message that is easily absorbed. Simplifying procedures, breaking tasks down into a number of easily identifiable sequential steps, sticking to routines, repetition—all of these can help to minimize the problem of forgetfulness.

Self-Care Problems

This is one of the aspects of behavior that deteriorates with dementia. Because of the memory problems, people with dementia forget whether they have bathed or eaten. They need to be tactfully reminded about personal hygiene and may need supervision during bathing, dressing, and eating. Nevertheless, it is important to continue to encourage independence and allow them to carry out whatever aspects of self-care they can still manage alone. Simplifying each task and introducing a series of clear steps can help. For example, dirty clothes can be removed from sight and clean clothes laid out in the order that they are to be put on. Talking the individual through a procedure can also help. Replacing buttons and zippers with pieces of Velcro, and using slip-on shoes, can make dressing easier. A variety of aids for bathing and eating are available, details of which are given in Chapter 9.

Incontinence, which is embarrassing for the individual and unpleasant for the caregiver, is a problem in a proportion of those with dementia. It may become necessary to remind the individual to visit the toilet at intervals during the day. At night, cutting down on liquids just before bedtime, and the use of continence devices such as disposable pads and a waterproof cover over the mattress, will minimize the incontinence problem and the caregiver's workload.

Language and Communication Problems

Initially, the person with Parkinson's disease and dementia may have only mild communication difficulties. *Dysarthria*—slurring of speech because of problems with articulation—may make his or her speech less easily understood, and there may be difficulty in finding the correct words. As the disease progresses, the individual will find it increasingly hard to communicate: to say what he or she feels and wants, and to make sense of what is being said. He or she may forget the drift of the conversation midway and start talking about a totally unrelated issue; a nonsensical phrase or a single question may be continuously repeated. All this can be very unnerving for the caregiver, and patience and tact will be required to deal with it.

Occasionally, the person may be completely confused and disoriented, and mentally regress in time. For example, he or she may want to take the children to school even though they are now grown up and married, or ask for someone who died many years ago. Because of the cognitive deficits, communication needs to be kept simple. It is important to speak clearly and slowly, using short sentences. To facilitate communication, if the individual uses sensory aids such as a hearing aid or glasses, these should be worn and kept in good working order. Since memories of the past are often better preserved, they can be more reliable topics of conversation. The caregiver may find that body language such as facial expression, eye contact, and touching may enhance communication. When speech becomes very incoherent, holding the person's hands, or giving a hug or a cuddle, can convey warmth. Music and dance can sometimes be alternative means of contact and communication.

A number of ways have been developed of enhancing communication between the person with dementia and the caregiver or other family members. The aim of *reality orientation* is to help the person, who is continually making mistakes with the date, time, places, names, and so on, to obtain as good an awareness as possible of his or her surroundings. This is achieved by using memory aids such as clocks and calendars and correcting the individual when places, times, or names are misperceived, keeping him or her informed about matters that are going on in the house or about major world events, and by repeating the information several times. When appropriately phrased and delivered with empathy, to emphasize strengths rather than highlighting weaknesses, such correcting can help to preserve the individual's remaining abilities. However, it's important not to correct whenever a mistake occurs—this may be perceived as too confrontational. Correcting should be done and information given in a sensitive manner to coincide with times when the person is most receptive and more likely to absorb and benefit from it.

Another approach, *validation therapy*, aims to help the caregiver or other companion to understand what the person with dementia is trying to express. Gaining a sense of his or her feelings and experiences can open up a channel for communication. *Reminiscence therapy* is another technique. Here, photographs, music, accounts of everyday or historic events are used as a basis from which to reminisce about the past, of which the person with dementia has a better-preserved memory.

Dealing with Potential Hazards

As the individual's memory, judgment, and reasoning ability deteriorate, everyday situations may become potential hazards. So it may become necessary, for example, to place medicines, bleach, and other cleaning fluids out of reach, to put guards over open fires and electric heaters with exposed elements. The house also needs to be made safe as far as access to gas or electrical appliances is concerned, and trailing wires or other obstacles that may cause accidents. The stairs can be made safer with good lighting and handrails on either side. Boiling water in the kitchen and bathroom can be hazardous. Get an electric kettle with an automatic cut-out and lower the temperature of the thermostat on the water heater. Handrails and a rubberized mat in the bathtub will help prevent slipping and falls. If the individual smokes, have plenty of ashtrays around and use fireproof material for bedding and armchairs to reduce the risk of fire. Locks on bathroom and bedroom doors may need to be removed if he or she is likely to lock him- or herself in. Driving should by now be a thing of the past.

While it is essential to take sensible precautions, whether the individual lives at home or in residential care, some risks will inevitably remain. Minute-to-minute supervision would entail restricting the individual's freedom, and is impossible anyway.

Mood and Emotional Problems

Although it is generally maintained that people with dementia have no insight into or awareness of their condition, for a significant number the gradual deterioration of their mental faculties is a source of anxiety and depression, at least in the early phases. Witnessing the disintegration of one's abilities can only be painful. It has been estimated that about 50 percent of people with dementia experience mood disorder. Disorientation, forgetting where things are when in new surroundings, or forgetting the identity of new people, can lead to panic attacks. Some people with dementia are emotionally unpredictable, breaking down and crying uncontrollably over trivial matters. Sympathetic listening and comforting can help them to vent their feelings, no matter how confused. Some individuals become suspicious, accusing others of stealing their purse or wallet, of trying to harm them, or of impersonating their husband or wife.

Loss of inhibition is another common problem—they may undress in public or make sexual advances to strangers. Accusations and loss of inhibition are very upsetting for the caregiver, but remembering that it is the disease, not the individual, who should be blamed for these behaviors will promote better coping. Confusion and hallucinations may also be experienced—the person may see things that are not there, such as someone sitting in an armchair. Reality orientation advocates that he or she be oriented toward reality and corrected when making such errors. Going along with hallucinations is likely to exacerbate them.

Agitation, Overreaction, and Aggression

Restlessness, agitation, and aggression can sometimes become problems with the person who has become demented. Agitation and overreaction may be associated with being in unfamiliar surroundings, with disorientation, disruption of daily routines, physical discomfort, or overstimulation. The person's anger may be magnified if the caregiver tries to interrupt or responds to it angrily. Since he or she has lost the ability to reason, attempts at reasoning are unlikely to be effective. Although it's not easy, it is often best to keep calm and let the angry outburst run its course. Forgetfulness means that the individual will usually forget the angry episode once it is over. It may be possible to prevent these bouts of aggression by avoiding touchy subjects or confrontation and reducing the demands made on him or her. If specific environmental contingencies that cause or contribute to agitation or aggression can be identified, it may be possible to prevent or control these behaviors. If problems of this sort occur frequently, it may become necessary to seek professional advice and help.

Aimless Wandering

Wandering is relatively common among people who have become demented. It results from disorientation, confusion, and perhaps partly from excess energy and a lack of stimulation. Day and night may be reversed, so that the individual gets up to go shopping in the middle of the night. Once outside, he or she may walk for miles in the hope of coming across a place that looks familiar. Installing locks to prevent wandering, getting him or her to wear an identity bracelet with a contact name and telephone number, may prove effective means of dealing with the problem. It has been recently suggested that the risks of wandering may be reduced by using electronic tagging devices. But while this may improve the safety of the person with dementia and reduce the inconvenience created for the caregiver, it also raises ethical questions to do with restricting the individual's freedom.

Financial and Legal Matters

In the later phases of the illness, the person with dementia will no longer be able to look after his or her financial interests, and it will become necessary for a relative to take over the decision-making on his or her behalf. For this reason, it may be appropriate to ask the individual to appoint the spouse or partner, or other relative or friend, as his or her *agent* or to give the chosen person a durable *power of attorney*. This is best done soon after the first symptoms of dementia develop, when the individual is still able to understand what it implies. This will make management of affairs, such as receiving pension and benefit payments, overseeing any investments or sale of property, easier to carry out. It is also sensible to encourage the individual to make a *will* early on and select a relative or a lawyer as the executor. This can prevent much confusion later on and make it easier for the spouse and family to manage the estate after the patient dies. Information about appointing an agent, giving power of attorney, and making a will can be obtained from your attorney (see also the resources at the end of this book).

Strategies for Preventing Problems

Each person with dementia is an individual and should be treated as such. Eventually, he or she may reach the stage of being unable to communicate needs and preferences. However, conversations with him or her in the early phases of dementia, as well as with members of the family, can help to build a picture of current needs and preferences within the context of his or her previous life history and style. There are a number of strategies that may prove valuable when it comes to minimizing problems:

❖ structuring the individual's daily routine so as to maintain a sense of familiarity and prevent confusion

❖ allowing him or her to engage as much as possible in enjoyable activities, such as listening to favorite music or talking about the past

❖ arranging visits from family and friends and outings to stores or restaurants or drives in the country

❖ avoiding fatigue and reducing stress

❖ ensuring that he or she gets regular exercise

❖ encouraging self-expression through such activities as painting and dancing

❖ at the first signs of disruptive behavior, resorting to distraction or talking to the individual in a soothing voice and making physical contact.

Moving in with Relatives or into a Nursing Home

Maintaining familiar routines and relationships is an important aim in the management of people with dementia. Living at home should be encouraged for as long as practically feasible. In the initial phases, the memory loss and impaired judgment may be mild enough to allow the individual to continue living alone. At this stage, a daily visit from a home care service may be sufficient to ensure that he or she is bathed, dressed, and fed adequately. Like Parkinson's disease, dementia is progressive and likely to get worse over time. The person with Parkinson's disease and dementia will eventually reach a stage when the physical and psychological symptoms are so severe that independent living is no longer feasible.

It is when the individual develops problems with self-care, is not eating properly, or is becoming a threat to his or her own safety or the safety of others that moving in with relatives or entering residential care may become necessary. The timing of such a move is very important. It should not be left so late that the individual becomes completely dependent on others for care and requires full-time supervision. On the other hand, a move that occurs too early may result in the loss of what remains of his or her capacity for independent function, as well as generating frustration and promoting dependence. As the nature and quality of care provided vary, a personal visit to any facility being considered should be done before choosing any residential placement.

With the deterioration of the person's condition, admission to a nursing home or other type of residential care becomes more or less inevitable. Such a move is invariably associated with experiences of guilt on the part of the caregiver, who may feel that it constitutes a betrayal of the loved one or be unable to reconcile the current situation with the memory of the personal dignity and personality that characterized him or her in healthier times. It is important to remember that the person with dementia is an individual, with the same needs and the same rights as anyone else. Residential care should therefore be of a kind that safeguards the individual's right of privacy and choice, his or her friendships and links with the outside world, and engagement in activities and entertainment. With increasing age, people tend to become more rigid, less able to cope with change. This lack of adaptability is magnified in dementia, so that frequent changes of surroundings are not ideal. Once a move to residential care has taken place, the surroundings should be made more welcoming by the addition of a few familiar items of furniture, a lamp, a favorite chair, framed photographs, and so on. Individuals should be allowed to wear their own clothing.

The Care of the Caregiver

Dementia not only causes profound changes in people with Parkinson's disease, but it also alters in many fundamental ways the life of the spouse or others living with them. Besides the psychological trauma of witnessing the gradual disintegration of a loved one, and the major changes that occur in the nature of his or her relationship with that person, the caregiver has to cope with the numerous additional daily demands that dementia presents. In addition to the practical issues, he or she may feel a sense of bereavement over the loss of companionship. There may be times when the person with dementia does not recognize the caregiver at all. Looking after someone with dementia can be physically, mentally, and emotionally exhausting. Surveys suggest that about 40 percent of caregivers experience depression. Care of the caregiver, looking after his or her physical and emotional health, is a major concern.

Given the virtual dependence of the person with dementia on the caregiver in the later stages of the illness, he or she may spend every hour of the day looking after that individual. It is important that the caregiver have frequent breaks from the task of caring so as to devote time to relaxing and pursuing personal interests. Each day a short time should be allocated to just being alone, to sit quietly, read, watch TV, or engage in whatever else may help him or her to unwind. For longer breaks, a relative or friend may be willing to look after the person with dementia, or a home care attendant can be used. Social ties should be maintained and strengthened—occasional venting of one's feelings to a friend or acquaintance can relieve the tension. Joining a self-help group, such as the ADRDA, which has many local chapters, can provide access to a group of people with similar problems. Most of the other strategies proposed for the care of the caregiver in Chapter 12 also apply to the caregiver of a person with Parkinson's disease who has developed dementia.

KEY FACTS 7

What is dementia?

Dementia is a progressive loss of intellectual abilities and impairment of memory to the extent that a person can no longer engage in the usual social and occupational activities or, later on, even the basic activities of daily living. When present alongside Parkinson's disease, dementia is initially mild, taking the form of forgetfulness, cognitive sluggishness, lethargy, and emotional apathy.

What percentage of people with Parkinson's become demented?

Some studies cite about 15 percent to 20 percent, others higher. The risk of dementia in Parkinson's disease is greater for people who are older.

What are the special problems of dementia in Parkinson's disease?

Initially forgetfulness, and later on severe memory difficulties, are major problems associated with dementia. Individuals become disoriented and may fail to recognize their relatives and friends, and even regress in time. They will become unable to look after themselves—to feed themselves, bathe, or dress. Incontinence may be a problem in the later stages. Their speech may be slurred and they may be unable to express what they want or how they feel, and may forget the drift of conversations in mid-course. Boredom, confusion, and disorientation may result in aimless wandering. The person with dementia may become unduly suspicious and make accusations or become agitated and aggressive.

Can dementia be cured or treated?

Unfortunately, there is no cure for dementia and not much in the way of medical treatment at the moment. When dementia is present, the mental state of the person with Parkinson's disease is often given priority, as far as medical treatment is concerned, over the physical state. Levodopa therapy can continue, but it may prove less effective, or only lower doses may be tolerated.

What strategies are there for managing people with Parkinson's and dementia?

The management of dementia concentrates on overcoming practical problems, minimizing risk, and ensuring the comfort and well-being of both patient and caregiver.

❖ In the early and milder stages of dementia, the individual may be able to continue living alone. In the later and more severe stages, moving in with relatives or going into a nursing home may become necessary.

❖ When dementia becomes more severe, the individual may need help in performing most daily activities; supervision and some help may be required when taking medication, bathing, dressing, and eating. He or she may need to be reminded to visit the toilet regularly during the day so as to reduce the likelihood of incontinence. Potential hazards (medicines, bleach, open fires, trailing wires, access to gas, boiling water, and so forth) may have to be eliminated or made safe.

❖ To reduce disorientation, a clock with large numbers and a calendar may be of value. In addition, individuals can be reminded daily of the date, corrected when they appear disoriented in time or place, and informed in simple terms of important family and world events.

❖ Display by the door a list of things to check and make safe (doors, windows, lights, electrical and gas appliances) or to pick up (money, umbrella, coat) before leaving the house. Choosing prominent and set places for frequently used items such as eyeglasses and keys can minimize the disruptive effects of impaired memory.

❖ Communication is best kept simple, using short sentences, spoken slowly and clearly. Eye contact, touching, and physical guidance may also enhance communication.

❖ There are strategies that can be used to prevent or reduce wandering, agitation, and aggression, including structuring the person's daily routine so as to maintain a sense of familiarity and avoid confusion, allowing him or her to engage in enjoyable activities, arranging visits to stores or restaurants or drives in the country, ensuring that he or she gets regular exercise but avoiding fatigue, and reducing stress; at the first signs of disruptive behavior, distracting or talking to the individual in a soothing voice, and using physical contact, should alleviate the situation.

❖ Looking after the emotional and physical health and the needs of the caregiver is also very important. Taking frequent breaks from caring, maintaining social ties and outside interests, can prevent the strain of caring from becoming a burden.

8

Young-Onset Parkinson's Disease

THE NATURE OF YOUNG-ONSET PARKINSON'S DISEASE

Since people with young-onset Parkinson's disease constitute a minority of those with the illness, they have not been widely investigated as a separate subgroup. Most of the medical research on young-onset Parkinson's has concentrated on certain specific issues:

❖ the family history of parkinsonism or essential tremor among the relatives of patients, the subject of interest here being the degree of genetic contribution

❖ the association of the illness with other disorders such as hypertension, diabetes, thyroid disorder, and pernicious anemia

❖ the natural history of the disorder, or the way the symptoms of the disease develop and change over time

❖ the short- and long-term effectiveness of levodopa therapy.

The main question underlying this research has been whether young-onset Parkinson's is Parkinson's disease manifested at an earlier age or a separate disease altogether. Whether the incidence of parkinsonism or essential tremor among the relatives of people with young-onset Parkinson's is higher than in the general population has not been firmly established, but more recent research suggests that it is. More recent data show no associa-tion between the young-onset illness and metabolic or systemic disorders. People with young-onset Parkinson's disease show the classic features of the illness, particularly resting tremor. Levodopa is clearly of benefit in most cases. Levodopa-induced dyskinesias and on–off fluctuations occur early and frequently in this subgroup. The incidence of dementia is low.

In summary, the general medical consensus is that young-onset Parkinson's disease is Parkinson's disease occurring at a younger age, rather than a different disease in many cases.

What has remained relatively unexplored is the effect of the illness on the patients themselves, and on their spouses or partners and their families. The small amount of research evidence that exists suggests that people who develop Parkinson's at an earlier age show a high rate of depression despite the slow progression of the illness—in contrast to those with late-onset Parkinson's who have a lower rate of depression, even though the disease may progress more quickly. Furthermore, while in those with late-onset Parkinson's disease depression is directly related to the degree of func-tional disability, no such association is found in people with the early-onset illness. This suggests that other factors may contribute to depression in young-onset Parkinson's disease. When people develop a chronic illness at an early age, it can be emotionally more devastating for them and for their families. We don't expect to fall ill in our youth or middle years, and the early onset of a chronic disorder brings with it the modification of our aspi-rations and expectations for the future, as well as the prospect of living and coping with disability for the rest of our lives.

THE SPECIAL NEEDS OF PEOPLE WITH YOUNG-ONSET PARKINSON'S DISEASE AND THEIR FAMILIES

Here we consider some of the special challenges faced by people with young-onset Parkinson's disease, and make some suggestions about ways of coping.

The Diagnosis

To be told that you have Parkinson's disease, a disorder associated with old age, when you are in the prime of life, can be emotionally devastating.

Recording his thoughts shortly after being given the diagnosis, Ivan Vaughan, a psychologist, wrote:

How could it be true? I didn't get ill. Anyway, I was young and fit and only old people got Parkinson's. It was cold comfort that it was pretty extraordinary to get the disease at my age and that at least it supported my desire to be different and unique.

In his book *A Shadow over My Brain* psychiatrist Dr. Cecil Todes, another person who contracted the illness at an early age, wrote about his inability to apply the image of the elderly person with Parkinson's disease to himself:

For me, Parkinson's disease recalled the shuffling, drooling and speech-affected old men and women in the outpatients' departments at hospitals where I had worked. I couldn't imagine myself in this role. From the viewpoint of a healthy thirty-nine-year-old there remained a vast distance to cover.

The diagnosis of young-onset Parkinson's disease may produce almost as great an impact on the lives of the family members, and particularly on young children, as on the patient. The widely differing reactions of her two children to the diagnosis were described by Margaret, an optician, who had gradually developed symptoms since the age of 39:

My daughter, aged 17 at the time of diagnosis, was very upset shortly after, but she soon returned to her usual self (a typically selfish teenager) when after two weeks she realized that I was not going to die tomorrow. My son, aged 15, said very little, despite my gently and slowly providing him with basic information about Parkinson's disease. Early on he asked, very reluctantly, if he was likely to suffer from Parkinson's disease in later life. However, the shock might have exacerbated his already worsening adolescent "blues" that four years on have manifested themselves as depression, which raises its ugly head every 10–12 months.

Medication

Levodopa therapy produces a clear benefit for most people with young-onset Parkinson's disease. However, a high proportion of patients tend to develop levodopa-induced dyskinesias and on–off fluctuations relatively early in the course of treatment. As with those who develop Parkinson's at a later age, the first appearance of these drug complications may be related to the rate of the illness's progression as well as to the duration of the levodopa therapy. (Levodopa-induced complications and their management have been described in detail in Chapter 3.) The complications are probably distressing for all who experience them, but their implications may be more drastic for someone who is in the prime of his or her personal and professional life. The dyskinesias and on–off fluctuations may disrupt daily activities, force him or her to stop work, and make socializing difficult. In Chapter 3, we noted that medical opinion is divided about whether levodopa therapy should be started early on or later. As may be imagined, the decision about when to start therapy is even more significant in the case of young people, who will have to live and cope with the illness for a longer period of time. Such decisions are usually taken after considering the life situations and needs of individual patients, and discussing the pros and cons with them and their families.

Work

In most modern societies, work serves many purposes other than enabling a person to earn a living. A considerable portion of our lives may be spent training for a particular profession or job. Subsequently, for most people work takes up a large part of the day, and many constitute a major aspect of an individual's identity and self-esteem. Work contributes to a person's self-esteem partly because it is through work that he or she takes on particular responsibilities, plays an active role in society, and achieves financial independence. In addition, the workplace is a social environment that provides the opportunity for interaction and friendship with colleagues both during and outside working hours. Active participation in the workplace has become such a fundamental feature of most people's everyday life that those who cannot fulfill such a role may sometimes feel like outcasts. Unemployment can be associated with feelings of depression. The inability to work because of physical disability may be equally distressing.

If they are employed, people with Parkinson's disease should try to continue working for as long as possible, until the disability makes it impossible.

One of the immediate concerns associated with the diagnosis may be the fear of being seen as incapacitated and, as a result, losing one's job. For this reason, as with later-onset patients, mentioned earlier, some attempt to keep the illness a secret. In recounting his experiences, Ivan Vaughan commented:

I was absolutely determined to conceal from friends and colleagues that I was ill and, when I could no longer keep it secret, to minimize the seriousness of the illness. . . . During the first few months, keeping the illness secret from other people was fairly easy. I could not stand the thought of having to put up with people feeling sorry for me. The last thing I wanted was to be regarded as "invalid": I wanted to go on being seen as a person to be reckoned with. I did not want to fall into the position where allowances or excuses had to be made because of difficulties of one kind or another.

Besides personal preference and the unwillingness to be considered less able, the need for secrecy may also be generated by the problem of convincing employers that, at least in the initial phases when the disorder is mild, Parkinson's does not affect the individual's ability to perform his or her duties efficiently. In *A Shadow over My Brain*, Dr. Cecil Todes describes the pressures on him to resign when he developed the illness:

Demands for leadership in the clinic were coming to a head, as there was repeated talk of closure and/or merging of the clinic with a neighboring one. Unfilled sessions were left unfilled and voluntary redundancies were being sought. I appeared a vulnerable candidate and the pressure on me from my colleagues to resign, on the grounds of ill-health, was mounting. A meeting was convened by the fellow consultants in my clinic, to which they summoned me and told me that my presence at the

Paddington Centre was negatively affecting the clinic in its struggle for survival, and that therefore I should resign or submit myself to the scrutiny of the Three Wise Men. This is a body of doctors drawn from a pool of consultants who would make an objective assessment of a doctor's fitness to work.

Depending on the nature of the job, in the early stages when the symptoms are mild, it is reasonable to expect colleagues and employers to make allowances for slowness and for the need to pace activities because of fatigue, and to accommodate the soft voice and the difficulty with and illegibility of handwriting. Such a degree of understanding and tolerance is to be justifiably expected if the individual has informed them about the nature of Parkinson's disease and the ways in which the symptoms may alter performance, and pointed out the areas of functioning that remain unaffected.

As the concerns and the degree of understanding and sympathy shown by employers are likely to vary considerably, it is difficult to recommend a standard way of approaching them or of breaking the news. But since the anxiety associated with secrecy can be as harrowing as the threat of losing one's job, it is generally best to inform employers about the diagnosis. The Americans with Disabilities Act (ADA) protects you against unfair dismissal, and readers should familiarize themselves with its provisions. Jobs very often can be modified or adapted to the patient's declining abilities. It is also important to remember that, besides having rights, each employee also has particular responsibilities toward the employer and in the workplace generally, foremost among them being the optimal performance of his or her duties. To give an extreme example, none of us would like to be operated on by an eye or brain surgeon who has the tremor and slowness of movement associated with Parkinson's disease! The performance of many other skilled professionals may be hampered if they have the symptoms of the disease: actors, teachers, architects, typists, or hairdressers.

So the interests of the individual with Parkinson's disease should be balanced against those of clients and employers. When the point is reached at which the symptoms interfere with the performance of an individual's duties or threaten clients' confidence in his or her abilities, retirement may be the best course of action for all involved.

It is hardly surprising, since work allows financial independence, the fulfillment of professional roles, social interaction, and a sense of positive self-esteem, that stopping work is often associated with a sense of withdrawal from society. This is particularly true for those with young-onset Parkinson's disease; young people who are unable to work because of physical disability or are forced to take early retirement often have a sense of premature social aging.

Fortunately, much can be done to prevent such a reaction. Even if no longer able to hold an outside job, the person with young-onset Parkinson's may be able to work from home. The development of new interests may prevent the mental and physical decline that is sometimes associated with early retirement and spending time alone at home during the day. Another option is to engage in a new hobby for which previously there may not have been time. Learning to play bridge, photography, a correspondence course, adult education classes in modern languages— these are just some of the possibilities. In her book *An Old Age Pensioner at Eighteen: My Life with Parkinson's Disease*, Helen Rose describes how, despite never having been very academically minded, she decided to learn how to use a computer.

The computer entered my life at a crucial time and has, I believe, kept me sane. It did most definitely change my life.

Alternatively, playing an active role in running the home can help the individual, man or woman, to maintain a relatively structured daily routine similar to that provided by most workplaces. As any full-time housewife can attest, running a household is an enterprising, demanding, and time-consuming affair. Freedom from outside work can allow a person to concentrate on being a parent or a wife or husband. Within the restrictions imposed by Parkinson's disease, it can still be satisfying to manage a family. Given the sex-role stereotypes inherent in most people's upbringing, older men with Parkinson's disease, as noted earlier, may be resistant to the role reversal involved in switching from being the breadwinner to running the household. But if the concept of the "new man" means anything, then younger men with Parkinson's disease should have no problem adapting.

Sidney Dorros, who recounted his experiences of young-onset Parkinson's in his book *Parkinson's Disease: A Patient's View*, wrote about the need to adjust to retirement by focusing on its benefits:

> *Accepting retirement at age forty-eight was as difficult as accepting the diagnosis eleven years earlier that I had Parkinsonism. It took Debbie [his wife] and me quite a while to acknowledge "permanent disability" as really permanent, but eventually we did. . . . As we learned to adjust to retirement we found some advantages in my relief from the pressures of time and responsibility. Retirement enabled us to enjoy our lives more, to cope more effectively with any ailment, to improve our relationships with our children, and to render increased service to others.*

See "Work and Leisure" in Chapter 5 for a discussion of work and leisure activities that includes aspects of equal relevance to the younger Parkinson's patient.

Finance

People with young-onset Parkinson's disease are still in the productive phase of their lives when the illness strikes. The financial burden of the illness is therefore likely to be higher than for those with late-onset Parkinson's. Besides meeting the costs of daily living, keeping up mortgage payments, and having a car, many have to accommodate the financial needs of children, including the cost of clothing, leisure activities, and sometimes school fees. These may pose less of a problem in the initial stages, when the individual is still in employment, but when he or she has to stop work, financial hardship may be experienced. Financial problems are likely to be less severe in families in which the person with the illness is a woman who has never worked or has made a smaller contribution to the family income. Conversely, when a man who was the main or sole breadwinner develops Parkinson's, it may become necessary for his wife to seek outside employment if she does not already work. The unmarried person with young-onset Parkinson's is usually in a less favorable financial situation. Contact with a social worker who can provide advice on benefits may prove useful (we discuss the various benefits available in Chapter 9). In addition, shortly after the diagnosis, a financial adviser may be able to suggest ways of maximizing income through investment of any savings that the couple may have.

The Spouse and the Marital Relationship

Coming to terms and living with the chronic illness of a husband or wife, particularly when it develops early in life, affects the other person in as many ways as it affects the patient. Besides the emotional impact of the diagnosis, the spouse or partner has to cope with the prospect of being less able to rely on the ill person to share life's burdens with. The disruption of future aspirations and expectations, the possibility of loss of social life and outside activities, and the likelihood of financial insecurity may all provoke anxiety in the partner. We all have conscious and unconscious images of how we hope our future will turn out. Like the person with Parkinson's disease, his or her partner has to come to terms with the disruption of their future plans. The daily routines of both may be drastically altered by the illness. And when the ill spouse has retired, if the partner does not go out to work there may be concern about the likely effects of being "thrown together all day long." Sidney Dorros, who retired at the age of 48 after developing young-onset Parkinson's when he was 37, wrote:

Like many other couples, Debbie and I had feared that too much togetherness might break our already strained marital relationship. However, within a year after retirement our love and respect for each other began to increase. After more than twenty-five years of frustration over differing attitudes and habits on a few crucial matters, we began to adjust to each other.

A range of mixed feelings often accompanies the news that a loved one has Parkinson's disease. These may include sadness, helplessness, and hopelessness. No matter how willingly a partner or spouse or other relative takes on the role of caregiver, there are likely to be periods of frustration, resentment, and anger, now and later, about the additional responsibilities, the practical demands, and the restrictions that the illness imposes on the lives of everyone concerned.

Such feelings may also be experienced by the ill person. Loss of independence and the need for role reversal can bring on feelings of helplessness and frustration. Right from the start, it is important to allow him or her to do as much as possible within the limitations imposed by the symptoms and the associated disability. The spouse should bear in mind that being unrealistically demanding can be as harmful as being overprotective. And it is equally important that the person with Parkinson's disease acknowledge the major impact that his or her disorder will inevitably have on the lives of spouse and family. Ivan Vaughan talks about his initial resistance to taking medication, and the implications of this and other unilateral decisions for his wife Jan:

The trouble was that Jan was highly implicated in the consequences of any decision I made concerning the illness. I decided this to myself for a long time and exaggerated the degree to which I was succeeding in maintaining my independence for coping from day-to-day. . . . In truth, I couldn't hope to have a more sustaining companion. I wanted her to support my desire to be self-determining and independent. What an impossible paradox! And what an uncomfortable role for Jan.

In *The Spaces in Between*, the graphic artist John Harris writes about the effect of his illness on his wife Caryl:

The other type of side-effect, and one that should not be underestimated, is the effect that my illness had on the family, and especially Caryl. First, there was the worry, for it is far worse to worry about someone other than oneself. Then there was Caryl's feeling of added responsibility and her extra work: taking on more of the domestic chores (Caryl would say she did these anyway). However, even one or two more are an added burden. Most of all there was the difficulty of knowing how to act towards me and my symptoms. Finally, there was the unease of not knowing how I would deteriorate in the future.

Love, understanding, communication, mutual respect, and above all give and take and compromise—the usual essentials of a happy marital relationship—are even more important when one partner suffers from Parkinson's disease. In his book *Heading for Goal*, Paul Baynes, who developed young-onset Parkinsonism following a football injury, says:

This story is dedicated . . . mainly to someone who has stood by me through it all. Through thick and thin, she has always been there when I most needed her and has also brought up two tremendous young boys through the difficult years. Through it all she has shown me the most love and affection that anyone could expect. That person is my wife, Margaret.

In the epilogue to the book, Margaret writes:

As Paul's wife I have shared the trauma of this period of his life. My role has been primarily to keep as normal a life as possible for our two children. . . . I could not have done this without the support of our families and friends. . . . There have been some very difficult periods for both of us. These have, however, made me appreciate better those things which I may have taken for granted, and it has made me stronger and more self-sufficient.

To an extent, the onset of a chronic illness such as Parkinson's disease can make or break a marital relationship. As discussed in Chapters 5 and 6, the quality of the relationship before the onset often determines how well the couple cope. But there are also a few basics that both patient and partner can do—or avoid doing—to guard their relationship against the stresses of the illness.

❖ Try to strike the right balance—give the individual the necessary help, but don't take away his or her autonomy and independence by doing everything for him or her.

❖ When there is a problem, discuss it openly.

❖ Allow each other space.

❖ Don't nag or criticize. Instead, make positive comments that motivate and help the other person to change.

Sexual Relations

Until recently, the topic of sex in relation to people with disabling disorders has been relatively taboo, avoided by those with chronic illness and by medical professionals alike. To overcome this, we recently conducted a study of sexual function in a group of people with young-onset Parkinson's disease. Their spouses or sexual partners also participated in the study. The majority—about 57 percent of those who took part—were satisfied with their sexual relationship. So we concluded that having Parkinson's disease does not mean that sexual problems are inevitable. A 41-year-old man whose wife of 12 years had had Parkinson's since the age of 32 wrote:

The only slight problem we have had is adapting to the various physical handicaps that PD presents—i.e. involuntary movements, tremor, rigidity, etc.—but these have been overcome by varying slightly our techniques of love-making. Neither of us is sexually inhibited, so we have great fun experimenting—patience is a virtue!

Partners tended to agree as to whether their sexual relationship was satisfactory. About one-third of those who took part reported that it was *un*satisfactory. More problems were reported by couples when it was the man who had Parkinson's disease. As described in Chapter 5, when a sexual problem exists, it isn't any different from the corresponding sexual problem reported by other people. Other factors that can contribute to the development of sexual problems, besides slowness, rigidity, and tremor, such as increased fatigue, and difficulty in nonverbal communication, need to be mentioned here too. Paramount among these are the stress of coping with the illness, worry about physical health, anxiety over job redundancy, financial concerns—as well as the possible need fundamentally to restructure family life, with individuals taking on new roles as provider or housekeeper or caregiver.

Lack of communication, or the inability to talk about it, was often mentioned as a stumbling block by couples who were dissatisfied with their sexual relationship. Acknowledging that a sexual problem or dissatisfaction exists is the first step toward addressing it. There are many ways in which people with Parkinson's disease and their sexual partner can avoid or overcome sexual difficulties:

❖ Finding out more about the sexual response, and understanding it, can help promote better adaptation. (Most people have a relatively rudimentary knowledge of sexuality and the human sexual response, often based on very elementary teaching at school combined with what they have picked up from friends in their youth.)

❖ Examining attitudes to sexual behavior may reveal where any inflexibility or anxiety stems from.

❖ Being relaxed, seeking to give as well as to receive pleasure, being considerate of the needs of your sexual partner—all of these are associated with good sexual relations.

❖ Communicating what you like and don't like, what gives you pleasure and what does not, is the only means of obtaining pleasure.

❖ Being open to experimentation and trying new positions and techniques can add a spark of novelty and excitement. Altering positions and adopting different sexual roles may improve your sexual satisfaction. As described later, such adaptation is necessary in any case to accommodate the symptoms of Parkinson's disease.

❖ Adequate contraceptive protection reduces the anxiety that may be associated with the risk of contracting AIDS and other sexually transmitted disorders or the problem of unwanted pregnancy. See p. 216 for details on suitable contraceptive methods.

A word about physical attraction is relevant here. We are all exposed to idealized images of the male and female bodies through the media and advertising. Although very few of us in fact possess bodies that match such images, years of exposure result in "internalization" of these images as norms; we adopt them as a sort of reference against which to measure ourselves and others. Feminists have made us aware of the pitfalls and psychological costs of "the beauty myth." If we don't measure up against the image, the feeling is there must be something wrong with us.

The damage that these fantasies do to a person's self-esteem and sexuality can be even greater for someone with a physical disability than for the rest of us. The person with Parkinson's may well feel less physically attractive and fear rejection by his or her partner. This negative body image was reflected in the accounts of some of the people in our study. There is no doubt that symptoms such as increased salivation and drooling, oiliness of the skin and hair, and involuntary movements may make the individual appear less attractive to his or her partner. Physical attraction is undoubtedly important for sexual arousal, performance, and satisfaction. However, in any long-term relationship people learn to love and appreciate different aspects of the person who is their spouse or partner. For many, particularly those with decades of marriage or companionship behind them, it is the "person within" rather than the "physical appearance" that matters most.

If the problem is not merely one of diminished contact or general dissatisfaction, but something specific, it needs to be addressed. Some difficulties can be dealt with relatively easily:

❖ It may be possible to partly overcome problems of arousal through longer periods of foreplay.

❖ If the man has problems obtaining a full erection, or if it is lost before intercourse begins, rhythmic stimulation may help maintain it. A relatively limp penis may still be stimulating when rubbed against the clitoris.

❖ Premature ejaculation can be prevented or delayed by gripping the area close to the tip of the penis and gently pressing it between the thumb and forefinger.

❖ In the woman, insufficient lubrication may result in discomfort or even pain. Lubricants such as KY Jelly can help to overcome this.

❖ Most people are unwilling to use sexual aids because they tend to be seen as kinky. But none of us has any reservations about using aids where other functions such as seeing or hearing are concerned—we willingly correct them with glasses and hearing aids. Sexual function is no different. Aids such as the energizing ring, which can help to overcome incomplete erections, or a vibrator that can substitute for a penis if erections are impossible, can enhance sexual performance and pleasure.

Specific sexual problems such as premature ejaculation may require professional treatment if they are severe or disruptive. But the main challenge faced by a couple one of whom has Parkinson's disease is to compensate for any problems produced by the symptoms of the illness, and there are a number of strategies that may prove useful:

❖ With diminishing physical capacity, a change in sexual roles may become necessary in which the partner with Parkinson's disease, whether it is the man or the woman, plays a more passive role.

❖ A shift in the timing of sexual activity may be called for to take advantage of the period when the motor status of the individual is at its best. So the time of taking medication may need to be altered.

❖ Since the person with the illness is more prone to fatigue, it may become necessary to take brief breaks in the course of sexual activity. Or the well partner could adopt a more active role from time to time.

❖ Instead of the standard man-on-top, or missionary, position, other positions may reduce the pressure on the joints of whichever partner has Parkinson's.

A sexual relationship is not just about sexual intercourse, and orgasm is not the only goal. Besides obtaining and giving pleasure, the aim of the relationship is to create intimacy between two individuals. The sense of intimacy can also be created by embracing, kissing, caressing, and fondling. The need for human warmth is a primary one. For most people, expressing warmth is embodied in the sense of touch: holding hands, touching and caressing, giving a hug, having a cuddle, holding someone in an embrace. Even if there are problems with full sexual intercourse, or if there is anxiety associated with having to "sexually perform," all these other means of communicating warmth can be rewarding.

Family Planning

A concern of many young couples when one partner has Parkinson's disease is whether they should have children, if they do not already have any. Or they may be hesitant about whether they should have any *more* children. The central worry here is the question of whether children will inherit a predisposition to Parkinson's. Obviously, this risk will differ according to the particular circumstances. In the very unlikely event that both parents have Parkinson's, the risk is relatively high. And there may be some risk if, besides the partner with Parkinson's disease, a primary or secondary relative has the illness or a related disorder. Conversely, there is no risk if the person has secondary Parkinson's disease, which has developed after injury. Both partners need to be reassured that, *in the majority of cases,* Parkinson's disease is not an inherited disorder and that their present or future offspring are not at any greater risk of developing it than is the general population.

A more important consideration for the young couple may be whether the individual with Parkinson's will be able to give his or her best to the parental role—and this should be evaluated in the long term as well as the short term. As discussed earlier, it is difficult to predict the likely course of Parkinson's disease. People have to consider five, ten, fifteen years hence. Providing for children's emotional and financial needs can be demanding not only during infancy and pre-school years but also later, in adolescence and even into adulthood. The joys of parenthood have to be weighed against the responsibilities, burdens, financial strains, and daily practicalities that go with the role of parent.

Parkinson's disease does not affect fertility, either in men or in women. If the couple do not wish to have children, or wish to have no more, safe methods of contraception have to be considered. Besides the more permanent and irreversible options of vasectomy and hysterectomy, other safe methods of contraception are available such as taking the contraceptive pill or having an intrauterine device (IUD) or a cervical cap inserted. Each couple should select an appropriate method by first discussing their particular needs with a doctor. The effects of the contraceptive pill on Parkinson's disease are unknown. The IUD may not be appropriate for some. For others, tremor and rigidity may make it difficult to insert caps.

For men and women of child-bearing age who are planning to have a family, another concern is the possible effects of anti-Parkinsonian medication on the unborn child and during breast-feeding. The medications commonly used in the treatment of Parkinson's are not believed to damage the unborn child. If it is the woman who has Parkinson's disease, it is usually best not to discontinue the medication during pregnancy, because this may result in increased muscle stiffness, with a risk of premature delivery or problems with labor and natural birth. Possible difficulties are best discussed with the doctors concerned—the neurologist and the obstetrician. When it is the man who has Parkinson's, neither the illness nor the medication should have any effect on the sperm or hence on the unborn child. A further concern for a woman with young-onset Parkinson's disease may be the likely effects of pregnancy on the symptoms and course of the illness. At the moment, there is no systematic information available about the possible influence of the hormonal changes associated with pregnancy on the symptoms of Parkinson's.

The onset of the *menopause*, which is sometimes accompanied by symptoms such as hot flashes and mood changes, can place an additional burden on the woman with Parkinson's disease. Hormone replacement therapy (HRT) is an option available to postmenopausal women that can help alleviate some of the symptoms and reduce the risk of others such as osteoporosis, a condition in which the bones become porous and brittle and less dense. An informal survey of British women with Parkinson's disease indicated that about half of those who participated were on HRT while receiving levodopa therapy, with only one person complaining that HRT worsened her Parkinson's disease.

Children and Their Reactions to Parental Illness

An often difficult issue after the diagnosis for people with young-onset Parkinson's disease is the question of telling the children. Parents can be uncertain about whether or not to tell young children about the illness and, if they decide to, how much to tell. As noted in Chapter 5, as a general rule it is best not to try to keep it a secret. The more dramatic conclusions that a child may draw from silence on the subject can have devastating effects on his or her emotional well-being, general behavior, and academic performance. Remember that the responsibility lies with you, the parent, and not with your child to open the topic for family discussion. Choosing a suitable time to be alone with the child or children to explain in simple terms and in ways that are appropriate to their age and maturity what Parkinson's disease is will alleviate fears and prevent unfounded speculation. Upsetting news may not be registered easily, so to avoid overloading the child, offer information gradually, maybe over several occasions. It may also help to describe the ways in which you or your partner may no longer be able to contribute to your child's upbringing as you have hitherto—all the time reassuring him or her, of course, that you would love to be able to. You might consider something along these lines:

Dad/Mom has Parkinson's disease. Parkinson's is an illness that affects a small part of the brain that controls movements. Because of this, Dad/Mom has difficulty moving, can only walk very slowly, talks in a soft voice, and his/her hand shakes. You may notice other things, such as that he/she can't swallow his/her saliva or do up buttons. These are all caused by the illness. It doesn't affect the mind, so he/she can think and feel normally. Doctors don't know why people get Parkinson's, but it's nobody's fault that Dad/Mom has got it. He/she is not going to die, but the disease is likely to get worse over the years, so that he/she will need more and more help in doing things. The fact that Dad/Mom has Parkinson's doesn't mean that you or the rest of the family are going to get it as well. It isn't an infectious illness like flu. You can't catch it from other people. Because of Parkinson's disease Dad/Mom can no longer spend as much time playing with you, or may not be able to play football or race with you. There will be times when he/she will be upset or irritated and snap at you, but this doesn't mean that he/she loves you any less.

Children should be encouraged to ask questions and to express their feelings and reactions to the news. They should also be given lots of reassurance. It is important to paint a realistic picture—not to be too dramatic, but not to minimize the meaning and implications of the illness either. The aim is not to frighten them, but to inform them. Such explanations can also help children to provide explanations to their friends about the ill parent's reduced participation in their upbringing or social life.

Besides the question of whether to tell the children about the illness and how much to tell them, parents with Parkinson's disease often have other related concerns. The parent with Parkinson's disease may be worried about his or her inability to spend more time with the children or to interact with them. Because of the physical restrictions imposed by the illness, there may be feelings of missing out on the children's childhood. The on–off fluctuations, the increased susceptibility to fatigue, and the need to take more frequent rests may make the ill parent less able to participate in play, more irritable, and less tolerant of noise or misbehavior. On occasion, the well parent may become the "mediator," preventing the needs and demands of the children from impinging on the other parent, or, on the other hand, shielding the children from the negative impact of parental illness by means of compensatory strategies, such as trying to be both mother and father. In some cases, so as to allow the well parent to go out to work, the children may take on a greater proportion of the household chores. This may interfere with their homework or limit the time spent with friends.

When confronted with a parent's illness, children may experience a wide spectrum of feelings. They may have a sense of grief, brought on by the evident changes in their ill parent and the fact that, compared to their peers, they are missing out on input from and interaction with this parent. Fear may be associated with thoughts that the illness may cause the family to split up. They may feel rejected, in the sense that they are no longer the center of attention in the family. Embarrassment may result from the fact that, despite being an adult, the ill parent is no longer able, in the more advanced stages of the illness, to do basic activities or look after his or her own needs. Older children may become particularly embarrassed by the parent's more evident symptoms such as tremor or rigidity, and ask them not to come to parent–teacher meetings or accompany them on shopping trips; or they may refuse to bring friends home. This can be upsetting for the parent, but the first rule of tolerant parenting is to make every effort to bridge the generation gap and view life from the adolescent's perspective. Making time to discuss the embarrassment openly, and finding ways of overcoming it, may well prove helpful for all concerned.

Children show diverse reactions to the changes that living with an ill parent may entail. Some become very upset and tearful. Others become stubborn, lazy, and self-centered. Yet others withdraw from family life and spend more time in their room or away from home.

Besides practical help, children, particularly older ones, sometimes provide emotional support for the caregiver-parent as well as for the ill one. Parents tend to worry and feel guilty about this burden of care falling on their children's shoulders. Certainly, even if they are willing and although circumstances may seem to necessitate it, children should not be expected to take on major responsibilities or to perform the role of sole caregiver. This would be unfair—they would miss out on their childhood and the responsibility might be too great for them. On the other hand, many children willingly take on new duties to help the ill parent. In her book, Helen Rose expresses her appreciation of the help given to her by her son Stuart:

Now that I have to use the wheelchair every time I want to go out, I quite often feel that I am more of a nuisance than a wife or a mother to my family. Ashleigh [her older daughter] no longer lives at home, so poor Stuart has it all to do, along with his Dad. Stuart is thirteen and does a lot more than Ashleigh did at thirteen. Of course I was much more able then than I am now. Apart from the weekly shopping trips in the car with Peter [her husband], Stuart pushes me in the wheelchair to the village and quite often he will take me and the wheelchair on the bus to the shopping center ten miles away. The first time he did this an old man was so pleased to see someone his age taking his mum on a shopping spree that he patted him on the back and gave him fifty pence.

Helen Rose's book helps to illustrate other problems that may have to be faced by children when one parent has Parkinson's disease. In their search for fun or a good laugh, children can sometimes be incredibly insensitive and cruel. Lack of understanding and misinterpretation of symptoms such as tremor, slowness, and involuntary movements can result in classmates making fun of the ill parent, maybe calling him or her "drunk," "mad," or "bizarre." Others may not understand why it is necessary for the particular boy or girl to spend more time at home with the ill parent, and make fun for this reason. This was the case with Helen's son:

[Stuart] arrived home from school one afternoon in tears. I comforted him and we had a heart-to-heart. It appeared that two boys taunted him by calling him a sissy because he chose to come home after school to help his mum.

On this occasion Helen intervened and talked to her son's teacher, who spoke to the boys concerned, who then apologized to Stuart and to her.

With experience and maturity, children can learn not only to cope with the day-to-day needs of the ill parent, but also to attain a better understanding of the challenges faced by him or her and the sacrifices made by the well parent. Ashleigh, Helen Rose's daughter, writes:

I suppose after fifteen years you just get used to the fact that you have a disabled parent. I could not imagine my Mum any other way than the way she is now. I do know she gradually becomes worse, but I have watched this since I was about two years old when she had her first symptoms. . . . But no matter how bad she gets, I will always love her and she will always be my mum. . . . Now that I am older and understand more of what Parkinson's disease is, I realize how much my Dad has gone through. It is not only the disabled person who suffers, and it has made me love and respect him even more. There are a lot of men who wouldn't stay with their wives and children with such responsibility, as he has. Only a few years after they married he had to dress her, bathe her and sometimes toilet her at bad times, and knowing her pride has all gone, you can see in his face at times the pain he is feeling.

As mentioned earlier, children's expectations for their own future may be colored by the parental illness and by the burden of increasing dependency. Older children may feel responsible, and may be concerned about what will happen to affected ill parent or how the other parent would cope alone if they were to marry or simply move out of the family home. These concerns shape children's decisions about their future and should be openly discussed.

Within the framework of the new *holistic approach* to health and illness, the family is considered as a *system*. Within this system, the inter-action of individual members has implications for their collective func-tioning and well-being. When one person falls ill, the functioning of the whole system is affected and its previously well-balanced working may be disturbed. To compensate for this imbalance, individual members such as the spouse or partner and children, and even members of the extended family such as grandparents, aunts, and uncles, may take on new roles. Such attempts may not always be successful, and friction and tension may develop. When this happens, family get-togethers to enhance communica-tion, allow the airing of discontent, and clarify roles, joint aims and means of achieving them, can prove helpful. Such informal "lay therapy" can often nip a problem in the bud.

However, if difficulties are not resolved by such informal *family therapy*, it may be appropriate to seek outside help so as to promote the necessary adjustments. Formal family therapy from a trained *counselor* or *therapist* need not be lengthy. Depending on the precise nature of the problems, six to twelve sessions, or even as few as three or four can prove useful. When problems with communicating and relating to each other develop, family therapy may help reestablish communication, unmask hitherto unvoiced or unrecognized feelings or problems, and help people to develop insight into the ways in which difficulties have developed in the past or escalated from minor to major. The therapist can also help the family create alternative ways of behaving or relating to each other that may stop difficulties from developing and explore realistic ways in which family members may adopt new roles or help each other. In this way, the family system as a whole can cope better with the daily strains and stresses posed by the challenges of Parkinson's disease.

In a British study to assess the impact of Parkinson's disease on chil-dren, some of the families interviewed expressed a need for specific help in relation to children. They said that an exploratory booklet or contact with other children in the same situation would have been valuable. As far as we know, no such booklet is available and no kind of formal network between children whose parents have Parkinson's disease has been orga-nized. But, where there's a will—and a need—there's usually a way! Such a network could be instigated by two sets of concerned parents—that's all it would take. In the United States, some support groups have "spinoffs" for young adult children of people with Parkinson's disease.

Single People with Young-Onset Parkinson's

Much of the preceding is written on the assumption that the young person with Parkinson's disease has already formed a long-term intimate relationship, whether inside or outside marriage. However, this is likely to be a gross stereotype, particularly since the available statistics suggest that during the last two decades there has been a tendency for women to concentrate on their careers in their twenties and thirties, waiting until later to form lasting relationships or family units. So the onset of Parkinson's disease before the age of forty is likely to strike a proportion of women and men before they have had the opportunity to "settle down."

The sexual and relationship problems that may be experienced by those with young-onset Parkinson's disease who are not married or in a stable relationship need to be considered. Those who have already left home may have to cope with the isolating effects of the illness. Those still living at home may be very aware of the burden of care falling on their elderly parents. Single people with Parkinson's may find it harder to cope than the "attached," as they may feel that their illness has deprived them of the possibility of lasting human contact and warmth, or that it cannot fail to limit their experience.

It is true that people with disability may have additional difficulty in finding and attracting a partner. First impressions do count, but appearance and physical attraction are not the only factors when it comes to establishing relationships. Certainly, staying at home and blaming the illness and disability is unlikely to be helpful. And there are in fact many people with Parkinson's or other kinds of physical disability who have no problem in establishing and maintaining relationships. Everything in life is relative, even misfortune. In comparison with some illnesses and disabilities, Parkinson's disease may appear benign! Instead of withdrawal and giving up without a fight, the first step may be *self-acceptance*. If you have gotten to know and accept your strengths and weaknesses as a person, understood what you can give and what you can expect from a relationship, you will be much more able to convey these important facts about yourself to another person when the occasion presents itself. One complaint may be lack of opportunity. The answer is make your own opportunities. Instead of social isolation, choose social networking. Anyway, even among those not hampered by a chronic illness, not everyone develops a long-term relationship or gets married. Not every marriage is happy or lasts—statistics tell us that one in three ends in divorce. So, if it's any consolation, it's worth remembering that as far as ability to establish and maintain satisfying relationships is concerned, even people who are not disabled by illness have problems in this department!

KEY FACTS 8

What is young-onset Parkinson's disease?

A person is said to have young-onset Parkinson's when the symptoms develop before the age of forty. Although Parkinson's is usually a disorder of old age, about 20 percent of people develop it at this earlier age in their lives. From available evidence, most doctors are of the opinion that the young-onset illness is Parkinson's occurring at a younger age rather than a different disease.

What are the considerations in the medical treatment of people with young-onset Parkinson's?

Levodopa therapy produces symptomatic relief, but for those with young-onset Parkinson's disease it is associated with on–off fluctuations and dyskinesias relatively early on in the course of treatment. As discussed in Chapter 3, for the individual who will have to live with the disease for 30 to 40 years, the decision about when to start medication is best taken after considering his or her present disability, if any, and quality of life as well as longer-term needs. Decisions such as this must take into account the particular circumstances and needs of each person.

What are their special needs?

As the illness strikes at an early stage in life, its disruptive effects are likely to be felt more acutely and for longer. The need to give up work sooner or later and the ensuing financial problems are a major concern. If the individual is married or in any other kind of stable long-term relationship, the marital/sexual relationship may be adversely affected by the stresses of the illness. Parkinson's disease affects the whole family, not just the ill person. The illness has major implications for the present and future life of the spouse or partner. Children react in diverse ways to parental illness: for example, by showing greater cooperation and taking on new responsibilities, or by withdrawal from family life and spending more time outside the home, or by becoming lazy, stubborn, or self-centered. Fear, sorrow, and embarrassment are commonly experienced by children of whatever age. If a couple are planning to have a family, they may be concerned about the effect of anti-Parkinsonian medication on the unborn child or the effect of the pregnancy on the symptoms of Parkinson's.

What strategies promote better coping?

Many of the recommendations in Chapters 9 to 12 also apply to those with young-onset Parkinson's disease. The strategies that follow may help you to deal with the specific challenges that you face:

❖ Continue working for as long as physically possible. When it becomes a major burden and source of stress, or when duties can no longer be reliably performed, it's best to stop.

❖ Stopping work does not mean becoming idle. Explore possible ways of working from home. Alternatively, whether you are a man or a woman, running a house and looking after the needs of your family can be challenging and rewarding.

❖ Secrecy is often motivated by fear—fear that in this instance may relate to losing your job or being considered different or incapable by others. As the symptoms of the illness will become noticeable sooner or later, secrecy only deprives you of the understanding and help that others would probably offer if you were to let them know the situation. By far the best strategy is to tell family, friends, and colleagues about Parkinson's disease and how it affects you. Only then will they be in a position to help.

❖ If you are married or have a partner, remind yourself from time to time that your spouse or partner is also affected by your illness and that it is a burden that you need to share and cope with together. Making time to talk, to share concerns, and to vent emotions will prevent the build-up of frustration, discord, and emotional outbursts.

❖ The symptoms of Parkinson's and the stress associated with the illness can adversely affect sexuality. Communicating with your sexual partner, being open to experimentation, and exploring new ways of coping with the problems created by the illness can be productive strategies. When marital or sexual problems develop that you cannot deal with, it's time to seek outside help. A short course of marital and/or sexual therapy may resolve or at least lessen the problems.

❖ Parkinson's disease does not affect fertility, and there is no reason why you should not have children if you wish. No clear scientific evidence yet exists about the effect of anti-Parkinsonian medication on the unborn child or about the way in which pregnancy affects the symptoms of the illness. Both you and your spouse or partner need to weigh the joys of parenthood against your ability to perform the parental role adequately in the long term, and the likely effects of the additional burden of child-rearing on your symptoms.

❖ The fact of the illness should not be hidden from children—otherwise they may reach more worrying conclusions about the changes they observe in the ill parent. It is parents' responsibility to adequately inform their children about the illness, and the explanation should be simple and appropriate to their ages. Children need to be reassured that they will not develop the illness and that the family will not split up as a result of it.

❖ Joining self-help groups will bring you and your family into contact with others who are facing and coping with similar life challenges.

PART III

Coping with
Parkinson's Disease

9

Getting Help from Others

Marjan Jahanshahi
Brigid MacCarthy

This chapter considers the various sources of help available to the person with Parkinson's disease and his or her spouse and family members, and the exact ways in which each resource can help them cope better with the illness. These other resources—referred to as *adjunctive therapies*—can help to alleviate symptoms and delay the onset of disability and handicap; they are adjunctive, or additional, to the standard treatments such as medication and surgery. Adjunct therapies and other sources of help fall into several broad categories:

- ❖ The main types that are aimed at alleviating the symptoms of Parkinson's disease are speech therapy, physical therapy, and conductive education.

- ❖ Other kinds of adjunctive therapy that can help prevent or reduce disability and handicap, or promote ways of coping better with emotional reactions to illness or with the psychological burden of caring, are provided by occupational therapists, social workers, the nurse practitioners, dietitians, and psychotherapists or counselors.

- ❖ Day care, respite care, and residential care are other sources of help that may be necessary to relieve the burden on the primary caregiver.

- ❖ The various procedures under the label *alternative medicine* constitute another option aimed at promoting health and combating disease.

❖ Voluntary organizations such as the various Parkinson's disease groups can also be of value.

When considering the range of services available, a few points are worth remembering:

❖ Don't be too proud to ask for and to use available services—they exist to offer help to people in your situation.

❖ As we have already noted, the needs of the person with Parkinson's disease and his or her caregiver vary at different stages of the illness; so the resources required and the frequency of contact with each source of help will vary similarly. Even though you may be able now to shop, clean, cook, and look after yourself or your relative with Parkinson's disease, a time may come when you will appreciate even a few hours of outside help.

❖ Some of the adjunctive services are home-based and require health care aides to attend to your more private functions. Initially you may find this intrusive, but as you get used to it you will find it more acceptable and worthwhile.

ADJUNCTIVE THERAPY: IMPROVING THE SYMPTOMS

Many people with Parkinson's disease do not take advantage of possible helpful therapies and do not have basic aids that would significantly enhance their comfort and function. Physicians do not always refer people with Parkinson's disease for adjunctive therapies, and you may find better information through the various Parkinson's disease organizations.

Speech and Language Therapy

About two thirds of people with Parkinson's disease complain of some sort of speech problem. In addition, about 40 percent suffer from drooling because they have difficulty swallowing. A speech and language therapist can help improve all aspects of communication, which include the following problems:

❖ weak and monotonous voice, delay in speech initiation, slow speech, speech that starts off at a normal rate and then speeds up

❖ blank and masklike facial expression, infrequent blinking, lack of gestures

❖ handwriting that gets gradually smaller or that is spidery and difficult to read

❖ difficulty in swallowing, choking, drooling.

A speech and language therapist will start off by assessing the precise nature of the speech and related problems. Then, advice will be given and particular exercises will be demonstrated and practiced, as appropriate:

❖ Exercises that can be practiced in front of a mirror, for achieving general relaxation or for reducing the rigidity of the facial muscles.

❖ Optimal methods of breathing using the diaphragm (the muscle separating the upper and lower parts of the chest) and ways of moving the mouth and tongue to prevent you from "running out of air" when speaking and to enable you to pronounce all sounds clearly.

❖ Intonational exercises using equipment that records and then plays back speech so as to provide feedback. This allows a person to monitor the volume, rate, and changes in pitch and rhythm of his or her own speech. A metronome may be used for teaching rhythm and timing of speech and a tape recorder for providing auditory feedback.

In addition:

❖ The individual is taught to overcome the delay in initiating speech by mentally counting 1–2–3 and then starting to speak. To make it easier for others to comprehend the person's speech, he or she is encouraged to utter each word slowly by opening the mouth widely, using short and precise sentences, and varying the way a request is expressed when repeating it. To help increase volume, the individual with Parkinson's disease will be reminded to speak loudly at all times, as if addressing an audience in a large room.

❖ The speech therapist is the best source of advice about mechanical aids such as portable microphones and amplifiers that can be worn around the neck. Remember that voice amplification will be of value only if the speech is intelligible. Other equipment that may improve communication are telephones with microphones and amplifiers, and small typewriters or computers with specially adapted visual displays for giving easily recognized messages, thus bypassing altogether the need to talk.

❖ The speech therapist will recommend various strategies for combating swallowing difficulties. Maintaining a good posture when eating and drinking can reduce both swallowing problems and the risk of fluid entering the lungs. Never swallow with the head tilted backwards. Instead, take a mouthful, lower the chin toward the chest, and then swallow. Yawning a few times before the start of each meal and drinking very cold fluids can help, too.

❖ Writing on lined paper can help maintain a constant size of script, and illegibility can be overcome by typing your messages or using a computer.

❖ The speech therapist may advise family members to be patient and not to rush the ill person when he or she is speaking or eating, as this can only complicate matters and result in mounting frustration.

Physical Therapy

The aim of physical therapy in Parkinson's disease is to use specific exercises to prevent or relieve musculoskeletal problems. Although most patients are referred to physical therapy when moderate to severe disability has already developed, it may be more useful at an earlier stage to prevent problems becoming severe in the first place. The aims of physical therapy exercises are:

❖ to reduce joint stiffness

❖ to increase the range of joint movements

❖ to prevent muscle weakness

❖ to improve posture and balance

❖ to retrain gait with a view to preventing falls

❖ to teach methods of counteracting "freezing"

❖ to promote relaxation

❖ to teach techniques for getting up from a chair or out of bed

❖ to teach strategies for rolling over in bed.

Physical therapy focuses on some of the symptoms and associated problems of Parkinson's disease. The course usually starts with an assessment of what the person can and cannot do—how posture, balance, and walking are affected, to what extent rigidity and slowness affect movements, and whether pain or discomfort are present and if so, where. Then an individualized treatment plan will be drawn up. This may include passive movements of body parts carried out by the physical therapist, as well as active exercises performed by the patient. Hydrotherapy—exercises in a swimming pool—may also be used to overcome some of the musculoskeletal problems.

Posture

The physical therapist advises on ways to improve posture while sitting or standing or walking. Practicing in front of a mirror will provide visual feedback and allow you to make adjustments and corrections where necessary. You can practice standing straight by standing against a wall with your heels, shoulder blades, and back of the head actually touching it. Sitting on a high-backed upright chair with a cushion to support your back can prevent stooped posture while you are sitting.

Walking

Because movements such as walking that are usually performed automatically—that is, without much effort or conscious planning—are affected most in Parkinson's disease, physical therapy concentrates on breaking movements into smaller component parts and teaching the patient to consciously control each part in turn. To improve walking, the physical therapist can teach you to strike the heel down and to reinforce the action by thinking to yourself "Heel first" with every step. A military-style heel strike, in particular, will improve gait. In addition, you will be asked to counteract the forward-leaning, or flexed, posture—which results in the displacement of the center of gravity, shuffling, speeding up and freezing—by trying to stand straight or by holding the shoulders slightly back. Keeping the feet a few inches apart can improve the stability of walking.

Falls

If falls have become a major problem, your physician may be asked to check your blood pressure in order to exclude postural hypotension—a sudden drop in blood pressure when standing up from sitting—as a cause. If most falls occur when you get up first thing in the morning or after an afternoon nap, postural hypotension is likely to be the main cause. For falls that have other causes, the physical therapist can give advice; equipping yourself with sensible shoes and a walking stick, for instance, may help. Soft slippers can result in falls and should be avoided, even at home. Solid shoes with hard soles are best.

Turning

Those who have difficulty with balance and turning will be taught to turn slowly in a large semicircle, to consciously lift their feet higher than their natural tendency, and to lengthen their pace at every step.

Freezing

The physical therapist may suggest a number of steps for unfreezing. First, learning to put the heel down first. Second, straightening up to correct the flexed posture. Third, using "trick" movements such as walking over imaginary lines or marching on the spot, which can get you moving from the stationary position.

Getting Up from a Chair

A suitable chair for a person with Parkinson's disease is a high one with arms that make it easier to rise and a high back that provides back support when sitting. To get up from a chair, patients are taught to move to the edge of it, tuck the feet back, then throw their body weight forward—for example, by rocking themselves forward and then pushing up with their hands on the arms of the chair.

Rolling Over in Bed

This can be made easier by teaching a number of steps. First, with the feet flat on the bed, bend your knees. Second, clasp your hands together and raise your arms into the air with the elbows straight. Third, turn your head and arms to one side—this can flex the hips sufficiently to allow you to roll onto your side. Fourth, use your arms and upper trunk to complete the movement. Rotational exercises such as twisting the trunk alternately to the left and right while sitting or standing, or rotating your legs from side to side while lying on your back, can make rolling over in bed easier.

Home Exercises

The ultimate goal of physical therapy is to achieve functional improvement in the patient's everyday life. To this end, in addition to the exercises carried out during an office visit, you will be taught a range of exercises to do regularly at home. These include breathing and relaxation exercises; exercises for the neck and head, the facial muscles, the shoulders and arms, hands, legs, and back; and exercises to help with rolling over. They should be done for between 10 and 20 minutes once or twice a day to prevent muscle weakness and to maintain a good range of movement in the joints.

Advice About Remaining Active

Because of fatigue, reported by about half of all those with Parkinson's disease, there is a tendency to be inactive. The fear that tiredness caused by exercise can cause setbacks is unfounded. Despite disability, you should remain as active as possible. It's a good idea to go for a walk every day, even though this may be only for a short distance in the later stages of the illness. Sports such as golf or swimming should be continued for as long as possible.

Advice to the Caregiver

The physical therapist can teach the caregiver the best methods for lifting the patient and for helping him or her to get up from a chair or out of bed, and how to support him or her while walking. These methods involve strategies that produce no damage to either the back muscles or the spine, and are safe for both parties. Caregivers need to be encouraged to take regular exercise and to look after their general physical health and fitness.

Conductive Education

Conductive education is a technique developed in Hungary after World War II by Dr. Andras Peto, a doctor with a special interest in rehabilitation, and was originally developed for children with motor disabilities. It is used in the rehabilitation of children with cerebral palsy, and adults with stroke, multiple sclerosis, or Parkinson's disease. The technique involves teaching people with a motor disability how to control their movements and is modified to fit the symptoms and meet the needs of each disorder. The courses are intensive and are often carried out in groups of up to 12, led by teachers who lead their pupils through the process of learning.

There is firm emphasis on four principles:

1. The active participation, but independence, of the patient.
2. The breaking down of motor tasks into small steps to make them more manageable.
3. The use of rhythm, music, and harmonic chanting—called *rhythmic intention*—to help the patient regulate his or her motor skills.
4. The use of speech to control motor tasks. When a sequence of actions is being learned, the conductor verbalizes the action as it is happening and the student repeats it out loud. As the action becomes automatic, the student can reduce the use of audible verbal regulation.

In addition, the teacher recommends daily practice of the exercises and inspires the student to strive to surpass yesterday's achievement. The conductor facilitates this process by fostering a positive attitude, encouraging effort, reinforcing progress, and structuring tasks so that failure is prevented or minimized.

Conductive education exercises target the types of motor activity that are particularly impaired by Parkinson's disease, such as doing two things at once, controlling posture, and performing sequential or repetitive movements. The aim is to facilitate everyday activities such as getting up from a chair or from the floor and rolling over in bed, as well as to alleviate writing and speech difficulties. The exercises are performed in different positions, such as while lying on the back or stomach or while standing or sitting. In the course of a session most muscles of the body are stretched and relaxed to some extent. During each exercise, the patient is encouraged to repeat the instruction given by the conductor— "I raise my left arm," "I lower my right leg," and so on. The verbal instruction is considered to create the intention of performing whatever action it may be. Rhythmic counting aloud—for example, 1–2, 1–2—is also used frequently when actions are being performed.

ADJUNCTIVE THERAPY: PREVENTING OR REDUCING DISABILITY AND HANDICAP

The services of occupational therapists, social workers, nurse practitioners, dietitians, and psychotherapists or counselors are all geared to reducing disability and handicap.

The Occupational Therapist

An occupational therapist (OT) focuses on improving an individual's motor skills and mobility, as well as his or her ability to carry out the activities of daily living, including work. First, the OT assesses the patient's daily activities to find out what he or she can still do efficiently as well as which activities are adversely affected and in what ways. In light of this assessment, the OT will recommend the use of particular aids and equipment, or alterations to the home. When necessary, training is provided to modify the way in which the patient does things or to teach alternative skills. The activities of daily living are usually assessed during a home visit to determine the special needs of the individual within the context of his or her environment. This also enables the OT to appraise the practical and physical demands made on the primary caregiver.

The degree of disability experienced by the patient in the course of daily living is only one factor considered in the choice of aids and equipment. The lifestyle of the individual and his or her family, the home setting, and the ability of both patient and family members to cope with the equipment as well as the effects of that equipment on them are other important considerations, as are safety, comfort, and convenience.

There is a wide range of daily-living aids and equipment, covering the requirements of eating and drinking; kitchen, bath and toilet activities, and dressing; walking and mobility in general; sitting, getting up from a sitting or lying position, getting in and out of bed, using the phone and television; reading and other leisure activities. Other aids and equipment may be provided to meet employment demands. Some kinds may require structural change to the home, such as the installation of stairclimbers and elevators; overhead hoists, showers, extra baths, toilets, or bedrooms; kitchen extensions, ramps and rails; changes to gates, garden paving, paths, garage and car ports; door-locking and -opening, and alarm systems. The OT may also suggest changing the arrangement of furniture and other objects in the home so as to improve safety and access and generally facilitate getting around the house.

The various types of aids and modifications that people with Parkinson's disease find valuable are listed in Table 9-1 and briefly described subsequently. But don't rush off to get them all! To be of value, aids must match the individual's disability and the activities with which he or she has trouble, and be introduced at the correct time. If they are acquired before disability indicates, they are likely to be left unused or lead to loss of self-confidence and of skills. If supplied too long after disability sets in, it may become difficult for the individual to incorporate them into his or her routine activity. The importance of the correct timing is illustrated by the following passage from John Williams's pamphlet, *Parkinson's Disease: Doctors as Patients: Eleven Autobiographical Accounts*, in which Dr. A., a psychiatrist, says:

The occupational therapist at the center for old people was most helpful. She visited our home and swathed the tops of corner posts of the banisters with soft material, fearing that I might fall. In fact I can manage stairs without too much trouble: we have a stair-lift, but we seldom use it. Likewise, the OT supplied me with a plank and steps for getting into the bath, but since having a bar fixed to the wall at the side of the bath I do not use them. The OT also fitted Velcro to one of my shirts, but I can still

Table 9-5   Sources of help for people with Parkinson's disease

Source	Nature of help
Physical therapist	Exercises to improve posture, balance, and walking, and to reduce rigidity and pain
Speech therapist	Exercises with feedback to improve monotonous and low-volume speech,reduce swallowing and drooling problems
Occupational therapist	Assessment and alteration of the home with a view to safety; provision of aids and advice to improve mobility and performance of daily activities
Social worker	Advice on available benefits and access to other services; discussion of personal and family problems
Psychotherapist/ counselor	Someone to talk to and get expert advice from when depressed or anxious
Nurse practitioner	Information about Parkinson's disease and available sources of help; referral to other resources; advice about practical problems; someone to talk to
Home care nurse	Home-based care: help with bathing, dressing, feeding, changing dressings; advice on lifting and incontinence
Dietitian	Advice on diet to avoid constipation, weight gain or loss
Health care aide	Help with bathing, dressing, feeding, shopping, and cooking; to give caregiver time off
Day care	Provision of lesiure activities and a meal at a day center or hospital; a break for the caregiver
Respite care	Temporary breaks to give caregivers a rest
Nursing home	Possible long-term accommodation for patients
Parkinson's disease organization	At local chapter, opportunities to meet others with the illness; help-lines and many other services; information booklets and tapes about Parkinson's disease

manage the buttons. However, a built-up spoon for the left hand is particularly valuable to me, and as my left side is still relatively good I can eat soup and other soft food with this spoon.

Once the appropriate aids and equipment are obtained, it may be necessary for the OT to come and demonstrate their use. Similarly, as the degree of disability progresses, the OT will need to pay follow-up visits to reassess the individual's needs and abilities, on the basis of which he or she will be able to recommend new aids or suggest the modification of those already in use.

Mobility Aids

The disturbance of balance and the walking problems associated with Parkinson's disease, particularly in the later phases of the illness, mean that the provision of walking aids is a major focus. Wheeled walkers, crutches, and canes make the gait more efficient by transferring weight-bearing to the arms, thereby reducing the need for support. Arm-strengthening and gait training may be required to use these devices safely. Wheeled walkers, particularly if fitted with hand-operated brakes, are best suited to the walking problems of Parkinson's disease patients. Shoes that lace or have Velcro closings should be appropriate for walking, and loose-fitting loafer-type shoes that might cause tripping and falling should be avoided.

For most people, using a wheelchair signals loss of independence or is somehow akin to being officially declared disabled. For this reason, many try to postpone using one for as long as possible. There is no denying that there is some difficulty attached to using a wheelchair, especially in public places, many of which still do not allow easy access. However, a wheelchair is a walking substitute—it permits mobility and independence to someone who may otherwise be confined to sitting in one spot. Before you buy a wheelchair, it is essential to have it assessed by your OT, who will be able to take into account your particular circumstances. The relevant factors are whether it needs to be used inside as well as outside the home, whether modifications to doors or paths are necessary, whether it needs to be foldable to fit in a car trunk or lightweight to be handled by an elderly caregiver, and whether it will be self-operated or pushed by others.

Washing and Toileting Aids

A shower cubicle is easier to get in and out of than a bathtub and can reduce the risk of slipping and falling. The danger of falls while bathing or showering can also be reduced by installing handles or rails on the wall near the bathtub or shower, as well as by using bath seats and a bath mat; a bath step can help you to get in and out. A toilet seat raiser and an adjacent handrail can help with getting up from the toilet. A stool of medium height in the bathroom allows you to rest while washing or shaving or putting on makeup. If tremor makes shaving with a razor hazardous, substitute an electric shaver. Similarly, an electric toothbrush may prove useful.

Dressing Aids

Clothing and footwear should be selected for ease of dressing and undressing as well as for washability. As already mentioned, dressing can be made easier by using Velcro or large-tabbed zipper-fasteners instead of buttons, which people with Parkinson's disease have difficulty doing and undoing. Wearing loose-fitting clothes—skirts and trousers with elasticized waistbands, cardigans instead of pullovers—can also make dressing and undressing easier, as can front-fastening bras and front-buttoning dresses. Hems can be adjusted to counteract the effects of stooping, and drooping shoulders can be boosted with shoulder pads. Slip-on shoes or shoes with Velcro closings eliminate the need for tying shoelaces, and leather soles are less likely than rubber ones to catch on the ground. A footstool can make it easier to put on socks, tights, and shoes, and a long shoehorn can also be useful. Suggestions for other adjustments to clothing can be obtained from a variety of suppliers to which your OT or other health professional can refer you.

Cooking and Kitchen Aids

Thoughtful reorganization of utensils and working surfaces in the kitchen will improve access and reduce fatigue. Safety can be improved by the use of electric appliances such as an electric crockpot and kettle, and a pot/pan safety-guard. Special peelers and electric jar- and can-openers are available. A tap-turner can be fitted on to kitchen taps to make them easier to turn on and off. A stool in the kitchen can provide support while cooking or washing dishes, or for periods of rest, and a small trolley or a basket attached to a wheeled walking-frame can be handy for carrying objects between rooms.

Eating and Drinking Aids

Eating can be made easier with the help of cutlery with large handles that are curved at angles; cups with special handles, a lid, and a spout to provide a firm grip and prevent spilling; plates made of unbreakable Melamine or other tough plastic and with a rim to prevent food escaping; Dycem mats to ensure that dishes remain stationary on trays or tables. A straw can make drinking from a glass or cup easier and prevent spilling.

Getting In and Out of Chairs and Beds

To facilitate these procedures, leg raisers can be added to increase the height of chairs and beds to a level that suits you. A seat with a stand-assist feature can help with getting up and out of a chair, and you can make getting out of bed easier by having a rope attached to the bed frame, to pull yourself up with. Satin sheets and bedclothes can help with turning over in bed—and they feel nice too. Alternatives are an electric bed and an overhead triangle, as Cecil Todes found:

Mobility in bed was much less of a problem since a friend gave me an electric bed which jacked me up from a horizontal to a sitting position and, combined with an overhead monkeyhold, helped me in turning from side to side and getting out of bed. I feel I know every corner of my bed and how to get to it.

Communication Aids

As mentioned earlier, telephones with voice amplifiers may improve communication over the phone; large push-buttons for dialing and hands-free telephones can also be useful; speech amplifiers may overcome a low-volume voice. Writing problems can be dealt with by using a typewriter or computer. For more information, see under "Speech and Language Therapy."

In addition to the OT and the physical therapist (PT), *home care attendants* can also provide information about such aids. Some kinds of equipment are occasionally loaned by voluntary organizations, but most will have to be purchased. Your OT or PT and some of the voluntary organizations listed in Appendix II can provide information about obtaining equipment. Many of the aids listed in Table 9-4 are available through local hospital supply stores. This kind of equipment is also sold by mail order companies (catalogues can be sent for). You should contact your tax advisor about structuring deductions; if you are a veteran, call your local chapter of the Paralyzed Veterans of America (1-202-USA-1300), which will often provide architectural advice (see Chapter 14).

The Social Worker

Social workers are part of many comprehensive care centers and offer a variety of help and advice:

❖ They are often the best source of information about welfare and Social Security benefits. If necessary, the social worker can help you to apply for benefits. For example, because of the changes in mobility associated with the on–off syndrome in Parkinson's disease, the social worker may advise keeping a diary of such changes to support an application for a handicapped parking permit.

❖ They can offer practical advice about ways of reducing some of the pressures of the illness on the family or the caregiver. They do this partly by arranging referrals to other services. For example, by arranging for home help, a home care nurse or an aide, or organizing attendance at a day care center, some of the burden of caring can be lightened. A social worker can also arrange for meals-on-wheels, a service that provides the patient with a hot meal every day or several times a week.

❖ Social workers can offer advice about local residential care and nursing homes and arrange short- or long-term admission if appropriate.

❖ As part of their training, social workers develop listening and coun-seling skills, so both patients and caregivers can discuss their prob-lems with them.

❖ They can also give advice on leisure activities and vacations.

Nursing Services

Most people associate nursing care with hospitalization, but there are several other types of nursing services.

Home care nurses provide a range of help and advice including:

❖ practical help with bathing, dressing, eating, changing dressings on pressure sores

❖ advice on the best ways of eating, such as ensuring good posture to prevent choking or the aspiration of liquid

❖ advice for the caregiver on the best ways of lifting and turning the ill person in bed

❖ advice on the management of incontinence, when present—the nurse may first recommend charting the pattern of the incontinence.

The involvement of *nurse practitioners* in the management of chronic neurologic illnesses such as Parkinson's disease is a relatively new idea. A nurse practitioner has background training in nursing and a specialist expertise in dealing with Parkinson's disease patients and their families. A specialist nurse practitioner is often your main contact at a comprehensive Parkinson's disease center, and he or she may contact you in follow-ups over the phone. The nurse practitioner can play several important roles in the management of Parkinson's disease:

❖ Immediately after diagnosis, he or she can provide the patient and the family with support and help them come to terms with the diagnosis.

❖ Supply information about the illness and the various medications used in its treatment; help the patient to monitor changes in his or her drug regimen and to cope better with the difficult side effects that can sometimes accompany drug therapy.

❖ Assess the needs of the patient and arrange for adjunctive therapy such as physical therapy, speech therapy, and occupational therapy; arrange consultations with a dietitian, a chiropodist, or a dentist.

❖ Be easily accessible to both patient and caregiver so as to offer them practical as well as emotional support.

Patients and their families particularly appreciate the opportunity to talk to someone about the illness and the problems caused by it, as well as knowing that the nurse practitioner could be contacted if problems arise.

These responses reflect the patients' perceptions of the services normally available to them. Few patients or their family members feel comfortable calling their primary care physician or neurologist for this type of help or advice. The attraction of the specialist nurse practitioner to people with Parkinson's disease and their families appears to be in his or her accessibility, specialized knowledge of their condition, and possession of a network of contacts in the other health professions. Nurse practitioners also are ideally placed for crisis management, particularly if patients feel that they can call them at such times.

Counseling and Psychotherapy

Even today, in most Western societies there is still some stigma attached to seeing a therapist or psychiatric social worker. The stigma derives partly from the assumption that everyone should be able to cope effectively with all the hardships that life throws their way, and that if they can't then there's something wrong with them. This is a false assumption. No one can be expected to cope all the time, particularly with the long-term and changing kinds of problem typical of chronic illness, without any help or support. Counseling or therapy is often used for crisis intervention—when problems have persisted for a long time or when they have built up to crisis point. Instead of waiting for a crisis to build up, consulting a therapist shortly after the problem is first experienced could actually prevent that crisis.

Regardless of the nature of the therapy or counseling provided, a counselor or therapist is not there to judge, to provide a personal opinion, or to give direct advice or practical help. Instead, the aim of most types of therapy or counseling is to establish a therapeutic relationship based on understanding, warmth, genuine concern, and respect. This allows the individual to vent his or her emotions, voice concerns, and sort out thoughts and feelings about specific matters. Clarifying the exact nature of the problem and gaining some insight into its source and the factors that contribute to the problem make it easier to work out ways of dealing with it within the context of the individual's special circumstances and abilities, and allows him or her to set him- or herself both short- and long-term goals for change. The particular type of therapy or counseling selected depends on the nature of the problem.

Individual Therapy

The onset of Parkinson's disease requires a major change in a person's view of what he or she can and cannot do and in his or her expectations. Some find it difficult to accept the reality of the illness, even after years of living with it, and experience depression or anxiety. As noted earlier, feelings of helplessness and hopelessness may also be experienced by the family members whose lives are affected by the illness in fundamental ways. Contact with a psychologist or counselor on a one-to-one basis may help both the patient and the family members to examine their worries and fears and the roots of their depression by exploring their thoughts and feelings about the illness and its implications for their lives.

Family Therapy

When someone in the family falls ill, the previously balanced functioning of the family system may be disturbed. When communication problems develop, family therapy may help reestablish positive rapport, provide insight into why the difficulties have occurred, and explore ways in which family members can help each other. This can enable all concerned to cope better with the daily strains and stresses posed by the challenges of Parkinson's disease. Family counseling can help children caught in the web of the family living through stress to come to terms with the implications of the illness both for their parents and for themselves.

Marital Therapy

This form of therapy can help couples to work through a difficult period in their relationship. The therapist is there as an impartial mediator to help them to learn to listen and talk to each other more effectively, sort out their feelings about each other, objectively examine what is happening in their relationship, establish a more realistic view of their expectations, and develop more productive ways of relating to and interacting with each other. As with most problems, it is best to seek help when they first arise, rather than leaving them to fester.

Sex Therapy

We discussed sexual problems and strategies for overcoming them in some detail in Chapter 8. During the initial assessment sessions of therapy, the nature of the sexual problem and the circumstances under which it occurs, will be discussed. Once the problem itself and the factors that may contribute to it have been clarified, methods for dealing with it will be discussed, and simple "homework" tasks set to be carried out by the couple in the privacy of their home. The aim is to improve sexual awareness and communication, induce sensitivity to the other partner's needs, and improve sexual performance within the context of a relaxed and pressure-free relationship. The "home exercises" recommended by the therapist are tailored to the particular problem that the couple are experiencing. There are specific techniques for helping with impotence or premature ejaculation, and for orgasm problems in women.

A referral for any of these kinds of therapy often can be arranged through your health care team.

The Dietitian

Dietary factors are relevant to the management of Parkinson's disease, and a consultation with a dietitian may be helpful in many ways. The information and advice offered by a dietitian include the following:

❖ As mentioned previously, a high-protein meal taken at about the same time as the levodopa dose has been found to interfere with the absorption of the drug. To optimize the absorption of levodopa, it is best to take the drug one half to three quarters of an hour before meals. If nausea occurs, soda crackers and sips of a carbonated beverahe usually help.

❖ The dietitian may also advise on the intake of certain dietary *minerals*. With age, bones tend to lose their calcium, becoming brittle and thin and more likely to break if you fall. Taking calcium is recommended. Iron supplements are sometimes recommended, especially to women, who lose a proportion of iron through the menstrual flow. Small amounts of these supplements are not harmful, but all the same, consult your physician before starting any vitamin or mineral supplements.

❖ Constipation is a common problem in Parkinson's disease. The long-term use of laxatives is not advisable, and the dietitian will be able to suggest other ways of dealing with it. Increase your intake of dietary fiber by eating more cereals, fruits, and vegetables. Frequent physical activity and exercise, as well as drinking six to eight glasses of water a day, can facilitate bowel movements. Going to the toilet at a regular time each day and when bowel movements are more likely, such as after a meal or exercise, may also be effective.

❖ Given this reduced mobility and reduced physical activity, it is easy for the person with Parkinson's disease to gain weight. Obesity can exacerbate the sense of imbalance and difficulty in walking and make it more difficult for caregivers to help the patient to get up and move about in the later phases of the illness. Obesity can be combated by cutting down on starch and fatty foods and by taking regular exercise.

❖ Instead of gaining weight, some people with Parkinson's disease lose it. Weight loss may be partly caused by the fact that, because of their slowness, some individuals manage to eat only half of what was their normal amount in the course of a mealtime. If this is a problem for you, it can be overcome by allowing yourself longer to finish your meals and serving them in two portions on two plates, one of which you keep warm in the oven. In other cases, weight loss may be related to the excessive sweating or the physical effort associated with the dyskinesias. Here, dietary supplements such as Ensure may be necessary to promote weight gain.

❖ Alcohol in moderate amounts does not interact with medication and can be enjoyed at mealtimes. Although the tremor in Parkinson's disease is not responsive to alcohol, by creating general relaxation it may to some extent alleviate tremor and rigidity.

❖ If problems with incontinence develop, advice about what to eat and drink may be crucial to preserve dignity and to allow the person with Parkinson's disease to continue living at home.

SOCIAL SECURITY RIGHTS AND BENEFITS

As a result of disability your capacity to work full-time may be reduced, as may that of your primary caregiver. Consequently, your household income may be much reduced as well. Disability also entails extra costs, as you may already have discovered. Besides aids and equipment, and possible modifications to your house or apartment and to your car, the extra costs of transportation, and of obtaining extra help with caring, household work, laundry, or gardening, all add up. Many people will have difficulty meeting these extra costs solely from their income. Some with disability who may be entitled to benefits that will help meet these extra costs are often unaware of the range of benefits available and so fail to apply for them.

Handicapped Parking Permit

This permit allows you to park in spaces reserved for disabled drivers. It is applied for through your local Department of Motor Vehicles office.

SERVICES FOR THE MIDDLE AND LATER PHASES

Day Care

In many communities, day care is available in centers that the person with Parkinson's disease can attend several times a week. Centers usually provide meals as well as various types of social activities and games. Appropriate and good quality day care can be stimulating for the patient and provide an outside activity to look forward to. It also provides family members with a break and may make it possible for the primary caregiver to continue in part- or full-time employment. Lily Warren, whose husband has Parkinson's disease, writes in her book *The Road Beyond*:

> *As time went on and to give me a break, it was suggested my husband spend one day each week at a day center. He quite enjoyed the change and I enjoyed the freedom. He was picked up by ambulance in the morning and returned about tea time.*

Respite Care

Like day care, respite care aims to provide the caregiver with a break from caring. This type of care may be available through a local voluntary organization, a comprehensive Parkinson's disease center, or directly through home health care agencies.

Residential Care

In the later stages of the illness, when the symptoms have become acute and are no longer well controlled by medication, the person with Parkinson's disease may become severely disabled and incapacitated. The loss of independent functions will mean that constant care is required for all daily activities such as bathing, dressing, and feeding. Although most caregivers and families try to postpone the need for residential care and want to look after the patient at home for as long as possible, a time will come when the demands of caring make nursing home care an option to be considered.

Assisted living accommodation combines independent living with access to help when required. It consists of a number of independent residential apartments, with communal facilities such as a laundry, a store, and a social activities lounge, and a supervisory staff that can be contacted when needed.

Residential and *nursing homes* provide more intensive care for their residents. In choosing a suitable home, visit as many as you can, assess the premises and ease of access by car or public transport, talk to the staff, try to judge the quality of care offered, the social and leisure activities, and the interaction between staff and residents.

VACATIONS

Like all of us—or perhaps more than most—the person with Parkinson's disease and his or her spouse or other caregiver will undoubtedly benefit from vacations away from home. In the initial phases of the illness no additional arrangements may be required, other than ensuring that an adequate supply of medication is available. (Carry these with you; don't pack them in luggage to be checked.) When disability sets in, both patient and caregiver may desperately want a break but be unable or unwilling to do so—for several reasons:

❖ The unpredictability of the illness, the fact that it may be difficult to foresee the physical condition of the person with Parkinson's disease over longish periods or even from one day to the next, makes advance booking relatively risky.

❖ The many modifications that may have been introduced into the home to cope with disability, such as wheelchair ramps, wider doorways, and handrails in the bathroom are not available in some resorts or hotels. Since passage of the Americans with Disabilities Act, this is becoming much less of a problem.

❖ The difficulties associated with mobility and transport may seem insurmountable at first sight.

❖ The additional financial demands made by the illness on limited resources may mean that a vacation is not easily affordable.

But all of these are problems that can be resolved with some forward planning and effort. Most travel agents offer vacation insurance that reimburses clients if the arrangements have to be canceled because of ill health. Vacation insurance is also a sensible option for other eventualities, such as the cost of medical care that might become necessary while away, or loss or damage to special equipment. There are a number of travel agencies that specialize in travel for people with disabilities, and several excellent travel guides (see Appendix II).

When you are selecting a hotel or other accommodation, it is important that access to and circulation around it should suit the level of abilities of the person with Parkinson's disease. For someone who uses a wheelchair, wheelchair access to all public areas is essential. The attitude of the hotel staff and their willingness to help if problems arise is another consideration. Off-season vacations are not only less expensive, but also may ensure friendlier and more helpful service from staff.

ALTERNATIVE MEDICINE

When a person is ill, it is a natural reaction to want to try any and all paths that may lead to a cure, or at least to the control or suppression of the symptoms. Yoga, meditation, hypnosis, and acupuncture and the Alexander technique are some of the alternative, or complementary, therapies that are available and that have been tried by some people with Parkinson's disease. Meditation and yoga, techniques to achieve relaxation, may be useful for the reduction of muscle stiffness, as may hypnosis. Acupuncture, which involves the insertion of special needles at specific points of the body, has been used for a variety of ills, and in Parkinson's disease it may be tried for the relief of pain. The Alexander technique is a method that teaches awareness of balance and posture in everyday activities, so that the individual learns to get rid of unnecessary muscle tension.

Although no systematic information about the value of these approaches to the treatment of Parkinson's disease exists, it is important to at least consider them. In individual cases they may prove helpful, largely by reducing anxiety and inducing relaxation and a sense of self-control in the patient. However, caution is necessary when investigating these techniques:

❖ Obtain full information about the aims and procedures of each technique before trying to ensure that at least no harm is done and that money is not wasted.

❖ Consult an accredited practitioner.

❖ Maintain an open mind and a balanced approach and know when to stop—being overzealous in a quest for a "cure" or effective therapy can sometimes have serious emotional and financial consequences.

❖ Consult your physician before embarking on a course of alternative medicine—it may help you to keep a balanced attitude.

In his book, Ivan Vaughan gives an account of the various hypotheses to which an individual can fall prey, not only concerning the possible causes of the illness but also about what, other than the standard medical treatments, might help to control the symptoms. He describes using hypnosis, his investigations into meditation, his forays into yoga and shiatsu, his week on a diet to eliminate gluten and animal fat from his diet, and his fava bean period. None proved of much value in relieving his symptoms—and some left him with other problems:

I had beans on their own, beans in stews—enough beans, I felt sure, to provide the same amount of L-dopa as I took in the tablets. I was full of beans but still not jumping! The lack of any noticeable effect left us with the problem of how to use up the huge sack of beans in the cupboard.

KEY FACTS 9

There are many sources of help available both to the individual and to his or her caregiver.

10

Self-Help Strategies for the Person with Parkinson's Disease: Minimizing Disability and Preventing Handicap

Richard Brown

Your ultimate goal in facing the challenge of Parkinson's disease is to be able to continue to lead a full life despite the illness. As in Chapter 5, I cover in this chapter five main spheres of daily living: self-care, mobility, work and leisure activities, financial independence, and relationships with others. In particular, I discuss self-help strategies that can help reduce disability and prevent handicap, and promote better coping. But first, an important general principle that applies to all of these areas—scheduling your daily activities.

SCHEDULING YOUR ACTIVITIES

One of the most obvious ways to minimize the effects of the symptoms on your daily activities is simply to allow more time to get tasks done, rather than rushing to finish them in the usual time. Many people with Parkinson's disease find that the pressure caused by trying to do activities quickly makes the symptoms worse and means that everything takes even longer to achieve. But deliberately taking things slowly and steadily may take some additional planning if the extra slowness is not to interfere with other aspects of your life. This may mean starting the daily routine of washing and dressing slightly earlier than you used to or scheduling subsequent activities for a later time. But while such a strategy may work well for you, problems may arise when the extra time you take to do something impinges on the lives of others—particularly if you haven't prepared them for it.

Another approach centers on picking the best time to get tasks done. Once the early phase of the illness has passed, there will almost certainly be some daily variation in your symptoms and an accompanying difficulty in performing routine tasks. As noted earlier, for many, the period in the morning immediately after waking is the best part of the day—the so-called *sleep benefit time*. Fortunately, this fits in well with the daily routine of washing and dressing, preparing and eating breakfast. In contrast, getting ready for bed at night can be a more leisurely process, and it rarely matters if it takes longer than it used to.

During the day, there may be patterns in your functioning that reflect definite "good" and "bad" ("on" and "off") times. If possible, try to organize your day to take maximum advantage of your "on" periods and reduce the demands that you make on yourself during the "off" times. Again, this may require some flexibility, both in your life and in those of the people around you. Do remember that someone who insists on sticking rigidly to old routines may find that he or she has more problems than a person with the same level of physical impairment who is willing to change his or her daily schedule.

In the middle and late phases, one of your doctor's primary tasks in managing your illness will be to maximize the amount of time that you are on and minimize the time that you are off. However, you may decide that the timing of the "on" periods is more important than their length. In discussing your drug regimen with your doctor, it's a good idea to have a firm idea of what you want to achieve in your average day, or when you need maximum benefit from the treatment, and of when you are willing to accept a decrease in speed, mobility, and so on.

SELF-CARE

Make Use of Physical Aids

In Chapter 9 we talked about the ways in which clothing and eating utensils can be altered to make it easier for the person with Parkinson's disease to get dressed or undressed and to eat; we also discussed practical aids relevant to many other aspects of daily life. Three imperatives were mentioned:

1. Obtain and use appropriate aids *at the right time.*
2. Have *regular assessments* by your OT so that any aids you may have can be readapted to your particular needs at the time.
3. Be positive in your attitude to using aids.

Point 3 calls for elaboration. Some people view physical aids in a negative way and even refuse them. They may see them as outward signs that they are disabled or handicapped. They may prefer to struggle on with buttons and shoelaces rather than switch to zippers and Velcro. If they are eventually forced, by necessity, to accept such help, they may see it as a defeat—a confirmation that they have in some way "given in" to the disease. Although one may sympathize with this attitude, or even admire such individuals for their determination, it is not necessarily in their best interests. Aids and special equipment are really just extensions of the many things that we take for granted in making our lives easier or more convenient. Television remote controls, electric toothbrushes, and electric razors are all "artificial aids" that we accept and use without a second thought, and they are no different from the special aids for the "disabled." They are all simply tools—a means to an end—that increase our independence or the amount of time that we have available to fulfill other, more important, interests.

The value of simple aids is illustrated by Jim, a man who had had Parkinson's disease since the age of 51:

A collapsible stool/stick . . . enabled me to go on holidays where I couldn't stand about listening to the tour guides. This has since enabled

*us to continue our hobbies (e.g. bird-watching), and we keep it in the car
all the time. I also use it in check-out queues, at bus stops and in train stations and while waiting for taxis.*

Keep Your Actions Simple

In their informative book *Moving Ahead with Parkinson's Disease*, Meg
Morris, Robert Iansek, and Beth Kirkwood suggest a number of general
principles that can make it easier to carry out self-care activities:

- ❖ Consciously think about and rehearse movements in your head
  before doing them, especially actions with which you have particular
  problems.
- ❖ Pay attention to each movement as you are doing it. Talking through
  the actions as you perform them is a good way to focus attention on
  what you are doing.
- ❖ Try not to do two things at once. For example, don't walk around the
  bedroom while fastening the buttons of your shirt. Either your
  walking will suffer, or you will take longer with the buttons, or both.
  For someone with balance problems, even standing up can be a distraction, so try sitting down while getting dressed.
- ❖ As mentioned earlier, breaking down complex actions or movements
  into a number of steps will enable you to carry them out more
  quickly and more efficiently. Do one step at a time. For instance,
  with dressing:

1. Choose and set out your clothes in the order in which you are going
   to put them on.
2. Sit on a stable chair.
3. Pick up a garment and talk yourself through putting it on—for
   example, "I'll first put my right hand into the right sleeve, then my
   left hand and arm through the left sleeve, and then pull it over my
   head," and so on.

MOBILITY

Many of the preceding suggestions can be applied to problems of mobility as well. The following strategies for improving general mobility and aspects of *walking* have been mainly arrived at by trial and error by people in the early to middle stages of Parkinson's disease. Such tricks work well for some but not for others, but they are certainly worth trying. If they don't work, modify them or think up your own.

❖ Transform your shuffling steps into a normal stride by imagining lines on the floor, such as patterns on a carpet or marks on the pavement, then high-stepping over them.

❖ If you have problems starting to walk, or if you suddenly freeze, try rocking gently forward and backward before taking the first step on a forward movement; or hum a song or whistle, then start to walk in time with the tune; or step over a real or imagined object.

❖ Remember to put your heel down first, rather than walking on the balls of your feet or your toes. Achieve this by thinking "Heel first" to yourself. Also, try to walk with a longer stride.

❖ To make turning safe, walk in a large circle and avoid sudden changes in direction. This way you reduce the risk of falls.

❖ While walking, avoid carrying anything in your hands. Use a small backpack, which will leave your arms free to steady yourself if you lose your balance, or to hold on to rails on buses or trains or when you are going up or down stairs.

In his booklet *The Parkinson's Challenge*, Jan Peter Stern describes a number of other self-help ideas that have helped him to avoid *falls*, particularly in the home, and to minimize the damage if they do happen. This list of tricks and tips is adapted from his suggestions, with some extras of our own:

❖ If you feel unsteady, or when you are in a situation where you may fall, keep your feet about eight inches apart so as to give yourself a wider, more stable base.

❖ Walk without shoes when possible so that you can better feel the contact of your feet with the ground. Avoid shoes with high-grip soles. "Slippery" soles are safer if you tend to shuffle or suffer from freezing.

❖ If you feel light-headed or dizzy when you get up, sit down again and put your head between your knees for a short while before going on.

❖ Use automatic night-lights all over the house so that you can see any obstacles.

❖ Remove loose rugs, and don't let people place objects in the main traffic areas, even briefly.

❖ Get a phone with an answering machine so that you don't have to rush to answer it.

❖ If you have glass doors, replace them with plastic ones or cover them with a safety laminate.

❖ Learn how to relax and roll the body in a fall so as to reduce the impact and protect the head—Jan Stern learned to do this from a martial arts instructor.

❖ Learn how to get up if you do fall.

❖ When climbing stairs, focus on the steps one at a time by counting them. Always hold the handrail.

❖ When approaching an obstacle such as a curb, deliberately lift your foot extra-high—it will probably then be just about right.

❖ When opening doors, try to stand to one side so that you don't have to take a backward step.

If fear of falling prevents you from venturing far, you will find Jan Stern's recommendations for learning *how* to fall and how to get up again especially helpful. Other practical aids, such as a walking-stick or frame, may provide as much psychological as physical support. The important thing is to keep walking for as long as possible.

Getting Out of a Chair, Getting Out of a Car, Turning in Bed

As mentioned elsewhere, getting up from a chair often presents problems. So break the process down into simple steps:

1. Move toward the edge of the seat so that your feet are well stabilized on the ground.
2. Move your heels back.
3. Lean forward.
4. Use your arms to push on the arms of the chair, or clasp your hands and with your arms held straight push your hands in front of you.
5. Stand up.

In any event, avoid those tempting low, soft chairs and sofas that you sink into.

A sequence of movements similar to those outlined above can be used for getting out of the car, which, in addition, requires turning your body around and putting your feet out of the car and on to the ground. To achieve this, some people find it helpful to sit on a plastic bag—because it's slippery, it's easy to turn the body in order to swing the legs out. Purpose-made transfer boards are available to help people transfer from a car to a wheelchair.

Turning over in bed is another automatic action that may be lost. We all toss and turn throughout the night, shifting position many times so as to be comfortable. We don't usually need to wake to do this. The person with Parkinson's disease, however, may have to concentrate so hard on turning and use so much effort that he or she—and his or her partner—are wide awake at the end of it. Again, solving the problem can involve a series of strategies. For getting out of bed, bend your legs, swing them over the side of the bed, and then push yourself into a sitting position. Both turning over and getting out of bed are easier if you have a firm mattress rather than one that leaves you stranded in a valley in the middle. Satin sheets and pajamas are also very helpful. Finally, a device like a trapeze bar, or a rope, can be fitted, which will give you something to hold on to while turning.

Keeping Mobile Outside

Walking

If walking in and around the house presents problems, you will also have difficulty outside. While you may make your home "user-friendly," you have far less control over the outside environment. This makes it all the more important, when walking, to take things slowly and carefully. When traveling alone, you may need to rely on strangers for occasional assistance. *Self-confidence*, as much as physical ability, is the critical factor. Many of the strategies mentioned previously can be used here.

❖ Time your trips, where possible, to fit in with your periods of maximum mobility.

❖ Allow plenty of time so that you do not feel stressed. Stress and haste are the enemies of the person with Parkinson's disease—they make the symptoms worse and accidents more likely.

❖ Pay extra attention to possible obstacles and problems. Make your movements even larger than you think you need to—it's better to look a little ungainly than to risk a fall.

❖ Use physical aids and supports whenever you can. You might consider using a cane when you are outside, even if it's not necessary for most of the time. The extra support may be useful if you suddenly feel wobbly. Some people find that stepping over the handle of a cane held upside-down is useful to unstick feet that are "frozen" to the ground. And, of course, the cane can serve as a useful signal to others, such as car and bus drivers, that you may need a little extra time.

❖ Don't put off getting a wheelchair if you need one. Unlike, for instance, people paralyzed after an accident who use wheelchairs independently, you will almost certainly need someone to push it and to deal with steps, ramps, and so forth.

❖ Accept help from others when it is needed and offered—don't be too proud to ask.

Driving

In both urban and rural areas, driving is an important means of transportation and a prime feature of independent living. Don't give up driving without careful thought, but do take these precautions:

❖ As with any activity, think about the timing—allow more time for your trip and avoid rushing and other causes of stress.

❖ Take extra care. Think about your actions.

❖ Regularly review your capabilities. There may be special courses in your area for "older" drivers, for refreshing skills and testing ability.

❖ Above all, do you feel confident driving? If you don't, then it may be time to stop, or to start relying less on the car.

❖ If you do decide to give up, don't necessarily do it overnight. It may be better to phase out the car gradually while building up alternative means of transportation, so that your life can continue with the minimum of disruption.

❖ If you have particular difficulty with walking for any length of time, you can obtain a handicapped parking permit.

❖ If you need specific adaptations to your car in order to continue to drive, you can obtain detailed information about specialized centers that carry out such adaptations from one of the Parkinson's disease organizations.

For more on cars and driving, see pp. 130–131.

Using Public Transportation

If you don't drive or have given up, public transportation may be your main form of travel when you go anywhere further than walking distance of your home. Public transportation can help you lead an active and independent life, and a few tricks and tips will make using it easier.

Buses   Getting on and off a bus, particularly during rush hour, can be a problem for anyone. A cane, as mentioned before, serves as a useful reminder to others to be a little more patient, and may help the individual with Parkinson's disease to feel less rushed. Don't be embarrassed to accept a seat if one is offered. The sudden stops, starts, and turns of buses seriously test the balance of us all—let alone that of someone whose mobility is impaired. And do stay in your seat until the bus has stopped, before standing up to get off. Ask someone else to request a stop if necessary. If you use a wheelchair, some or most buses may be accessible. This varies widely in different cities.

Paratransit services   Even if you have no need of this most of the time, you should know how to obtain transportation if it is available in your area. If you use a wheelchair, this could be your main form of transportation.

Taxis and car services   The main form of transportation for some people. While expensive, they offer the advantage of door-to-door service. Some taxis in some cities are adapted for wheelchairs. It's a good idea to develop a good relationship with a local taxi company or car service. If you are a regular user, it may be possible to open an account. You will often be able to ask for a particular driver who knows your needs—and the advantage of a driver who knows you is that he or she is more likely to help you in and out of the car, carry your packages to your front door, and avoid driving the car around turns like a competitor in the Grand Prix.

Trains and subways   When aiming to catch a particular train, don't forget to leave extra time for "emergencies" or delays. If you are traveling to or from an unfamiliar station, try to check in advance on access to platforms—particularly if you use a wheelchair. There may be many stairs or escalators, and few stations in most cities have elevators. During off-peak hours many stations are unattended, so there will be no one available to help at those times.

WORK AND LEISURE

Work

It is difficult to offer detailed advice, given the vast differences in the work people do. Also, Parkinson's disease affects people's ability to work in different ways. When problems with mobility develop, arranging to work from home, if possible, will allow you to avoid the journey to work.

The same advice for increasing mobility about the home can be applied to the workplace, although it will probably be more difficult to make physical changes there. However, it may be possible to reorganize your workspace so that everything is closer at hand and requires you to move around less. If you work at a desk, having a comfortable chair is important. Wheels on the chair may help you move around without having to get up all the time, but for someone troubled by leg dyskinesia, having the chair firmly anchored to the spot would be more useful. An occupational therapist may be able to help if particular adaptations such as wheelchair access are required at your workplace, to enable you to continue work. A word processor or computer is recommended—your typing speed may not be great, but errors can be corrected and the final product will always be legible. If you need to speak regularly—for example, in meetings, to clients or to customers—and have problems making yourself heard or understood, speech therapy could be useful; and you might consider using some sort of portable mini-amplifier/loud-speaker.

Several factors are important in determining a person's ability to continue working, including:

1. the need for a flexible approach to work
2. the central role of fatigue as a limiting factor and the need to accommodate it
3. the importance of other people at work, such as employers and colleagues

Be Flexible

When looking at the pros and cons of a job in the light of Parkinson's disease, there are four main options—to continue as before, to modify the existing job to fit in with your limitations, to change jobs, or to stop work altogether.

If your illness is having little impact on your ability to perform the job, then *working as usual* is the obvious answer. This will have several positive effects. It will maintain your self-esteem and sense of achievement, the feeling that you are making a contribution; it will permit continuing daily social contact with others; and it will enable you to remain financially independent. But many people try to work as before *despite increasing difficulty*. While this is an understandable response, such persistence may bring with it considerable costs, both to the individual and to others. John Williams's booklet *Parkinson's Disease and Employment* illustrates this. One person with Parkinson's disease recalled:

> *During the last two years it has been difficult to remain fully committed to my work: it takes all my resolve just to keep going, and giving top priority to my work has had a direct effect on my social and family life.*

And Dr. I., a family physician:

> *When I was first diagnosed I felt it was important to keep working for as long as possible, so, for the good of the practice, I kept the news to myself for two or three years. I worked for eight years after the diagnosis was made, and at first there was little difficulty and patients were unaware of my problems. . . . However, this being a small town, it eventually became common knowledge that I had PD. I was treated very sympathetically by my patients. Nevertheless, it became more and more embarrassing to examine patients with my tremor, which hardly inspired confidence. By 1987, being then 58, I realized the time had come to retire since I was also having difficulty with speech, driving and night calls.*

The pressure of trying to continue working as usual may increase the physical symptoms, which may increase the pressure, which may make work more difficult, and so on in a vicious circle. To avoid such a situation, you might consider *modifying your job.* If you are lucky enough to be self-employed, or if you work in an organization with a sympathetic management, it may be possible to decrease the number of hours you work each day. If your symptoms follow a reasonably regular pattern, you could try to negotiate working those hours when you are most able. Alternatively, you might ask to be transferred to a less demanding job, with less pressure—a *change of job*, in effect. Sometimes this will be a sideways move with no reduction in pay or status. Under the ADA, your employer is required to make "reasonable" accommodations.

The time may come when you have to ask yourself *"Should I stop work?"* When to stop is very much a matter of personal choice. Perhaps there is only a short time before you reach normal retirement age. If so, it may be worth continuing until that time is reached in order to receive full Social Security benefits. If you have longer to go, it is sensible to continually evaluate the pros and cons of working or not. In particular, do the benefits of working, both financial and personal, outweigh the disadvantages? Is there more frustration and failure than job satisfaction?

When you do decide to give up work, you may be able to negotiate a period of time to "wind down" the job, so as to avoid the abrupt jump from being fully employed to being "retired," and to give yourself time to plan your retirement. Do treat retirement as a *positive step*, not as "giving in" to the disease. Plan what you will do with your newfound time—don't leave it to chance or circumstances. Think of the activities that you enjoy, see it as an opportunity to rediscover old lost hobbies and pastimes and to discover new ones. The account given by Dr. G. portrays one approach to remaining active despite retirement:

It was not until I had retired that I appreciated how much the stress of trying to carry out my duties aggravated my symptoms. Once I had retired, my family and friends were very understanding in that they did not treat me as an invalid but were always ready to help me with any physical task I found difficult. Retirement does not mean that I have become a "couch potato," since I set myself small tasks every day: short walks, minor DIY [do-it-yourself] jobs and helping more around the house. To keep my brain active I attempt crossword puzzles and play weekly bridge. Despite my forebodings I am enjoying my retirement more than I dared hope, and as I am not yet too severely affected I am fully independent.

Coping with Fatigue

Neither physical nor mental fatigue is likely to be helped by medication. Appropriate scheduling and structuring of your activities will help you to minimize the effects of fatigue on your performance. Set yourself priorities each day or each week. Do the most important, urgent, or demanding parts of your work first thing every day before fatigue sets in, or allocate them to the times of the day when you are at your best. Regular short breaks may help you to work more efficiently and prevent fatigue from building up: just sit quietly and rest with your eyes closed, or, alternatively, have a cup of coffee or chat with a colleague. In preventing fatigue, a shift of attitude is as important as any practical accommodations. Avoid overloading yourself—try not to take on too many responsibilities or tasks at the same time. Don't expect to be able to work as fast or as hard as before you developed Parkinson's disease. Learn to make allowances for your illness, and don't drive yourself too hard to achieve deadlines or other goals.

Communicating with Employers and Colleagues

Although a few people work totally on their own, most of us work with others; these may be managers or supervisors, or other colleagues with whom we share the workload. You may be in a managerial or supervisory role with staff of your own. Even if you work alone, there may be clients or customers whom you meet regularly. As far as the options mentioned are concerned—carrying on your work just as before, modifying your present job, or changing jobs—clearly, much will depend on these other individuals.

To renegotiate your job or your working hours, or to plan early retirement, you will need the fullest cooperation and support of your employers. From a practical viewpoint, they may also help by modifying your working environment to accommodate any mobility problems or provide you with the equipment to make your job easier. Colleagues may provide either a formal or an informal support service; while you may arrange to transfer some duties permanently, it may be enough for them to take over as the need arises, from day to day.

However, none of this will happen unless you tell them about your illness. The importance of honest communication was discussed in Chapter 5. But it can't be emphasized too strongly that you should not put off telling employers and colleagues that you have Parkinson's disease. And tell them which tasks you do need help with and which you can manage on your own. It can be as frustrating to have to contend with colleagues who want to take over as with unhelpful ones.

Leisure and Social Activities

In Chapter 5, we underlined the importance of avoiding the phenomenon of *premature social aging*—that is, the gradual withdrawal from active participation in work, in personal responsibilities, and in social interaction that can be associated with Parkinson's disease. There are ways of coping with each of the difficulties—financial constraints, mobility problems, increased fatigue, unpredictability of response to medication, social embarrassment—ways that can help to some extent to prevent premature social disengagement. What is important is to guard against the isolation setting in in the first place. It may be that the particular symptoms that make social situations difficult and embarrassing will improve at some point; new treatments or modifications in existing drug regimens may reduce on–off fluctuations or dyskinesia. But remember that it is difficult to regain the habit of going out once it has been lost. Friends and relatives may stop inviting you, or even stop thinking of including you in social activities, if you have repeatedly declined previous invitations.

Perhaps social embarrassment is the single most important problem to overcome. The embarrassment associated with being stared at in public, with being considered as "odd" or "disabled," finally persuades many to avoid social situations completely. It's so much easier to say than to do, but it really is necessary to grow a thick skin. Be selfish and think about yourself, not what others may be thinking. Above all, force yourself to continue as long as it is physically possible for you to do so. Sidney Dorros offers a wise word on the subject:

I was so embarrassed I often closed my eyes, pretending I wasn't there. But as long as Debbie [his wife] and our friends were willing to drive me and to endure awkward situations, I decided to risk the discomfort we often experienced rather than withdraw into a private shell.

Describing their many trips to various locations in the United States and Canada, Dorros says:

We saw and did more than many healthier travelers. How did we manage? Through very careful planning. This included dividing the trip into several side trips of a few days each with a return for rest and recuperation to our home base, our son's house, between trips.

Even when life is at its most difficult, you *can* make it easier for yourself and for others. You may be able to "juggle" your tablets so that you have a good period when you need it. If you enjoy eating out, find a local restaurant and use it regularly. Get to know the staff, and explain Parkinson's disease to them. Order dishes that involve less cutting up and that you can eat with a minimum of help. To prevent spilling, put only a little in your glass at a time. If you use special cutlery, bring it with you. You may be able to choose times when restaurants are less busy—midweek, they are often practically empty in the early evenings. The same may apply to movies and theaters, where afternoon showings are less crowded and rushed.

Most of us tend to have a well-defined circle of friends with whom we spend the larger part of our social lives. As these are people we have known for some time, we share with them varying degrees of intimacy, friendship, and caring—which may well help to create enough understanding to make social situations, even in the later phases of the illness, less embarrassing and daunting. In John Williams's *Parkinson's Disease: Doctors as Patients*, Dr. F. wrote:

> *We continue to enjoy occasional lunch and dinner parties so long as we know our hosts and guests well.*

Hobbies, too, play a key role in keeping us mentally and physically active. But your symptoms may make it necessary for you to modify them. The need to give up old pastimes is reflected by Dr. H., a physician with Parkinson's disease, who wrote:

> *My fly fishing was inaccurate and I had a "twitch" at the end of each cast. I used to play snooker once or twice a week and I found that using the cue was becoming more difficult. I used also to sing in a choir and found that my voice was higher and weaker.*

But there is an endless list of alternatives: gardening, decorating; taking part in sports such as swimming; doing jigsaw or crossword puzzles, reading, knitting, building model planes; helping in charitable work, attending adult education classes. Whether your own particular bent is toward becoming an expert on eighteenth-century novelists, perfecting your appreciation of classical or folk music, learning a new language or games such as chess, backgammon, dominoes, or bridge, or learning to paint or type—now is your chance. Replacing the daily habit of work with new ways of passing your time will make the transition easier. As long as you keep yourself motivated and your curiosity and imagination alive, the range of leisure activities that you can still enjoy, despite Parkinson's, is infinite.

Above all, *keep yourself active*—mentally, physically, and socially. Set yourself targets that are realistic and achievable, but still challenging.

The aim is to keep a balance of activities, within the limitations of your illness but with you in control.

Set Yourself Targets

While it may be easy to say "I'll keep active" or "I'll look for a new purpose in my life," it is sometimes difficult to know where to begin and not to be discouraged by what might appear to be failures. Here are a few ideas that can be applied to everyday tasks or to the grandest scheme:

- ❖ Try to set yourself concrete targets—something that can be achieved in a single session of work or recreation. It might be anything from polishing your shoes to getting yourself to the movies and back. Avoid vague, open-ended goals, or ones that would take a long time to achieve. A "session" may be ten minutes or ten hours, depending on what you can deal with at the time. The aim is to have achieved what you set out to do. If an activity is too long to be done in one go, think of ways in which you can break it up into manageable chunks.

- ❖ As part of your target-setting, build in a few rewards. Promise yourself something that you enjoy—even if it's only a bun with your coffee—but *only* if you achieve your goal. No cheating! The bigger the achievement, the bigger the reward—which might just be having a quiet time doing nothing in particular!

- ❖ Although your aim is to set *manageable* targets, there will be times when you will "fail." Indeed, if you were to achieve a goal 100 percent of the time, you would probably be making it too easy, failing to push yourself. Setting your targets too low is little more use than setting them too high. And if you do fail, don't give up— try again another time. If you keep on failing, though, consider changing the target slightly.

FINANCIAL INDEPENDENCE

Careful financial planning is important—ideally, before any drop in your income. If you are working, it is advisable to start the ball rolling as soon as you learn that you have Parkinson's disease. You may be able to obtain advice through your employer, or through your bank or other financial adviser. If you are taking early retirement, it is essential to discuss carefully with an expert, or even two, any occupational or private insurance that you may have to consider the pros and cons of stopping contributions or continuing even after retirement, or taking some early payment. You may also consider other ways of generating capital, such as moving to a smaller house or apartment or one better suited to your physical needs. Even if you rent rather than own, there may be savings to be made to the monthly bill. If you no longer need your car or plan to stop driving anyway, you can save money there. As well as whatever you get for the car, there will be savings in insurance and operating costs—although these will have to be offset against the cost of alternative means of transportation.

It is worth doing some careful calculations of the likely change to your monthly income. Calculate current income and expenses, and what they will be after you stop working or reduce your hours. Don't forget to take into account savings that will be made through not working—travel costs, meals, special clothing, and so on, together with any new income through pensions or extra benefits. Clearly, if there is a major shortfall in your estimated future income and current expenses, some adjustment to your lifestyle will be required. The most obvious choice for most people is to cut back on "luxuries." Unfortunately, for many people luxuries include going out, be it to the movies or to restaurants. Financial constraints, therefore, may precipitate the social withdrawal discussed earlier. So it's important, in drawing up a budget, to allow enough to continue some of your previous entertainment and social life, or look for less expensive alternatives. Also, don't be too proud to claim any federal, state, or local benefits to which you are entitled. Remember that while you or your spouse or partner were working, you made contributions toward these benefits and are therefore entitled to them.

RELATIONSHIPS

Most of us have relationships with other people, such as a spouse or partner, other family members, friends, colleagues, and neighbors, all involving differing degrees of closeness and caring. Depending on the nature of our relationship with each of these various sources of *social support*, discussed in Chapter 4, they will be more or less able to provide you with practical help, empathy, and understanding. But they can only be that buffer against the stress of chronic illness if you tell them about it. And not only must you decide *who* to tell, but also *when* to tell them, *what* to tell them, and *how* to tell them.

To Tell or Not to Tell?

The issue of telling people about the illness has cropped up several times in this book—hardly surprising, since it underpins all the relationships that the person with Parkinson's disease has.

What are the advantages of telling and the disadvantages of not telling?

Inevitably, sooner or later your symptoms will begin to show, even if they don't yet interfere with your life. To put it at its most practical, there may come a time when you require help from the people around you. Clearly, if they are told about your illness in advance, they will be in a better position to offer you that help when it is needed. One consequence of keeping the Big Secret is that other people are unlikely to raise the subject themselves, even when it is obvious, and are therefore less likely to offer help. As mentioned earlier, there is also a risk that people may misunderstand some of the symptoms. The published writings of people with Parkinson's describe many instances of problems with walking and balance being taken for drunkenness, fatigue for laziness, tremor for nervousness, lack of facial and vocal expression for boredom or depression. Such misperceptions can seriously affect a relationship, whether at work or at home, with friends or with strangers.

What are the disadvantages of telling?

The main argument comes from the desire to keep everything the same—either from a wish to *deny* the disease and possible future problems or from a desire to *fight against* it. Either way, some people reason that it will be difficult to act as before if everyone knows. People may treat you differently, label you as "having Parkinson's disease" or "being disabled"; offer help when it is not required; avoid you because of embarrassment; or assume that you are unable to do tasks that you are perfectly capable of doing. You may be afraid that you will lose your job or be passed over for promotion.

Even if you don't tell, people will still treat you differently as the symptoms start to become evident. But if their attitudes and behavior are based on ignorance or misunderstanding, they will be very different from the attitudes they might have had if they had been able to base them on information about the true nature of the situation.

Sidney Dorros, in *Parkinson's Disease: A Patient's View*, comments:

> *Like many Parkinsonians, I was reluctant to tell people I had the ailment. However, when I thought that they were noticing and wondering about the symptoms, I did try to tell them the cause as matter-of-factly as possible. I learned that people often misinterpret some of the symptoms if they don't know their origin. When I told them about my illness and its effects, it eased some of their concerns.*
>
> *I also wish that I had discussed my illness earlier and in more detail with some people. Somehow, I took for granted that they knew more than they did. In later years, I found that I had failed to talk about my Parkinsonism with some of the people most important to me. My children, my parents and brother, certain close friends and associates at work have all told me that they didn't learn what was wrong with me until long after they had started worrying about me.*

When you have considered all the pros and cons of telling people about your Parkinson's disease, I believe that you will conclude that telling wins over not telling. Decisions about *when, what,* and *how* to tell may be more variable—they depend on your circumstances and the nature of the individual relationship.

Your Spouse or Partner

As already noted, the pattern of a couple's relationship before the onset of Parkinson's disease is likely to continue afterward. Relationships marked by communication, trust, and warmth will continue as such. Couples who have tended not to talk about their personal needs and feelings may find it difficult to adjust to the extra demands on them both.

While the gradualness of the changes that occur with Parkinson's disease can permit a smooth transition, it may also allow the slow build-up of dissatisfaction. Small irritations can become major sources of resentment if they are bottled up. Although it may seem obvious that the best way to encourage smooth adaptation is through talking to each other, it is surprising how many couples fail to communicate the small irritations, let alone any more important concerns. For some, it may be difficult to "complain" without feeling guilty—how can they criticize someone who is having to cope with the problems of Parkinson's disease? Or the person with Parkinson's disease may be afraid of offending his or her partner, who may have been working harder and taking on extra duties.

The most useful rule is probably this. Rather than criticizing your partner's behavior or the situation, say what it is that you would *like* to be happening. For example, rather than saying "It really gets on my nerves the way you sit around all day doing nothing," try "I think we both need to make more effort to get out and about." One very important aspect of such communication is that there should be *no blame*—remember that your annoyance or resentment comes as much from you as it is "caused" by your partner or by the situation.

Even better, make some concrete suggestions for dealing with the current problem.

Unfortunately, it's not always easy to be so open, flexible, and positive. Once problems build up, it may take the help of a third party (discussed in Chapter 9) to guide the couple through the situation.

How best to cope with problems in the *sexual relationship* was discussed in Chapter 8. And the advice for dealing with such problems is the same as for any other kind. Discussion and communication are essential. Avoid criticism and blame. The same sources that offer counseling on general relationship problems can help with specific sexual ones; and, more importantly, by facilitating discussion they can help to determine what both members of the relationship want from intimacy, then help to "negotiate" an arrangement acceptable to both.

If, either with the help of a therapist or on their own, a couple decide to stop having sexual relations, it is important that some substitute be found so as to maintain a level of physical intimacy in the relationship. It may be that they spend more time cuddling or they start giving each other massages. It is often the case that when the pressure of having sexual relations is removed by mutual agreement, a couple start to rediscover their sensuality. They are able to take pleasure in physical contact with their partner and may even feel a rekindling of sexual desire.

Other Family Members, Friends, and Colleagues

Close contact and intimate relationships with others are basic human needs. We feel part of the world when we care about others and receive care and love in return. As already mentioned, telling your family and friends about your illness is the first and most important step. Give them information gradually and at appropriate times, answering any questions they may have. Tell them what the disease means for you, about your medication and about your particular symptoms. Armed with information, they are going to feel more at ease and so, therefore, will you.

To make social situations easier and more enjoyable, think about when and where you meet. While, in the past, you may have met friends in the evening, it may be easier now to meet during the day if that fits in better with the times when you are most mobile. You may find crowded places physically difficult and stressful. Busy restaurants may present too many challenges and stop you from relaxing. Choose quieter places and less busy times. If your finances are strained, go to the movies rather than the theater, meet for a drink rather than for a meal. Even less expensive, go to their home or invite them to yours.

However willing you are to adapt your old patterns, though, there may be times when life becomes just too difficult. There is nothing wrong in saying you can't come to a party, for instance. But rather than just saying no or giving some tired excuse, keep them informed—say "Thanks, but I'm going through a bad patch at the moment with my Parkinson's—perhaps we could try to meet next week." This way they know that you want to continue contact. Treating people like this is a sign of trust and respect—important aspects of friendship.

And don't forget that work colleagues need to be taken into your confidence, too.

What to Say to Others

People's reactions to disability range from drawing attention to the symptoms, to ignoring the disability completely in situations where acknowledging it would be the preliminary to providing some necessary help, to treating the disabled person as if he or she is mentally incapacitated.

Such negative reactions are the product of ignorance—people feel uncomfortable with what they don't understand, and to hide this discomfort they resort to denial or draw absurd conclusions. Unfortunately, until such time that the public's understanding and acceptance of disability improve, the person with the disability and his or her companions will continue to bear the burden of such ignorance. As always, the best way to combat it is to inform.

Clearly, it is impractical and unnecessary to tell everyone that you meet about your illness. For those times when it *is* necessary, it's useful to have a plan or a form of words that suits the situation. For example, you may be subject to freezing episodes or to unpredictable "off" periods. If you are alone at the time, passers-by may come to your help or ask if you need an ambulance. So it's best to know what you need other people to do at such times and ask them. It may be that you don't need any help, in which case, briefly explain that you will be alright in a minute. Alternatively, they might be able to "unfreeze" you by gently rocking you from side to side—whatever you have found works. Having a prepared "speech" and advice to offer will reduce the stress and embarrassment of such informal encounters and make you better able to cope. Sidney Dorros dealt with off moments this way:

No, I don't need an ambulance. It's a neurological disorder that isn't dangerous. My medication needs time to work.

Jan Peter Stern lists in his booklet *The Parkinson's Challenge* a series of common questions that he has learned to deal with from a usually well-wishing public.

Question	Answer
"Do you feel all right?"	"Yes, this is normal for me—thank you for asking."
"Do you have a bad back?"	"Sometimes."
"Are you in pain?"	"Fortunately not."
"When will you get better?"	"Some days are better than others."
"Is it contagious?"	"Definitely not."
"Why are you so slow today?"	"My muscles are stiff."
"Did you have a stroke since I last saw you?"	"No, actually I'm learning to live with Parkinson's."

Don't forget that it may sometimes be helpful to prepare people in advance. Sidney Dorros describes how he prepared a tour guide before setting off on a walk:

Don't be concerned if you see me having difficulty walking. I take medication for a neurological condition that works very erratically. Sometimes I move too freely and sometimes I get very stiff.

KEY FACTS 10

Make use of all of the resources available to you.

Resources include your own personal strengths, the help and support of others close to you, and the expert help of professionals. In this way you will be able to minimize the impact of Parkinson's disease on your life.

Be flexible.

There will almost always be something that you can do to reduce the impact of the disease on any particular aspect of your life. Be willing to adapt and change, to make adjustments, to try new ways of dealing with your limitations, to accept assistance, and to look for new opportunities.

What self-help strategies are likely to be useful?

First, schedule activities that you find difficult for those times of day when you are at your best. Whatever you're doing, allow more time. Try breaking complex sequences of actions into manageable stages. Talk yourself through actions as you perform them. Try to avoid doing two things at once.

How can handicaps be minimized?

As well as the resources and support offered by others, make use of any available aids and be ready to make physical changes to your home and working environment. Even apparently small changes can have a significant impact on a particular problem—for example, with eating or dressing. Take an active attitude to such changes—don't see them as "giving in." Changing the way you do things, or when you do them, or using some "artificial aid," are all aimed at reducing handicap or removing it altogether.

Keep active, both physically and mentally.

This is central to maintaining health, enjoyment in life, and a sense of self-worth. Don't let your Parkinson's disease restrict your normal patterns of work, leisure, and social activities any more than absolutely necessary. Because things may be physically more difficult, too expensive, or embarrassing, individuals sometimes begin to turn in on themselves. Don't. Keep going with your existing activities, modify them as necessary, or find suitable alternatives.

Set yourself targets for your day.

Targets should be neither so easy that you can achieve them without effort nor so difficult that you continually fail. Keep each target concrete, rather than vague, and build in some reward for yourself when you've achieved it.

The more people know, the more they will understand.

People are crucial in our lives—our families and friends, our colleagues, even strangers. Tell them what they need to know about your illness. As well as being better able to help, if and when help is needed, they will not misinterpret your symptoms or other problems.

11

Self-Help Strategies for the Person with Parkinson's Disease: Maintaining Emotional Well-Being

In Chapter 4, we reviewed in detail the factors that affect a person's adaptation to stressful life events such as a chronic illness. How can knowledge of these factors be translated into ways of coping better with Parkinson's disease? In a sense, what this chapter offers is a list of *dos and don'ts* for maintaining emotional well-being and preventing depression and anxiety. But, as we have said from the start, bear in mind that each person's Parkinson's disease is different from the next person's. You will find no recommendations here that will be 100 percent effective in every case. But the suggested strategies have been found useful by other people in similar situations, and they may work for you. To find out whether they do, try them out for yourself.

ACCEPT THAT YOU HAVE PARKINSON'S DISEASE

It would be somewhat unusual not to be upset by the news that you have Parkinson's disease, that you are no longer completely healthy. But following this initial phase of shock and disbelief, a gradual acceptance of the reality of the illness usually follows. This means that you are beginning to accept the physical limitations imposed by the illness and to let go of lost function without anger or regret. The process of *accommodation*— or acceptance and adjustment—has started.

This involves achieving a balance between finding ways of working around the illness so as to overcome the limitations imposed by the symptoms, and at the same time learning to make allowances for your illness and disability. Achieving such a balance is the best way to remain socially active, for example. You need on the one hand *to push yourself* and motivate yourself to do and achieve despite the difficulties posed by Parkinson's disease, and on the other hand, *not to be hard on yourself.* It is only realistic *not* to expect yourself to meet your previous standards. Instead set yourself new and more achievable ones. This kind of realism about your illness, and giving yourself some "slack," make it more likely that you will not give up, more likely that you will achieve your goals. For instance, to accommodate fatigue, you need to adjust your daily routine by doing the most important tasks before fatigue sets in and alternating periods of activity with frequent short rests.

Active denial of the disorder, pretending that nothing is wrong and carrying on as before, may work in the short term, but it is likely to lead to poor long-term adjustment. The despair and depression that some people experience result from letting their imagination run loose and magnifying the possible implications of the disease for their health, their daily functioning, and their future prospects. Realistic acceptance of your illness means enjoying your mobility and physical abilities while they last and *dealing with problems as they arise.* Your attitude to the illness and your outlook on the future are perhaps the most important determinants of how you choose to live and cope with Parkinson's disease.

Remember that every individual has his or her own challenge in life. Some, such as having a life-threatening illness such as cancer or a handicapped child, are more demanding than others. As Alexander Burnfield, a doctor who has multiple sclerosis, writes in his book *Multiple Sclerosis: A Personal Exploration*, what is important is how one deals with such challenges:

I no longer need to fight because I know that I have the power in me to respond to whatever has to be. Although I cannot change the cards that life has dealt me, I do have some choice about how I play my hand, about how I answer my fate.

Cecil Todes, a psychiatrist with Parkinson's disease who has figured several times in this book, commented:

> *It has been said that we experience illness in the style that we live our lives.*

It is up to you and your family to decide how to face the challenge and what style you set yourself in coming to terms with and coping with Parkinson's disease. The importance of *choosing* how you react is succinctly put by Glenna Wotton Atwood in her book *Living Well with Parkinson's Disease*:

> *After my diagnosis in 1981, I realized that I could not control the fact that I had Parkinson's disease, but I could control the amount of time I might waste sitting around and wishing I didn't have it. I am passing this thought on to you: let your Parkinson's make you a better person, not a bitter person.*

She goes on:

> *You did not choose to have Parkinson's, but you can choose how to live with it. Find the right doctor, join a support group, start the exercise program, eat to live, build your family relationships and friendships, pursue the activities that have meaning to you, and you will find that, yes, there is a life with Parkinson's. Only you can decide to make it happen.*

INFORMATION PERMITS CHOICE

Obtain information about the illness and its medical treatment. People differ in how much they want to know—some try to find out as much as they can, whereas others would rather know as little as possible. But, in general, information allows you to make informed decisions. It also prepares you for what to expect and gives you a sense of control—both of which can help reduce anxiety and fear.

The information you need can be obtained from doctors, from reading books such as this one and any of the others listed in Appendix II, or by contacting one of the Parkinson's disease organizations. Most books on the illness produced for patients and their families can be obtained from major bookstores and public libraries. But do remember that books by people with Parkinson's disease may only reflect an individual's disease and his or her reaction to it. If something is unclear, don't be afraid to ask your physician for further explanation. You might, for example, want to find out more about current thinking as regards causes—maybe just to be clear about what did *not* cause your illness— or about the medication and its side effects, how the drug regimen might change over the years, how much disability to expect in the future, whether there are other symptoms that might emerge over time. Most of this information can be found in Chapters 1, 2, and 3 of this book, but you may want to ask your doctor about how a particular point applies to you.

AVOID NEGATIVE THINKING

What we think, how we feel, and the way we behave are very closely related to each other. Optimism breeds contentment and self-confidence, goal-directed and problem-oriented behavior. On the other hand, negative ways of thinking ruin self-confidence, create sadness, sap motivation, and paralyze a person into inactivity. Some psychologists and psychiatrists refer to self-defeating negative thoughts and attitudes as *mind traps* that undermine self-esteem and successful coping behavior. Such negative thoughts and attitudes immobilize the individual and prevent adaptive behavior.

Our thoughts reflect the way we see the world and how we interpret events. When people are depressed, they tend to think negatively about themselves, their future, and the world. Similarly, feelings of anxiety can be triggered by negative thoughts and unrealistic anticipation of danger. Such biased interpretations of reality occur because of distorted ways of thinking. See whether any of the following figure in your own streams of thought.

Overgeneralizing

You expand on a single experience or event to conclude that something unpleasant will always happen to you or that you will never have a pleasant experience. For example, after a fall you may think "I will *always* fall if I go out." This overgeneralizing will stop you from going out.

Personalizing

You consider yourself personally and solely responsible for unpleasant events, overlooking the part played by others or by external factors beyond your control. This unrealistic sense of personal responsibility gives rise to self-blame and guilt. For example, if you wrongly blame yourself for your Parkinson's disease, thinking that failure to look after your body has brought it on, you are personalizing an event that was completely out of your control.

Black-and-White Thinking

A tendency to evaluate yourself, your circumstances, other people, and situations in extreme terms either as good or as bad, with no room for in-between states. An example of this is the person who labels himself or herself as *totally* helpless, *completely* unable to cope, if he or she fails to cope with *all* situations *all* the time. With this style of thinking you will get caught in a "no-win" situation, because neither you nor anyone else will ever be able to meet the rigid and perfectionist standards you have set.

Driving Yourself by "Should" Statements

You drive yourself and those around you by ideas of what you "should do" or "ought to be able to do." Similar to black-and-white thinking, this results in rigid and inflexible codes of behavior that will probably not usually be met by you or by anyone else. This failure may in turn lead to frustration, anger, and guilt, or be interpreted as yet another example of personal inadequacy and so reinforce low self-esteem. Believing that you "should" be able to do everything as quickly and efficiently as before the onset of your illness is an example of this kind of thinking.

Jumping to Conclusions

Arriving at conclusions on the basis of little or scanty evidence can prevent you from dealing with situations in a positive manner. On occasion, this type of distorted thinking can result in your drawing conclusions—usually negative—about the future, as if you were able to look through a crystal ball and predict it. The bleak picture that you paint for yourself will only make you feel helpless and drain your motivation to meet the challenges of living with Parkinson's disease.

Catastrophizing

You are catastrophizing when you fail to see the positive aspects of your life or your personal qualities because you blow up the negative aspects out of proportion—thinking that your life is totally ruined by Parkinson's disease, that your situation is dreadful and unbearable, is typical of this frame of mind.

Disqualifying the Positive

This is similar to catastrophizing, but entails even more distortion. It involves not only ignoring the positive, but also changing the positive into a negative. For example, a stranger may take the trouble to be helpful and sympathetic when he sees you in trouble. But rather than regarding the helpful gesture in a positive light, you turn it around and see it as a sign that you are useless and dependent on the charity of strangers. This virtual reversal of reality and facts can lead to unhappiness because you are seeing yourself, your life, your experiences, and the world around you through perpetually dark glasses.

The first step toward dealing with such negative thoughts is to become aware of them and to perceive their role in creating your moods and determining your behavior. Over time, they may have become habitual and automatic. First, you need to catch yourself thinking these thoughts. Write each one down, together with the situation in which it occurred and the feeling that it triggered. See how such thoughts have made you feel sad or anxious, or have undermined your confidence. Identify the particular error of thinking that each negative thought involves. Then question yourself—examine the evidence for each thought and whether alternative interpretations of events or situations may be possible. Try to challenge these negative thoughts and replace each with an alternative positive statement to yourself. This is the basis of the method called *positive self-talk*, which challenges and changes your habitual negative thinking into positive thinking. But don't expect positive self-talk to work overnight. It is a skill that has to be developed over time. Practice it consistently, and it won't be too long before you are rid of your negative thinking pattern and able to regain your sense of well-being and your confidence.

LEARN TO DEAL WITH YOUR EMOTIONS

Anger

Like loss of any sort, the loss of mobility and independence in Parkinson's disease is associated with a range of emotions. Anger and the thought "Why me?" may be your first reactions after diagnosis. Later on, frustration and anger may be triggered by changes in your level of disability or increasing physical dependence. In *Living Well with Parkinson's Disease*, Glenna Wotton Atwood describes how she deals with her feelings of anger:

> *Anger, an emotion I have always tended to hide, reappears from time to time. I've never been good at expressing it. . . . In coming to terms with my Parkinson's, I needed to give myself permission to be angry at times, because the disease had upset my life. I needed to learn to express a healthy amount of anger without feeling guilty about it. I decided to try to deal openly with my anger in positive ways. I could go outdoors and walk it off. I could tackle the housework and allow myself to slam the cupboard doors. I could go to the typewriter and write about my feelings. What worked for me won't necessarily work for you, but the important thing is for you to admit you have normal emotions, to take a look at how you deal with them, and to allow yourself not to feel guilty about having them.*

Although some degree of anger can be useful if it relieves the pressure and helps you to feel better afterward, with some people angry feelings can take over. If *you* experience anger, work out what thoughts or aspects of your situation trigger it. Examine the evidence for and against such thoughts, and try alternative and more positive ways of evaluating your situation. Since it is difficult to think straight in the middle of a fit of rage, this is best done after a "cooling down" period. To contend with your anger, try distracting yourself, do something different, break off from whatever you were doing when the fit of rage took hold; take a walk, turn on the TV, read a book, phone a friend. Try the breathing exercises described on p. 289 to relax yourself. Above all, avoid venting your anger on innocent bystanders such as your spouse or partner or children.

Instead of cooling you down, angry outbursts can at times pump up your system to make you even more furious. Even if it is someone else's behavior that has provoked you, it's best to talk to him or her about it *after* you have cooled off, when you can put your point of view across in an assertive and constructive, rather than an aggressive, manner.

Anxiety

In contrast to the way that anger builds up to a peak, anxiety may be present throughout a person's waking day and even at night, interfering with sleep. Anxiety may have to do with worrying about your inability to cope in an emergency, fear of rapid progression of the illness, anticipation of helplessness and dependence, and of the need for assistance in performing most of your personal functions, the fear of becoming a burden on your family. Glenna Wotton Atwood describes her particular feelings about it:

Over the years, one of the hardest things to control has been worry. Worry, of course, uses a lot of energy. It is unproductive. It is useless. Despite these disincentives, I have to admit that I still do some worrying. Fortunately, in my set of mixed feelings there is a balance more positive than negative. . . . I resent all the limitations, but at the same time, I'm so thankful for all the things I can still do.

When it is intense and persistent, anxiety may be treated with medication. In severe cases, though, antianxiety drugs, or tranquilizers, are now seen as only a short-term measure. In Parkinson's disease such medication may make rigidity and slowness worse and should only be taken after consulting your physician.

It is better, if you can, to learn to combat anxiety with psychological techniques such as *changing your perception and outlook* or *using relaxation methods.* Try to prevent anxiety from building up in the first place by making a conscious effort to maintain a positive outlook and adopting a pragmatic approach. Convince yourself that you can tackle each problem as it arises, instead of expecting the worst from the outset. After all, you have evidence from previous episodes that you *can* cope effectively. Don't dismiss this. Use your successes to boost your confidence. The technique of *positive self-talk* is of value again here. As before, identify the negative thoughts that trigger your anxiety, challenge them, and replace them with positive statements. When applied consistently, this can neutralize the "poisonous" effect of such thoughts and change your outlook.

The best antidote for anxiety is relaxation, since neither the body nor the mind can be anxious and relaxed at the same time. The quickest way to achieve mental and physical relaxation is to engage in *deep, slow breathing* and to use *mental imagery.*

Sit in a comfortable position, where you will not be disturbed. Close your eyes. Focus your attention on your breathing—try to establish a regular rhythm, deep and slow. Count slowly in your head to pace your breaths. Breathe in, pause, and then breathe out. Once you have established this rhythm, try to relax mentally. Think of a relaxing scene. Imagine yourself by the sea, listening to the sound of the waves and feeling the warmth of the sun on your skin. Alternatively, see yourself, in your mind's eye, in the countryside—listening to the birds, smelling wild flowers, and feeling a gentle breeze.

Once you have practiced these relaxation techniques and have become proficient in using them, they are at your disposal anywhere and at any time. There are many excellent audiocassettes available to help you develop these skills.

Depression

In Chapter 5 we dealt in some detail with why and when depression may strike in Parkinson's disease, and the question of who may be vulnerable to it.

Apart from making you feel awful and making you difficult to live with, depression can be just as disabling as Parkinson's disease itself. As we noted earlier, it is probably most helpful to see it as a reaction to the disability and handicap caused by the disease. Viewing it in this way, as a reaction to real or anticipated handicap, offers the individual and his or her family the possibility of actively preventing depression or of dealing with it if it occurs—the strategy is to *minimize that handicap.*

❖ Obviously, effective medical control of your symptoms is crucial if your primary task is to reduce the level of your handicap. Handicap can also be decreased if you take steps to minimize the impact of those symptoms that remain. All of the strategies discussed in previous chapters— changing the times when you do things, taking things more slowly, avoiding stress, making use of aids, involving others—are aimed at reducing the impact of the disease on your life, at reducing your handicap. And, in turn, reducing the impact of the disease will guard against depression.

❖ Try to identify the aspects of your life that you most fear losing or most regret having lost. These are the areas where you should make maximum effort to find ways of maintaining or regaining roles, or looking for alternatives.

❖ The various negative thinking patterns that we described can play a key role in bringing on depression. The depressed person thinks negatively about himself or herself, about the world, and about the future. One of the most effective self-help strategies for combating depression is to *break the spiral of negative thinking* by learning to recognize the distortions that it involves. Catch yourself thinking such negative thoughts. Write them down. Identify the distortions that each thought contains. Then challenge them, and tell yourself more realistic and positive ideas, thereby building up a more constructive and balanced point of view. You'll be surprised how this disposal of your mental "dirty laundry" will liberate you and empower you to feel more cheerful!

❖ Although self-help techniques may be effective, there may be times when depression is more severe and you need to seek professional help. Changing aspects of one's life or one's outlook is never easy—and even less so for someone who is already depressed. When depressed, a person finds it difficult to see a way out of the current situation and may be poorly motivated to try. If your depression persists and appears intractable, do seek professional help. Psychologists, psychiatrists, psychotherapists, and counselors can all help with "talking therapy." If your depression is so severe that it requires medication, your doctor will prescribe a course of antidepressants to treat the main symptoms. Even then, it is likely that some additional psychological support will be useful to prevent further episodes. Friends and family can be invaluable in providing emotional support at such times.

❖ Be aware of possible *vulnerable times* for depression, when your handicap is increasing or there is a risk of its increasing. Discuss your fears or concerns with others—family, friends, colleagues. Even though, given your state of mind, you may find it hard to believe, they *may* be able to help alleviate the problem. Merely talking about your feelings with others at an early stage may prevent you from getting into the spiral of negative thinking.

As a general rule, never let your emotions build up to fever pitch. Learn to occasionally air your feelings with your nearest and dearest, with a friend or colleague, or with your doctor. Hearing their reactions and interpretations can also help you adopt a more balanced view. Above all, in dealing with your emotions, bear in mind President John F. Kennedy's comment, "We should not let our fears hold us back from pursuing our hopes," and remember that this is the only shot that you will have at living your life.

MAINTAIN YOUR SELF-ESTEEM

"Self-concept" is that familiar sense that each of us has of the "I" or "me" we refer to, the ways in which this "me" is unique and different from others. Our self-concept has many facets—our own evaluation of our personality and behavior; of our achievements at school, at university, or at work; of our performance as a spouse or parent; our interests in politics, arts, or sports; our feeling toward our bodies and our perceptions of how others perceive us; and, of course, our weaknesses. In addition, we expect people to behave toward us in set and familiar ways. Our self-esteem, or the respect we have for ourself as a person, partly comes from the constancy of others' behavior in their dealings with us. Furthermore, we are creatures of habit. Chronic illness interrupts our habitual ways of living and may alter the ways in which others interact with us. As a result, a profound threat to self-esteem may ensue, which may make us feel inadequate, unworthy, and incapable.

With the progression of Parkinson's disease, maintaining self-esteem despite increasing disability and handicap may be difficult. To protect your self-esteem, the core of your personal identity, from the assault of the illness, remind yourself that despite the physical changes, the real you, the person inside the body, has not changed. Parkinson's disease cannot reverse your past achievements or take away past happiness. Neither can it prevent you from achieving new goals, provided they are realistic.

Loss of self-esteem, which is also a characteristic feature of depression, has to do with negative self-critical thinking, particularly extreme black-and-white thinking. So the most effective strategy for preventing this is positive self-talk. Remember that you are more than your physical body. Perhaps, instead of merely trying to keep your inner core untouched, you could give it a chance to grow—by putting maximum effort into adapting to your new circumstances. To mold a more adaptive sense of your personal identity, your abilities, and your limitations, a degree of restructuring may be necessary. We are often our own worst critics. We tend to reserve compassion, appreciation, and encouragement for others. Why not indulge yourself by *acknowledging your efforts* in the context of your new abilities and your new limitations?

In her book, Helen Rose describes periods of negative thoughts and feelings, and how these undermined her self-esteem. From therapy sessions with a psychologist, she gained insight into her thinking about herself as well as into her reactions to outside help.

I was finding it hard to accept that I just wasn't as able as I used to be. This feeling not only applied to housework but to other things as well. He [the psychologist] said it was obvious that up to now I had always managed to fight the disease and that, now that it had finally got the better of me, I felt totally and utterly useless. And because of these feelings I rejected anybody who wanted to help me. Now that I knew what was happening to me, it seemed easier to handle. The situation is better now, although there are still the odd occasions when I find something difficult and these feelings return.

Although coping behaviors are generally similar, each new stress sets its own challenges and demands in unfamiliar ways. When challenging your self-critical thoughts, remember that it is not as if you have been in a training course on how to cope with Parkinson's disease and have failed. You may have had other difficulties in life to cope with, such as loss of a loved one, divorce, business or exam failure, but nothing in life could have prepared you for the onset of Parkinson's disease.

COMMUNICATION OPENS DOORS

We have already dealt with the importance of communication in Chapters 5 and 10. Since your psychological and emotional well-being is intricately linked with your relationships with others, it might be a good idea to remind yourself of what we said earlier.

❖ Remember that communication with doctors is a two-way process. Neither your primary care physician nor your neurologist will know that you are depressed, anxious, or angry, or that you need outside help, unless you tell them. Don't assume that, without any clues from you, they will automatically refer you to the available sources of help covered in Chapter 9. It is up to you to tell them how you feel and what your needs are.

❖ Honest and regular discussion within the family prevents frustration and conflict. Above all, remember that marriage and family life are about warmth, trust, and mutual respect. Show your spouse or partner and your children that you appreciate their concern and help. Express warmth with hugs and occasional treats and presents. After all, Parkinson's disease does not alter your ability to be kind or to give pleasure to others!

❖ Avoid secrecy with friends and colleagues. This undermines trust and leads to deterioration of your relationships. Honest communication can prevent misunderstanding. You cannot expect your employer or your colleagues to make allowances for your problems if you are not honest with them.

❖ One of the major subjective traumas of a chronic illness is the sense of solitude, the sense of being alone in one's experiences. But your experiences *can* be shared—and sharing them may go some way toward overcoming the feeling of solitude.

POSITIVE ACTION CAN BRING RELIEF

Helen Rose came to this conclusion:

There are two choices: give up or fight. I chose the latter.

These are some of the positive steps that you can take in your fight against the disabling effects of the illness:

❖ As part of adaptive ways of coping, ask your primary care physician or neurologist for referrals to the various sources of adjunct therapy, if you think you can benefit from them.

❖ Keep your social network alive. We have all heard the saying "A friend in need is a friend indeed." Remember, if the situation were reversed, you would want to help any friend or relative who had Parkinson's disease. At times, merely knowing that there are friends and family who care can make a difference. But friendships have to be nurtured, so take Glenna Wotton Atwood's advice:

Be very deliberate about keeping in touch with your old friends, and make time to see them each week, or as often as possible. At the same time, establish new contacts and make new friends through church activities, clubs, adult education classes, and volunteer work. You need to be stimulated by other people, to interact in meaningful ways with other people, to reach out and socialize with others. What you don't want or need is a life of sitting at home alone.

❖ Janet, a nurse who had gradually developed symptoms since the age of 41 and was moderately disabled by Parkinson's disease, writes:

I try to lead a full social life. I need to go out and meet people frequently. I often ask friends in or go to them in the evenings, as I am usually slow and stiff and unable to do activities, and being with others cheers me up. I continue to have dinner parties courtesy of [take-out] and a helpful husband. Guests help with serving (I have swallowed my pride) as I prefer this routine to not entertaining at all. When meeting new people, I ask friends to explain Parkinson's disease and especially dyskinesia to them beforehand, or I look for a suitable opportunity to explain the basics of Parkinson's disease. This makes it less embarrassing for everyone.

❖ Try to remain active. Over time, inactivity and lack of productivity may be taken by the person with Parkinson's disease as evidence of his or her "uselessness" and lead to depression. *Staying active* can keep depression away and prevent the sedentary lifestyle and social isolation that can be associated with Parkinson's disease. Activity can distract you from negative thoughts, give you a sense of being in control, and make you feel more motivated to do other things. It doesn't matter what the activity is as long as you find it enjoyable and it gives you a sense of achievement. In *An Old Age Pensioner at Eighteen*, Helen Rose describes her decision to learn to use a computer and take up word processing:

I would probably never have achieved what I have with the computer nor would I have been in the paper or on the television or nominated for an award if I hadn't been cursed with this thing inside me.

❖ Janet writes:

I have got myself fully occupied with activities which give me great pleasure, mainly handicrafts, but also recording many minor as well as major emotional experiences in the form of poetry.

❖ Keep the fight against the illness, even the treatment, within reasonable perspective. Although many kinds of complementary therapy (discussed in Chapter 9) may be of some help, irreversible treatments such as surgery should be undertaken only after serious consideration.

❖ Above all, be flexible. Don't resist change that may be to your advantage, such as role reversal within the household, seeking help from others, or obtaining state benefits.

BE WILLING TO ADJUST CONTINUALLY

An unfortunate aspect of a progressive disorder such as Parkinson's disease is that the stresses and strains are not "one-offs" but are recurrent, reflecting the changes that take place during the course of the illness.

Let's take the example of someone whose Parkinson's disease has progressed very slowly over many years. Initially the symptoms may have been very mild, requiring no treatment; subsequently they may have been well controlled by medication. Then this individual reaches the point when the disease becomes more severe, the medication loses some of its efficacy, and disability becomes more evident. This is a period that requires *readjustment*. Sometimes even a slight worsening of the symptoms may bring with it disproportionate increases in disability, so that the individual has to modify plans and ways of doing things. Periods when he or she and his or her family feel that they are adjusting well to their altered circumstances may be interspersed with times when they feel overwhelmed by the demands of the illness. In other words, coming to terms with change and coping with the demands of Parkinson's disease is *an ongoing process*.

Not knowing the precise course of the illness, how quickly it will progress, how long the medication will remain effective, how the later daily on–off fluctuations will affect you, all contribute to the uncertainty that is characteristic of Parkinson's disease. Added to this is the fact that you don't know how long you can continue working, driving, and enjoying your favorite hobbies. One way of coping with such uncertainty is to *live life one day at a time.* It may sound like a cliché, but if you really think about it, it makes sense. This was the conclusion that Dr. E., in John Williams's *Parkinson's Disease: Doctors as Patients,* arrived at:

> *Since my student days I have generally been on some committee or other, looking ahead and planning for the future. However, when I retired I determined to stop this and to "live each day as if it were my last." I do not worry about what the future may bring.*

KEY FACTS 11

There are strategies that can help you to adjust to the illness, maintain emotional well-being, and prevent depression and anxiety. Here is a list of dos and don'ts.

Accept that you have Parkinson's disease and develop a positive outlook.

Your attitude and your outlook are very important in shaping how you live and cope with Parkinson's disease. With time, you should come to accept the limitations imposed by the illness and find ways of working around them. Adjust your daily routine to accommodate slowness, fatigue, and involuntary movements. You are more likely to remain motivated and active if you set yourself realistic goals and standards.

Obtain relevant information.

At every stage, information about the illness and its treatment can be helpful in many ways. It shows you what is on offer and what choices you have available to you. It makes it easier to arrive at informed decisions. It prepares you for what to expect and gives you a sense of control that can help reduce anxiety and fear. Relevant information can be obtained from doctors, books, and the PD organizations.

Combat negative thinking styles.

Thoughts, feelings, and actions are closely related. This means that the way you think affects the way you feel and behave. While optimism brings about contentment and confidence, pessimism undermines confidence and motivation and creates sadness and inactivity. Distorted ways of thinking can result in biased interpretations of reality. To combat negative thoughts, first become aware of them and the part they play in how you feel. Catch yourself thinking negatively. Write down the negative thoughts. Identify the errors of thinking involved and then challenge their accuracy. Think of alternative ways of interpreting events. Banish the negative thoughts and speak positive statements to yourself. With practice, such positive self-talk can help you combat pessimism and make you feel better.

Learn to deal with your emotions.

Anger, depression, and anxiety may be experienced at different stages of the illness. Such feelings are counterproductive because they sap your energy and undermine your confidence. The first step toward dealing with them is to ask yourself what situations, events, or thoughts have brought them on. When feeling angry, give yourself time to cool off, and then deal with the cause of your anger in a calm and assertive but not confrontational fashion. The best antidote for anxiety is physical and mental relaxation through deep, slow breathing and relaxing mental imagery. The technique of positive self-talk can help you to combat depression. Learn to air your feelings to your friends and family—this can help you to develop a more balanced view. If depression and anxiety persist, seek professional help.

Maintain your self-esteem.

To protect your sense of self-esteem, remind yourself that despite the physical changes brought about by Parkinson's disease, the real you, the person inside, hasn't changed. The illness cannot change your past successes or prevent you from achieving new ones. But set yourself more realistic standards. Don't be your own worst enemy through excessively self-critical thinking. Acknowledge your current achievements in the context of your present abilities and limitations, and reward yourself from time to time.

Communicate with friends and family.

Talking openly and often with your spouse or partner and family about how Parkinson's disease affects your daily lives and how you can get around the problems and prevent frustration from building up. Also, if each person is clear about his or her roles and duties, your household will run more efficiently. Telling your friends and colleagues about the illness and how it affects you will prevent misunderstanding. Similarly, your doctor will not know how you are feeling if you don't tell him or her. Communication with those around you may also help to reduce the sense of solitude that can be associated with illness.

Taking positive action

There are many positive ways in which you can minimize the effects of Parkinson's disease on your everyday life and your emotions:

❖ Ask your physician for referrals to the various sources of help available if you think that you can benefit from any of them.

❖ Keep your social network alive. Knowing that there are people who care and who are willing to help can make you feel less alone in your fight against the illness.

❖ Try to remain active. Don't give up your professional or social roles prematurely. Take up new activities and hobbies. Not only is activity pleasurable in the short term—in the long term it gives you a sense of control and achievement.

❖ Be flexible. Don't resist change that can help you live and cope better.

Be willing to adjust continually.

The stresses and demands of Parkinson's disease are not one-time problems; they recur in different forms during the course of the illness. The periods when you experience difficulty coping with the symptoms will be interspersed with longer spells when they are well controlled by medication. These changing phases make different demands on your personal and emotional resources, so prepare yourself for a continuous and ongoing process of adjustment.

12

Self-Help Strategies for Families

Brigid MacCarthy
Marjan Jahanshahi

It is a popular misconception that families have given up their caring roles. This is not borne out by the facts. As we noted earlier, a high percentage of people care for a relative who is disabled or elderly. Increased geographic mobility and changes in family structure—fewer children, more women working, and so on—mean that care of a chronically ill person is less likely to be shared by an extended family network and more likely to become the responsibility of one or two family members. So in addition to his or her other duties such as going to work or looking after the household, each individual caregiver is more likely to have to cope with all the stresses and strains of looking after the ill relative rather than being able to share them with others.

In this chapter we describe the strategies that caregivers can use to optimize their coping with the new challenges and demands that Parkinson's disease imposes on their lives. Some of this information emerged in the course of our interviews and conversations with caregivers.

Remember that no single strategy is right for everyone. What is important is that both caregiver and patient feel comfortable and satisfied that they are achieving the best possible for themselves under the circumstances. A strategy that works for one of you, but leaves the other feeling guilty, overloaded, or exposed, will not help you to forge a smooth-running partnership.

STRATEGIES FOR COPING IN THE MILD TO MODERATE PHASE

During our interviews and conversations, family members demonstrated a truly striking resilience and an ability to discover ways of coping that alleviated both practical problems and emotional distress. We were impressed by the courage and humor with which difficulties were faced, as well as by the highly individual solutions arrived at. These strategies for coping that others have devised may or may not work for you. To find out, try them.

Your Attitude Toward the Illness

Developing a coherent attitude toward the illness is an important aid to well-being. We found that in the early stages older individuals and their spouses viewed the onset of the disease and its restrictions simply as one way of growing old. This kind of acceptance prompts people to review their past lives, recognizing and valuing their achievements and satisfactions, and encourages them to move to this new stage with different expectations. Seeing the illness as an event appropriate to their stage in life helps people to feel less alone, less singled out by misfortune. Others, who were able to accept that developing the illness reflected random misfortune, also tended to accept the consequences of the disease fairly tranquilly. Some, however, chose more personal explanations for its onset, or continued to ask "Why me?", "Why us?", and these were the ones who usually had more difficulty in tolerating the consequences. This is where obtaining accurate information about Parkinson's disease and its possible causes is particularly significant; knowledge can facilitate the process of coming to terms with it.

Some caregivers stressed the importance of holding on to realistic hopes for a breakthrough in treatment. Many of the people with the illness and their spouses volunteered to take part in scientific trials of new interventions and took an interest in all sorts of ideas about how to maintain health and well-being. This enabled both parties to take an active role in minimizing disability, which effectively combated any sense of helplessness. Yet another attitude, which seemed to be much less helpful, is that of a wife who expressed a kind of magical optimism:

I just hope one day he will change. He might change one day and it will all go away.

This strategy *appears* to maintain hope. But, in fact, with each day that passed, with her husband's Parkinson's disease neither improving nor "going away," she became more and more desperate. So keeping a hold on realistic hopes and an active interest in developments in the treatment of the disease, but avoiding wishful thinking, appears to be the most effective approach.

In order to establish a mutually acceptable attitude to living with Parkinson's disease, talk about the disease and its implications together, as much as you need to, particularly early on. Spouses who suspect the patient of not trying very hard, or who mistakenly perceive real disabilities as shamming, find it extra-hard to deal effectively with practical day-to-day tasks. Some couples reported that when one or another partner became preoccupied with the disease and had difficulty accommodating it, the disease came to dominate their lives unduly. Respecting one partner's desire to minimize the impact of the condition is helpful as long as minimizing does not involve denying its reality. As we noted elsewhere, the couples who believed that they had reached a mutually acceptable approach early on seemed to have found the initial adjustment least traumatic. They usually had arrived at that position by compromises built on plenty of discussion. Some spouses we spoke to found particular solace in religion, which helped them to deal with feelings of anger and futility about the onset of the disease and to keep faith in the future alive.

Choosing a Doctor

Those who had managed to find a doctor they thought they could trust and relate to early on felt better equipped to face the challenge of the illness. As soon as possible after the diagnosis, ensure that you choose a doctor both of you trust and with whom you feel comfortable. Because Parkinson's disease is a chronic disorder, you can expect to have a long relationship with whichever physician is going to manage your relative's medical care. It is important that you believe that the doctor is aware of your needs as a caregiver as well as those of the ill person, and is able to give you the information and support that you require.

Getting Relevant Information

As we have already mentioned, accurate information, sensitively given shortly after the diagnosis, is invaluable in helping families to manage the process of coming to terms with the disease. Fears that go unacknowledged can drive a wedge between people at a time when they especially need to depend on their close relationships. These fears often are groundless or exaggerated. Insight gained from a range of serious illnesses shows that being fully informed about the symptoms of a disease and its treatment, and about what to expect in the future, helps people cope more effectively, both practically and emotionally. You don't have to become an expert on Parkinson's disease, but make sure that you think you have enough information to make sensible decisions about your relative's treatment and that you understand everything you have been told. Some people prefer to find out just the basics and not to become too involved with the details. Decide what information you need to plan your present and your immediate future effectively.

Coping with Your Relative's Disability

Managing the disabling consequences of the disease effectively has a major part to play in minimizing family stress. In the early stages, relatives rarely need to take over specific tasks. But the person with the illness often needs to be encouraged not to give up activities that he or she is functionally able to perform because, unjustifiably, he or she has lost confidence. Several caregivers spoke of the difficulty their relative experienced in making choices—for instance, about what to wear, how to unpack the groceries, or choose the next job to do around the house.

Encourage the person with Parkinson's disease to take responsibility for his or her general health. The emphasis should be on wellness, not on illness. Encourage him or her to remain in full-time employment for as long as possible. Don't let him or her withdraw from engagement in daily responsibilities and decision making—this would only accelerate the process of "premature social aging." The focus should be on what he or she can still do, rather than on what is no longer feasible. The independence of the person needs to be respected at all stages of the illness. Allow him or her to do as much as possible—self-care, household duties within reason, and whatever else he or she can manage. Don't be frustrated by slowness, and don't nag or apply pressure. Remember that the more he or she carries on doing, the less *you* have to do. Also, as mentioned earlier, once skills are lost or your relative gets out of the habit of performing particular tasks, regaining them will be difficult. Later, when moderate disability sets in, you may find the fluctuations in the symptoms frustrating—he or she may be able to do certain things in the "on" phase, but become totally incapacitated "off." Remind yourself that such fluctuations are a feature of the illness— the best you can do is accept them and adapt your schedule accordingly.

Of course, respecting the individual's independence has to be balanced against other practical demands on the caregiver's time. Spouses spoke frequently about how difficult it was to achieve the right balance, stepping in at the right moment without taking over, and dealing with their own frustration too.

His slowness sort of frustrates me and I think, "Oh, if only he'd leave things alone and leave me to get on with it." But I still let him continue.

Some preferred to take over discreetly, and finish jobs off when the individual had done as much as he or she could.

I come to the rescue in a quiet sort of way, because I don't want to deflate him.

Others negotiated things much more openly, sharing tasks to ensure that the individual was making a contribution to their joint lives. Sometimes this entailed his or her learning new skills or duties, and when this was possible it was experienced as highly rewarding all-around. One woman spoke jokingly of having "banned" her husband from a range of tasks that he could no longer finish reliably. She admitted that she now stopped him from doing some things that he could do at least some of the time, but she thought that having clear rules was the only way she could keep worry within manageable limits. In contrast, one man had prioritized delaying his wife's disabilities for as long as possible:

I don't help a lot. It may sound mean, but I think in the long run it's in her interest to continue doing as much as she can do. Also, if you get people to do everything for you, you feel a damn sight worse.

Sometimes caregivers have discovered idiosyncratic tricks to help the individual overcome particular problems. One woman whose husband had had a military career found she could help him unfreeze by shouting "Left, right, left, right." Another man who had been very outgoing and had played a competitive sport professionally could be helped to speak more coherently if his wife spoke to him in the manner of a sports coach:

Calm down. Speak slowly, speak clearly. Calm, slow, clear. Calm, slow, clear.

Each of these strategies illustrates how personal the process of adjusting to living with the illness is. Choosing the right approach is so important. For some, managing uncertainty and worry is clearly a priority, and sacrificing some competence may be a small price to pay. Other couples find the challenge of continuing to perform tasks despite increasing disabilities very rewarding, and are less troubled by the risks entailed by that strategy. This approach is easier to adopt if neither partner has other pressing duties, such as work or children to care for.

Another factor worth bearing in mind is that there is nothing unique about dealing with illness. Chronic illness has many features in common with other situations with inherent stress. It may turn out that the most efficient way to deal with it is via methods that the family has successfully used to deal with other major difficulties. Falling back on old and tested ways also induces a sense of control and familiarity. If avoiding confrontation is important, introduce changes more discreetly. But if open discussion or even a good argument is the preferred means to a solution, then use them—provided they don't cause long-term distress.

Nurture Your Partnership

The quality of the caregiver's relationship with the person with the illness plays a major role in determining how stressful they each find the early to middle stages of the illness. Many spouses we spoke to had found great strength in respecting the individual's efforts to cope. For some, coping together had improved their relationship; acknowledging that the illness was a joint life event increased mutual involvement in its management. Appreciation of the fact that lack of facial expression, a monotonous voice, and apathy were features of the illness, rather than signs of the person's loss of interest in the spouse, helped caregivers to accept and compensate for them. Some spouses reported that the illness had made the person with Parkinson's disease gentler, more tolerant, and more easy-going. Similar expectations about the right level of care and some degree of reciprocity—the person with Parkinson's disease doing things for the carer, and vice versa—are valuable. Reminiscing about the past, sharing what can still be enjoyed together, remembering to express affection, maintaining mutual respect and trust, and talking about problems—all these strategies were used in households that were coping well.

Couples who took care to safeguard their personal relationship against the stresses of the illness often did well. Despite the physical limitations imposed on the individual and the burden carried by the caregiver, such couples had managed to keep the core of their relationship alive by expressing warmth and appreciation. One husband expressed his appreciation in this way:

> *Every evening in bed, I give her a cuddle and a kiss. It's my way of saying thank you for everything she does for me during the day. After all, she has a lot to put up with—me and my Parkinson's disease are not a bed of roses.*

A woman in her late fifties described how adopting a long-term perspective on her life with her husband of 35 years, who had had Parkinson's disease for eight years, helped her:

When it all becomes too much, I remind myself of my wedding vows: for richer, for poorer, in sickness and in health, till death do us part. It helps me accept the disease as just another part of our lives. I sometimes look through our albums and try to remember him as handsome as he was when we first met, and review all the good times we've had together. Then I know that I can go on and do my best for him and for me.

As already emphasized, if conflict and resentment do build up, there is no substitute for direct and open discussion. Some of the people we interviewed told us they had arranged to put some special time aside to talk about the awkward issues in detail, making a commitment to be as open and honest as possible, sharing feelings and talking together about their needs and preferences. Others found it easier to have a third person present, perhaps a grown-up child or a close friend, to help sort out exactly what the problem was. These sessions work best when all parties stick to concrete issues such as who is going to feed the dog or manage the household bills. It is important that a plan of action be agreed on before ending the session. If the relationship between partners has been under strain for some time, mere discussion may not suffice and outside help may be necessary.

Maintain Outside Contacts and Seek Social Support

People with Parkinson's disease often find it difficult to get started on things or make major choices. But if gently prompted to do things in their own time and at their own pace, they find old favorite occupations very rewarding. Developing a thick skin and being familiar with local resources can combat social embarrassment caused by the more noticeable symptoms. One couple had been active supporters of the local theater for all their married lives. Seats at the ends of rows, near exits, were always available, and for them, seeing half a play was a lot better than giving up this major interest entirely.

Caregivers need persistence and flexibility if they are going to maintain a level of interest and engagement with the outside world that suits both partners. They can so easily become isolated and feel that they have no life of their own. Keeping their separate friends and interests is not a selfish preoccupation but a vital lifeline to keep the carer–patient partnership in good shape. Maintaining an energetic involvement with their own independent interests was thought by some caregivers to be crucial for a variety of reasons—here are two:

I'm not a martyr—to be able to carry on I need to have a break.

I've started to go out more, which encourages him to try running things by himself, at least for a while. It seems to work.

Those who had built up close links with their extended family and friends to gain emotional support and practical help also fared well. One woman reported that her husband confided more in their daughter, and that was a welcome sharing of burdens.

It is also important for the caregiver to avoid secrecy, because insisting on telling no one about the diagnosis imposes a severe strain. In addition, openness allows you to seek support outside your relationship—from friends and family, or from your local chapter of a Parkinson's disease group—if you want to. All these alternatives will help to ensure that you don't feel isolated with the problem. It is better to build or reinforce links early on rather than allowing them to loosen while you cope alone—only to find later, when you need help, that you have lost your old network of contacts.

Look After Yourself Too

For the caregiver, chronic illness in a close relative means sleep disturbance, increased workload, change of future plans, the need for emotional and work-related adjustments, confinement, restriction of social activities, and financial strain. Unsurprisingly, research on a host of chronic physical illnesses has shown that the primary caregiver is also susceptible to major psychological stress and physical strain.

Unfortunately, caregivers often fail to look after themselves. One of the common worries of elderly caregivers is what would happen to their relative if they were to become ill. Obviously, such worries can best be handled by putting aside time to look after themselves so as to reduce the risk of ill health. Making contingency plans such as arranging for close relatives to come and look after the sick person at home if the need arises, or temporary admission to a nursing home, can also help to allay such fears.

How is the task of looking after yourself best achieved? The following strategies can help you maintain your physical and psychological well-being.

❖ Have *regular daily breaks*, no matter how short, from the chores of caring. You may just want to sit quietly and have a cup of coffee, look through a magazine, watch a favorite TV program, or call a friend to chat. Longer periods away from home can be a welcome break both for the person with Parkinson's disease and for the caregiver. Accept invitations to stay with grown-up children, relatives, or friends. Alternatively, use the methods for arranging vacations discussed in Chapter 9.

❖ Even though the task of caring for your relative may be physically exhausting, try to put aside some time every week for two or three sessions of *exercise*. Go for a swim with your relative or take the dog for a brisk walk. Take up ballroom or country dancing, which can be enjoyable as well as good exercise. Avoid pulling muscles or straining your back by learning proper ways of lifting from a physical therapist or nurse.

❖ Make sure you get a good night's sleep and enough rest during the day. If your spouse's or partner's illness disrupts your sleep, move to a separate bed or bedroom. Don't let sleepless nights build up—it becomes impossible to cope during the day when you are exhausted. Ensure that you and your partner are following a healthy and balanced diet.

Remember, in addition, all those other ways of keeping yourself emotionally and physically healthy that we have mentioned elsewhere:

❖ Socialize, with or without your relative. Accept invitations.

❖ Give yourself a break from looking after your relative. Get someone to fill in for you. Don't feel guilty about taking time off to recharge your batteries.

❖ Develop new interests—some of which you might share with your relative. Activities that take your mind off your duties as a caregiver are particularly worthwhile.

❖ Obtain all the benefits to which you and your relative may be entitled (see Chapter 9).

❖ Be flexible and adaptable. Don't hold on to old ways of doing things that no longer suit your altered circumstances.

Above all, don't try to be a martyr. Don't overdo stoicism. Strike the right balance between caring and meeting your own needs.

Join a Caregivers' Support Group

Among the caregivers we talked to, those who had joined a support group considered it to be a lifeline. They enjoyed the meetings and consequently felt better equipped to cope with caring and combating stress. Such groups perform many functions for them. They provide a place to exchange information about the illness and about the available services and benefits, as well as other practical advice. The social aspects of the support groups—the opportunity for conversation and for airing and sharing emotions and concerns, empathy, and understanding; the exchange of ideas and opportunities for joint problem solving; the development of friendships; the organized activities and outings—all these were considered equally important in reducing the caregivers' sense of isolation, served to relieve frustration, and helped them to develop a pragmatic approach to caring. Additionally, members may have experiences that can be shared with newcomers. Such assistance by necessity is beyond the scope of staffs of national organizations. One put it this way:

I have found that those in the support group I attend are the people I can relate to most. They all have been through similar experiences as me, and they seem to be the only ones who understand what I am going through.

Another spouse highlighted why the support group provided such an important break from the duties of caring for her:

The only time that I really relax is when I go to the meetings of the caregivers' group. I feel I am among people who understand my situation.

I have a chat with a couple of other people I have got to know well. We exchange news about the ups and downs, give each other tips about how to cope, but also manage to have a good laugh.

Contact your local Parkinson's disease chapter to find out whether there are any Parkinson's disease caregivers' support groups in your area. If there aren't any, and you know others in similar situations who may be interested in joining, why not start your own?

Live for the Present

Learning not to focus on the illness, mentally minimizing rather than magnifying its consequences, making the most of daily pleasures, and focusing on the present rather than the future are universally successful:

I don't treat him as if there was anything major wrong with him. Maybe it's very selfish and maybe the day will come when it will be different, but right now this seems to be what we both want.

I think everything is an attitude of mind. If you've got something and you can't get rid of it, then make the best of it. Be thankful you've got an arm—some people haven't got an arm—there's always someone worse off. When I wake up in the morning I say, "Oh, thank God I'm here," and carry on. I don't think of the future as such.

Keep Your Sense of Humor!

Some caregivers found humor a vital strategy in minimizing and deflecting tension. They were not afraid of seeing the funny side of the predicaments in which the disease sometimes leaves them. When humor is shared, people with Parkinson's disease are unlikely to experience it as belittling their difficulties.

We laugh at it. You have to, otherwise there would be tears. We just have a laugh and start again.

What's the good of keeping on bellowing? It only sets him shaking, then we're worse off than originally. We end up with a laugh, and so long as I can get a laugh from him, that's a reward.

STRATEGIES FOR COPING IN THE SEVERE PHASE

When disability has become severe, the *way* people cope makes an enormous difference to their sense of well-being and to their practical management of their individual circumstances. In our contacts with caregivers and patients, we were often moved and impressed by the courage and good humor with which they tackled overwhelmingly difficult situations.

Solving Practical Problems

Many of the strategies discussed earlier work equally well when it comes to severe disability, but the need to organize effective solutions to practical problems is more urgent at this stage. Evidence from other sources and the experiences of the caregivers we talked to indicate that no amount of effort expended in dealing with personal feelings, either with or without the help of others, can substitute for making good use of practical, problem-focused strategies. Only once the best possible practical solutions have been arrived at can working on personal feelings contribute to the caregiver's sense of well-being.

Those caregivers who put energy and enthusiasm into using any practical aid available seemed to gain something more than the simple mechanical advantage—it may be that a sense of increased control and mastery comes with the sense of efficiency:

Practical everyday things are just something to get around. At the moment I'm very much on top of it. I like to feel I will continue to be, but one never knows.

For example, one man with a severely disabled and totally dependent wife solved the problem of serving hot meals at times that fit in with his wife's unpredictable on–off periods by learning to cook with a microwave oven.

He reported feeling delighted at learning a new skill—something he had lacked the time or energy to do for several years—that also provided a solution to a major problem.

When the disease becomes incapacitating, it may be necessary to obtain appropriate eating utensils. Other self-care activities such as washing, bathing, and dressing may no longer be possible to perform unaided and may require the caregiver's help. The main priority here is to find ways to make these tasks easier (see Chapter 9 for available aids and equipment).

The person who uses a wheelchair or is confined to bed should be moved every few hours to prevent pressure sores (see subsequent section) and pneumonia from developing. You will need to learn ways of lifting or moving him or her without damaging your own back or pulling any muscles—an occupational therapist, physical therapist, or home care nurse can help here.

Communication problems will increase as speech deteriorates—give the patient time to communicate or develop alternative means of communication. Above all, be patient—frustration is not good for either party. In solving practical problems, you may often have to resort to the various sources of outside help discussed in Chapter 9.

Make Use of Outside Help

All the sources of outside help listed in Chapter 9—family physician, neurologist, physical therapist, occupational therapist, social worker, members of the various nursing services, psychotherapist or counselor, the Parkinson's disease groups, and so on—are available to provide guidance and help for the caregiver as well as for the sick person. When Parkinson's disease becomes moderately to severely disabling, drawing on these various resources can provide major relief for the caregiver.

In our interviews with caregivers, we discovered that the morale in households that were able to rely on paid help or on close and committed relatives for practical assistance was noticeably higher. When respite could be afforded by someone else providing the constant vigilance that many severely disabled people needed, caregivers felt more able to manage their daily routines and to snatch some time for their own interests. Households that assemble for themselves a package of practical sup-

ports from a variety of sources, formal and informal, are in a strong position to tackle both daily stresses and sudden crises.

Balance Your Partnership

With the progression of the illness and the sick person's increasing disability, the spouse may begin to feel that he or she is constantly giving but
receiving nothing in return. Although most people willingly undertake all
the practical tasks dictated by their partner's illness, the main complaint is
often lack of emotional support—particularly if the partner becomes
engulfed in the symptoms and the changes in disability or totally wrapped
up in his or her own emotions. The gradually increasing dependence of the
partner, if combined with a lack of communication and emotional give-
and-take, may make the other partner feel that he or she is reduced to the
role of nurse.

Many of the ways of coping used in earlier stages of the illness to
protect and nurture the partnership seem to be just as useful at this later
stage:

❖ Spouses emphasize the importance of still being able to shout and
   argue occasionally without feeling guilty. One couple kept to a
   firm rule that they would not "let the sun go down" on their bad
   temper, and it was agreed between them that they would argue but
   that no dispute should be allowed to last longer than the day it
   began. Bottling up anger or frustration can have serious consequences for both parties, particularly for the long-term security of
   their relationship.
❖ Acknowledging and promoting give-and-take within the constraints
   imposed by severe disabilities is also very important.

*I don't do anything with the bills, he deals with them. It's a respon-
sibility that he cherishes. It makes him feel he is making a contribution to
running our life.*

❖ Many caregivers find that the courage and good humor of the ill
person, in the face of all the problems, gives them the strength to continue.

❖ Not allowing the daily demands of Parkinson's disease to reduce life to a series of self-care routines is of paramount importance. Deliberately putting aside time, no matter how short, to gossip, to reminisce, to make decisions, to plan future activities, promotes interaction and involvement. At bedtime, expressions of warmth and appreciation through hugging, cuddling, or kissing can make a demanding day more tolerable for both.

❖ Humor remains an invaluable resource when there is little else to resort to.

Dealing with Your Emotions

Of course, Parkinson's disease evokes a range of emotions in a spouse. The feelings that are perhaps most unjustified, as noted elsewhere, are *self-blame* and *guilt*. Sometimes the healthy partner may feel guilty that he or she is not physically incapacitated and does not have to live through the ups and downs in mobility and dyskinesias that can characterize the late stages; another common source of guilt is simply taking time off. Caregivers may also blame themselves when things go wrong, even though there may have been nothing that they could have done to prevent accidents such as falls or the distressing side effects of medication. When one partner is ill, the other may feel guilty about becoming irritated or losing his or her temper.

These feelings are often rooted in a deep concern for the relative, but irrationality also contributes to them. Feelings of self-blame are misplaced in this context because they are based on the assumption that you as caregiver should have control over situations that may in fact be uncontrollable. Also, they do not allow for the fact that we all make mistakes or judge situations wrongly. Furthermore, they are based on the assumption that the caregiver should somehow be selfless. Only angels are selfless!

Whatever the nature of your emotions, don't lock them up. Don't feel guilty about talking about them with close friends or family. Don't think that you are betraying your partner. Airing your feelings will not only make you feel better, but also it may bring you a new perspective or useful insight or advice. If you don't, you are more likely to feel strained by the demands imposed on you and more likely to have outbursts when it all becomes too much for you to handle.

In learning to deal with your emotions as a caregiver, you will find that the techniques of mental and physical *relaxation* and *positive self-talk* described in the previous chapter can work equally well for you. If you catch yourself thinking negative thoughts, identify your particular errors of thinking, challenge your negative thoughts, and replace them with more positive statements—and with time you will feel better. Put aside time for doing the relaxation exercises. If you go through a particularly bad patch, when it all seems to have become too much for you, seeing a psychotherapist or counselor may help you to develop new perspectives and coping strategies.

Keep a Sense of Realism

Developing a realistic attitude about the future, without falling into pessimism, is a vital asset. Caregivers' individual efforts to deal with their feelings about their situation seem to focus on trying to achieve resignation while avoiding despair. The weariness brought on by coping with a very long-term problem can threaten to defeat people unless ambitions and expectations are adjusted.

I've always got the hope that he won't get worse—or depressed.

The caregivers we spoke to identified some helpful strategies in trying to strike the right balance: recognizing that major improvement is out of the question, being committed to maximizing the use of functions that remain intact, leading a healthy lifestyle, hoping for plateaus to last as long as possible, and participating in trials of new treatments when opportunities come up.

Recognizing the strengths of the ill person helps many caregivers to accept the daily difficulties they face. It is important to appreciate whatever abilities are preserved; for example, several caregivers emphasized the value to them of the intactness of their partner's mental capacities. Yet others stressed the patience or good humor of the ill person, preserved despite extensive physical deterioration.

Prepare for the Time When Your Caring Role May End

The time may come when your relative becomes so severely disabled that you can no longer look after his or her needs at home. This is the point at which you need to give careful consideration to some form of *residential care*. Discuss the pros and cons with your relative and with other members of your family. View potential homes and decide which is the most suitable for his or her particular needs (see Chapter 9).

When the time comes for the separation, you will need to have mentally prepared both yourself and your partner for the changes that are going to occur in your living circumstances and your daily routines. Discuss the likely changes together so that you can both start accepting them. It is even more important to talk about your feelings so that you don't end up feeling guilty because you think you are abandoning your relative. The reality will be that you have done your best in caring for him or her up to now, but with the current level of disability, his or her needs are going to be best met by an alternative arrangement. You are doing what is *best for both of you.*

The other commonly expressed feeling is a sense of uselessness, of no longer being needed, now that you have given up those caring duties that may well have dominated your life in the last few years. Feelings of loneliness may also prevail. One man in his mid-seventies put it this way:

After living together for 50 years, the last 15 of them with her Parkinson's disease, my wife is now in a nursing home. Life is certainly less chaotic for me, but the house seems very empty, and at times I don't know what to do with myself now that she is no longer here to look after every day.

With time, you will learn to care for the person with Parkinson's disease in your new capacity. Frequent visits, taking with you news of friends and family and a supply of favorite foods and magazines, will be much appreciated. And now, if you have managed to keep up your contacts with friends and maintained your outside interests, you can pick up your own life again.

CAMPAIGN FOR SERVICES THAT WILL MEET YOUR NEEDS

In their leaflet "Carers' Needs—a Ten-Point Plan for Carers," the Carers' National Association in Britain has set out the criteria for ensuring that caregivers and the people they care for can lead full and independent lives. According to this, caregivers' needs are:

1. Recognition of their contribution and of their own needs as individuals in their own right.
2. Services tailored to their individual circumstances, needs, and views, agreed upon through discussions at the time help is being planned.
3. Services equally accessible to caregivers of every race and ethnic origin, reflecting an awareness of differing racial, cultural, and religious backgrounds and values.
4. Opportunities for a break, both for short spells (e.g., an afternoon) and for longer periods (a week or more), to relax and have time to themselves.
5. Practical help to lighten the tasks of caring, including domestic help, home adaptations, and help with transportation.
6. Someone to talk to about their own emotional needs—at the outset of caring, while they are caring, and when the caring task is over.
7. Information about the available benefits and services, as well as about how to cope with the particular condition of the person cared for.
8. An income that covers the cost of caring and that does not preclude caregivers' taking employment or sharing the caring with others.
9. Opportunities to explore alternatives to family care, for both the immediate future and the long-term future.
10. Services designed, at all levels of policy planning, through consultation with caregivers.

Reflecting on your own experiences, you may think that there is a large gap between this "ideal" list and the actuality of being a caregiver. As a first step in bridging this gap, consider joining a lobby to campaign for the provision of better services. Groups often can voice their needs more effectively than individuals. Join a support group if you haven't already. Also, as an individual caregiver, you may find this list useful as a guideline for obtaining the services that will help you to cope.

KEY FACTS 12

No single strategy works for everyone. Select and try out strategies that may work for you.

When the Illness Is Mildly to Moderately Disabling

Establish a shared approach to living with Parkinson's disease.

You and your relative need to arrive at a common approach to living with Parkinson's disease. Talk about the disease and its implications with your relative and with other members of the family. Accepting the reality of it while maintaining hope for new treatments will help you develop ways of accommodating it with minimal disruption and distress.

Choose a doctor.

Early on, you and your ill relative should choose a doctor—whether primary care physician or private neurologist—whom you both trust, feel comfortable with, can talk to easily, and consider able to appreciate your particular circumstances and needs. Continuity of care from such a doctor is likely to be beneficial for the medical management of the illness.

Get relevant information.

Knowing about the symptoms and about their impact on your relative's daily activities will help you to understand the limitations imposed on him or her and the fluctuations in ability. Accurate information about possible causes, likely courses, and available treatments will prepare you for what to expect and so prevent unnecessary anxiety and irrational fears. Information also allows both of you to make sensible decisions about treatments, about stopping work, and about giving up driving or changing residences.

Cope with your relative's disability.

Knowing about the illness can prevent you from feeling frustrated, from pushing your partner too hard, and from nagging. For as long as the illness allows it, encourage him or her to continue work, to exercise, to take on new or different responsibilities, to do household tasks, to drive, and to socialize as before. Even when disability sets in, let him or her continue to do as much as possible. Show appreciation for efforts made.

Nurture your partnership.

When the disease becomes moderately disabling, you and the ill person may be spending a considerable amount of time together. How you treat and interact with each other will be very important for the quality of your lives. Major setbacks and new pressures can be faced more effectively if you pool your resources, rather than fighting alone or in ways that would undermine your individual efforts. Respect each other's wishes and learn to compromise. Express affection and warmth and show your appreciation of your partner's efforts.

Maintain your social contacts.

When you are faced with the daily demands of the illness, keeping in touch with friends and family and pursuing your hobbies may seem your last consideration—but it should be precisely the opposite. It is now, perhaps more than ever, that you need to make social activities a priority. Don't deprive yourself of the practical help and emotional support that your friends and family can give you. Don't let social embarrassment turn you and your partner into hermits. Live for yourselves—don't be bothered by what other people—mostly strangers, anyway—may think. Explain to people in simple terms about Parkinson's disease and how it affects your relative.

Look after yourself.

- ❖ Take regular daily breaks from caregiving.
- ❖ Put aside some time every week for exercise.
- ❖ Make sure you get a good night's sleep and that you are eating healthily.
- ❖ Take time off.
- ❖ Be flexible and adaptable.
- ❖ Don't try to be a martyr.

Join a caregivers' support group.

Meeting other people who are in your situation will help reduce your sense of isolation; provide you with important sources of information about services and benefits and with practical advice; furnish opportunities for airing and sharing feelings and exchanging ideas; and offer social support, organized activities, and outings.

Live for the present.

Enjoy life *now*. This does not mean that you shouldn't plan for the future. Simply don't postpone what you can enjoy now until some indefinite later date.

Keep your sense of humor.

Having a good laugh can often help to relieve tension and lighten the burden for both of you.

When the Illness Becomes Severely Disabling

Solve practical problems.

When the disease becomes severely disabling, the person with Parkinson's disease may need much more help with everyday activities. Making these tasks easier by obtaining appropriate equipment and by seeking help from available resources will be critical in lightening your workload. Remember that the various external resources—doctors, nurses, therapists, and so on—are there to be used. Instead of fighting alone, ask for whatever services you think will benefit both of you.

Achieve a balance in your partnership.

Despite your partner's disability, building some form of reciprocity into your relationship will be most gratifying. Allow him or her to do things for you, no matter how small. Express appreciation of his or her patience, tolerance, and efforts to cope—this will in turn encourage him or her to show appreciation of your hard work.

Deal with your emotions.

Try the techniques of mental and physical relaxation and positive self-talk described in Chapter 11—they can work equally well for you. Catch yourself having negative thoughts, identify your errors of thinking, and replace your negative thoughts with more positive statements. Banish any feelings of guilt—you cannot expect yourself to be completely selfless or to be able to control situations that are beyond your control. Don't lock up your emotions—share them with friends and family. It may help you feel better and bring you a new perspective or useful insight or advice.

Maintain a sense of realism.

Developing a realistic attitude to increasing disability, and to the implications for you and the rest of the family, is difficult. But don't let pessimism and despair take over. The most adaptive coping strategies at this stage are realistic acceptance, a pragmatic attitude to problem solving, living for the present, and not worrying about the future.

Prepare for the end of caring.

A time may come when your partner's needs are best met in residential care. Accepting this as the best course of action may be difficult partly because you have unjustified feelings of guilt at "abandoning" him or her.

Discuss the practicalities, as well as your feelings, so as to prepare both yourself and your partner for the changes in your daily routines. After his or her departure, you are likely to feel a void. It is easier to pick up your life again if you have kept in contact with friends and maintained outside interests.

Campaign for Better Service Provision

Your needs should not be overshadowed by those of the person with Parkinson's disease. Familiarize yourself with the list of priorities for meeting the needs of caregivers. Ensure that you obtain access to services that will allow you to fulfill these needs. Join others in campaigning for better service provision.

Financial and Legal Issues

Lanny E. Perkins, Esq.
Sara D. Perkins, Esq.

Having Parkinson's disease is not against the law. But given its progressive nature and its common occurrence later in life, legal problems do frequently arise during the course of the illness. Common nonmedical issues faced by people with Parkinson's disease include health care costs, insurance, employment, disability benefits, taxes, debts, and estate and probate matters. Although it is beyond the scope of this chapter to fully discuss any of these topics, a brief introduction may help you to take steps to lessen their impact.

CHOOSING PROFESSIONALS

Your ability to handle legal and financial problems will be greatly improved if you already have a good working relationship with your doctors and other health care professionals and have access to the appropriate attorneys and financial experts. Without the assistance of these professionals, you may be unable to achieve your legal or financial aims.

It is generally easier to find the medical, legal, and financial help you need in large metropolitan centers. Even in cities, however, it is not always obvious which professional you should choose and for what purposes. For example, although an internist or general practitioner may be able to manage much of your ongoing medical care, a neurologist who is experienced with Parkinson's disease should be better able to assess your employment capabilities. Furthermore, if you need or want to apply for either private or government disability benefits, the opinion of a neurologist (preferably board certified) should carry more weight with the person who is evaluating the disability claim. In any event, you need to be routinely seen by health care professionals, and it is imperative that your records be well maintained so that if a question does arise about employment, mental competency, or insurance payments, the written evidence to support any desired action is readily available.

The local chapters of the several national Parkinson's organizations (see Appendix II) should be able to provide useful information about the Parkinson's disease professionals and services in your particular locale. Support groups, whether affiliated with a national agency or not, can be another referral source.

Your family lawyer, if you have one, may be the first source of counsel for any legal problem that occurs as a result of the illness. However, he or she may not be experienced or interested in such matters as Social Security disability, Medicare and/or Medicaid, or tax and estate planning. In some cases, you may think you cannot afford to hire an attorney. Fortunately, in many areas of the country there are free or reduced-fee resources for people who meet certain qualifications. Many law schools provide such services to the community through legal clinics, although these clinics often take cases because of their teaching value and are therefore not open to every potential client. There are also state and local legal aid societies, but they are generally accessible only to the indigent. Your local, county, or state bar associations are more practical referral sources. Although these referrals are not a guarantee of professional quality, they often have the advantage of offering extremely low-cost initial visits (for example, $20 for the first half hour), so that whether you decide to proceed with some legal action, you can at least get a professional opinion about your problem. The bar associations should also be able to provide information about areas of legal specialization.

You may want to obtain professional financial advice in arranging assets to ensure a certain retirement income or to provide care for a spouse or children. Attorneys and some certified public accountants (CPAs) can help in tax and estate planning matters. Certified financial planners affiliated with national associations, bank trust officers, insurance agents, and stockbrokers can offer valuable services, although the potential for a conflict of interest may exist because in many cases these professionals are paid through commissions from sales to their customers. They are rarely a substitute for appropriate legal and/or accounting assistance.

Ideally, the medical and nonmedical professionals who work with you and your family should be available to interact as a team when circumstances warrant. Such cooperation will greatly help you achieve your goals and cut down on misunderstanding and confusion. For example, suppose a doctor or therapist suggests certain physical modifications for your home, but you are concerned about costs. An attorney or CPA may be able to suggest tax planning strategies to minimize costs, or a social worker may be able to direct you to public programs that will pay for all or part of the modifications as long as certain regulations are followed.

Sometimes professionals in one field are not accustomed to dealing with those in another area and do not understand how important joint efforts can be to their patient and/or client. Unfortunately, many health professionals have had unhappy experiences with lawyers in particular and are suspicious of their motives. Then, too, suspicions sometimes are directed toward patients and families, for instance, that they are "giving up" too soon on employment by seeking disability benefits. An interdisciplinary approach can help allay such doubts while simultaneously allowing everyone to work together to meet your needs. You can then plan for future events, not simply react to sudden crises.

EMPLOYMENT

Although many people with Parkinson's disease are over 65 and retired by the time the illness is diagnosed, many are still working when symptoms become apparent. Many want to continue to work as long as possible, and with improved treatments, the stages of illness during which they can remain active and independent have been extended. Notwithstanding this progress, employment concerns remain. People with any serious condition worry about the effect working will have on their health. You may also be uncertain about whether and how long you will be able to continue at your regular job. Many people are fearful that, irrespective of their level of performance, they will suffer discrimination from their employers, perhaps even termination.

Fortunately, federal legislation protects individuals from employment discrimination on the basis of disability. Most states and even some cities also have such statutes. Although it is not identical to the civil rights laws that protect people from race, sex, age, and other forms of discrimination, the federal disability legislation is similar in its intent and application.

The key piece of federal law that protects most employees of private employers, state and local governments, employment agencies, and labor unions from discrimination on the basis of their physical or mental limitations is the Americans with Disabilities Act (ADA), which was signed into law in July 1990. The ADA both standardizes and expands federal protections against discrimination in employment, public accommodations, transportation, and telecommunications, although its provisions are being phased in over a number of years.

The ADA covers employers with 15 or more workers. It forbids discrimination against "qualified individuals with disabilities" in all employment practices and activities, including hiring, firing, promoting, training, pay, working conditions, and benefits. An "individual with a disability" is defined by the ADA as an individual who has "(A) A permanent or temporary physical or mental impairment that substantially limits one or more major life activities of such individual; (B) A record of such an impairment; (C) Or being regarded as having such an impairment."

A person with Parkinson's disease is covered under the ADA. However, whether he is deemed to be a qualified individual with a disability depends on his ability to perform what the Act refers to as the "essential" or key functions of a job with or without "reasonable accommodation." "Reasonable accommodation" might include such actions as restructuring a job, modifying work schedules, making the workplace more usable or accessible, acquiring appropriate equipment to aid performance, or reassigning a worker to another position if he is no longer able to do his original job. The ADA only requires an employer to make an accommodation to a "known" disability, that is, one known to the employer; it does not require the employer to hire or retain a worker who cannot perform a job safely.

This point about a "known" disability may raise the question: Should a person with Parkinson's disease disclose his diagnosis when the symptoms may not be apparent to employers or coworkers? Under the ADA, there are restrictions on preemployment inquiries and physicals that should offer some protection to the person with Parkinson's disease, particularly one with "hidden" or controlled symptoms who changes jobs. An employer is forbidden under the ADA to ask if a prospective employee has a disability, although he may inquire whether the employee is able to perform the essential functions of the job for which he is interviewing. An employer may require a prospective employee to take a medical examination but only if such an examination is required for all would-be employees in that job category, the examination information is maintained in confidence as mandated by the Act, and a conditional offer of employment has first been made. The prospective employee may volunteer that he has a disability so that the employer can request what accommodation, if any, to this condition is required. Volunteering such information should be done with discretion, however, especially if the effects of Parkinson's disease are not readily apparent; notwithstanding the disability statutes, an employer may well not hire a person with Parkinson's disease simply because of his diagnosis.

Another related problem for the person with Parkinson's disease (as it is for people with many other chronic illnesses) is accurately assessing his ability to perform his job or any alternative suitable to his training and experience, particularly as symptoms progress and treatment efficacy changes. Once again, a regular pattern of visits to health care professionals who keep a well-maintained record of your condition can be crucial in fairly evaluating whether the time has come for health or safety reasons to alter your job or stop work altogether.

In actual practice, however, the decision to continue working is often not made by the person with Parkinson's disease. Whether through intentional discrimination—for example, to remove you from public view or to get you out of the group insurance plan, or because it is sincerely believed that you can no longer adequately or safely perform your job duties, your employer may take steps to terminate you. Unless you are working under an express or implied job contract, in most states there is little you can do about this unless you can show that your employer is in fact engaging in a prohibited form of discrimination—that is, one based on disability, age, race, or the like. Of course, with a condition such as Parkinson's disease, job performance may in fact be impaired, If this is the case, and even if your employer does not fire you, you may still be encouraged to cut your hours or change your job, possibly by moving to a lower paying position. In any case, you may find yourself at a turning point.

If you are currently employed, you should be especially wary about taking any action that might jeopardize your employee benefits. For example, cutting back your schedule and working part-time may allow you to remain in the work force longer, but if this is done at the cost of losing health or disability benefits (such benefits are often only offered to full-time employees), it is of questionable value. You—and your health care providers—may suddenly have to reevaluate your ability to work if you are faced with the prospect of early retirement, a job cutback, layoff, or firing. However, if you believe you have suffered discrimination and want to take legal action, what are your options?

Under the ADA and similar federal and state laws (which may cover you instead of or in addition to the ADA), you may file a complaint with the appropriate government office. Depending on the violation alleged, this may be the Equal Employment Opportunity Commission, another federal department, or a state human rights agency. The complaint will be investigated, and remedies may include hiring, reinstatement, back pay and benefits, and court orders prohibiting further discrimination by your employer. With certain exceptions, an ADA complaint must be filed within 180 days of the date of the alleged act of discrimination; after investigation by the government agency, the complainant may bring a private suit against the employer.

Although antidiscrimination statutes have been helpful to many people, the enforcement process can be long and stressful. Because Parkinson's disease is a progressive condition, you should give considerable thought to what you stand to gain before starting any action. A complaint or suit can be expected to last at least many months and more commonly several years.

In addition to the ADA, the Family and Medical Leave Act (FMLA) of 1993 may offer flexibility and job protection to people with Parkinson's disease who are still in the workforce. To be eligible for FMLA leave, you must work for a covered employer—meaning local, state, and federal agencies and schools, and private sector employers who employed 50 or more workers—for at least 20 workweeks in the current or preceding year.

You must have worked for that employer at least 12 months and 1,250 hours in the 12 months before requesting leave. You must also work at a location where the employer employs at least 50 workers within a 75-mile radius.

Leave can be taken all at once, intermittently, or by working a reduced schedule.

The employer may require you to take any accrued paid leave to cover some or all of FMLA leave. Similarly, you may elect to substitute accrued vacation or personal leave for FMLA leave, as provided by the employer's policies for such substituted leave.

A serious health condition means an illness, injury, impairment, or physical or mental condition that results in a period of incapacity. But this does not mean that you have to be receiving inpatient or residential care in order to qualify for FMLA. You can take leave to treat a serious chronic condition such as Parkinson's disease.

An employer may require you to obtain a medical certification from a health care provider to support the need for the leave.

One of the most important features of FMLA is the requirement that an employer maintain group health insurance (if any), including family coverage, on the same terms as if you were still working. So if you pay part of the health insurance premiums, you must continue to pay them while on FMLA leave. But note that an employer's obligation to maintain health benefits stops if and when you tell the employer that you do not intend to return to work at the end of the leave. The employer's obligation also stops if you are late in paying premiums, and in some cases an employer can recover the premiums paid to maintain the health benefits.

When you return at the end of leave, you must be given your original job or one with equivalent pay and benefits. But FMLA has some special provisions for "key" or highly paid employees who may be denied restoration to their jobs if that would cause substantial economic injury to the employer. Likewise, FMLA places some restrictions on how school district employees may take leave near the end of a school term.

You are protected from discrimination for taking FMLA leave. This includes hiring, promotions, or disciplinary actions. You do not have to be disabled to qualify for FMLA. If you are eligible, you can take FMLA leave, with its insurance and job protections. It is also possible to be protected by the ADA at the same time. So it is important to consider both the ADA and the FMLA in planning strategies to ensure job protection, unwanted transfer, maintenance of health benefits, and reasonable accommodations.

The U.S. Department of Labor (DOL) Wage and Hour Division enforces FMLA. If you believe you have suffered discrimination, you can file a complaint with DOL; you also can bring a private civil action against the employer.

For more information on FMLA through the Internet: www.dol.gov; telephone: (800) 959-FMLA.

DISABILITY BENEFITS

A person who is employed at the time of diagnosis should anticipate the possibility that he may one day have to stop working because of Parkinson's disease. Under both the Social Security system and most private and employer-provided disability policies, an eligible individual under the age of 65 may apply for disability benefits. Upon one's reaching age 65, Social Security disability payments are automatically converted to old age benefits. Benefits from private or employer plans may terminate and/or be coordinated with pension income.

Most people who have worked have paid premiums to the Social Security Administration (SSA), and some are covered by a disability policy through their employer. You also may have purchased a private, individual disability policy before diagnosis, but once you are diagnosed with Parkinson's disease, it is unlikely that you will ever be able to buy such insurance.

There are many misconceptions about disability benefits, particularly about how one qualifies. Private or employer-provided policies vary significantly, but because many require that a claimant eventually file for Social Security Disability Income (SSDI), it is important to summarize the key points of the government system.

Two Social Security programs make cash payments to disabled individuals and, in some cases, to their spouses, ex-spouses, minor children, widow(er)s, and dependent parents: SSDI and Supplemental Security Income (SSI). Supplemental Security Income is a welfare program for people with extremely low income and resources (assets). Work history and payment of Social Security taxes (FICA) are not at issue for SSI; however, the standard for determining whether a claimant is disabled is the same for both SSDI and SSI, as is the claim process, with some exceptions. When a request for an application form for disability benefits is made, the SSA representative who receives the request should try to determine if the claimant is eligible for SSI; if not, the claimant should raise the matter himself.

Social Security Disability Income is paid to eligible disabled workers who have worked the requisite number of three-month periods or quarters. Although there are some exceptions (and those most likely would not affect the typical person with Parkinson's disease who becomes disabled sometime well into his working life), any worker who has been credited by SSA with a total of at least 40 quarters of work and who applies for benefits within five years of the last quarter worked will be deemed an insured worker for SSDI. This does not mean that you must have worked full-time for 10 years (40 quarters), but you must have earned enough and paid in enough to Social Security in FICA taxes to receive "credit" for one quarter. In 1999 a worker who earned $740 received credit for a quarter of coverage. To find out how many quarters have been credited to you and what your estimated benefits are, call SSA and request Form 7004. Within certain limits, errors discovered in your SSA record can be corrected.

A claimant must file a claim for disability with SSA in order to obtain benefits. This lengthy form asks for information about both your personal life and your work life. The point of these questions is to provide a fuller picture of your lifestyle and thereby aid SSA in determining your work capacity. You will also be required to furnish medical information about your disability. This information includes the names and addresses of treating physicians, clinics, and/or hospitals. They will be contacted directly by SSA for additional reports and records.

If you are deemed to be insured for SSDI, your claim (the application plus information from your health care providers) will be evaluated according to medical criteria set forth in the SSA regulations (called the

Listings) for the particular disability alleged. In the case of parkinsonian syndrome, the Listing—1 1.06 of 20 CFR Pt 404, Subpt P, App, 1—is brief.

> Parkinsonian syndrome with the following signs: Significant rigidity, bradykinesia, or tremor in two extremities, which, singly or in combination, result in sustained disturbances of gross and dexterous movements, or gait and station.

A claimant found to have a serious impairment that meets or exceeds the requirements of the relevant Listing(s) will be given disability benefits. However, in all cases, and irrespective of the particular disability alleged, the standard for SSDI is one of *total* disability, defined in the SSA regulations as "inability to engage in any substantial gainful activity by reason of a medically determinable physical impairment, which can be expected to result in death or has lasted, or can be expected to last for a continuous period of not less than 12 months." Both laypeople and health professionals are sometimes confused about what this standard really means. Although it is in fact a strict measure, generally much more stringent than the disability standards contained in many private or employer-provided policies, it does not mean that you must be, for example, comatose or completely bedridden. But your disability must be so severe that you are unable to perform work for which you would earn more than a small amount of money—currently up to $700 a month. It does not mean that you can no longer perform your regular job or a former job. However, such factors as age, experience, and education levels may be taken into account to help determine disability and your "residual functional capacity" (remaining capacity for work) when the medical evidence of the disability is not incontrovertible.

It is of the utmost importance that a person with Parkinson's disease who is applying for SSDI have the full support of his health care team, whose records will provide the key evidence for a finding of disability. Social Security Administration may request that you see a doctor(s) of its choosing for a second evaluation; however, SSA must give greater weight to the opinions of your regular physician(s). Fortunately, there is little work involved in assisting you in your application for disability—a few SSA forms to be filled out, perhaps an affidavit if the claim must be appealed. Although it is by no means unusual for an applicant with

Parkinson's disease to be approved for SSDI on his initial application, you frequently must be willing to appeal a denial of disability in order to secure his benefits.

If your application is denied, you have the right to request a Reconsideration, which is a "paper" review of the initial application plus any additional medical information you supply. If this review is unsuccessful, you may request a hearing before an SSA Administrative Law Judge (ALJ). Although you may represent yourself or have nonattorney representation throughout the claim process, the ALJ stage is the first level at which most lawyers become involved, and you would be foolish not to seek professional representation at this juncture. By law, all attorney's fees must be approved by SSA and generally come out of back benefits that have been withheld during the appeal of the application. The ALJ stage of appeal is the point at which most claimants have the best chance of getting a denial overturned. Evidence in the form of written affidavits from your doctor(s) is extremely effective in making the case for disability, and a lawyer can obviously assist in this effort. Other evidence, such as written or personal testimony about job performance from coworkers or employers, can also be presented to the ALJ, but it is often unnecessary.

If the claim is denied by the ALJ, you can appeal to the Appeals Council of SSA. This is the final level of review within SSA. Beyond this point, a claimant must file an action in federal district court. The court is limited to a review of SSA's application of the law to the evidence already presented in the case; new evidence by the claimant usually is not permitted.

Because there are significant restrictions on a claimant's ability to offer new evidence in the upper levels of the disability appeal process, it is imperative that you prepare a careful application and ALJ appeal, as necessary. It is also imperative that all appeals be timely filed (within 60 days of the date of notice of each SSA decision). *Note:* The disability review and appeal process is undergoing trial changes in some parts of the country. Check with your local district office of SSA for more information.

Many employer-provided and private disability policies have more liberal standards for defining disability than SSA, at least for some period of time, such as the inability to perform one's regular job for two years after onset of disability. Some private plans have attractive cost of living adjustments (COLAs), whereas others do not; SSDI benefits have annual COLAs. Many private and employer plans require that a beneficiary apply for SSDI if eligible and also require a complete or partial offset of any SSDI income against benefits received under the policy. Some private plans allow a beneficiary to earn a small amount of income, at least for some period of time, without jeopardizing disability status. This is a point you as a beneficiary should fully investigate by examining a copy of the actual policy, which you are entitled by law to see. Because an earnings test may be a part of the disability standard under an employer-provided or private policy, just as it is with SSA, work of any kind should be undertaken with extreme caution. For example, a person who receives SSDI may now earn up to $300 a month and still be deemed to be disabled. Such earnings may also need to be offset against some policies; if they are reported by an IRS 1099 form, both SSA and the insurance company and/or employer may learn about them. In any case, earnings may cause more problems than they are worth by raising the question of continued disability status. *Note:* Unearned income (interest or dividends) is not a factor in qualifying for or maintaining benefits from either SSDI or most private or employer policies.

The disability process is one area in which a team approach by the health and legal professionals working with you can make an often difficult crossroads less anguished, This is especially true if the principal parties, namely, the patient with Parkinson's disease and his doctor, understand and agree in advance of a crisis that disability status may be not only unavoidable, but also preferable to impaired physical and psychological health or financial upheaval resulting from lost benefits

MEDICARE, HEALTH INSURANCE, AND MEDICAID

Because of the need for regular medical treatment and the high cost of such care, it is absolutely essential that you retain or secure the health insurance benefits to which you are entitled. These benefits can be both public and private. In time, they may also include benefits related to long-term, custodial, or nursing home care. Following is a brief discussion of some of the major health care financing issues facing people with Parkinson's disease and their families.

Medicare

Most people are aware that Medicare is the federal health care program available to individuals over age 65 who have become eligible to receive Social Security, Railroad Retirement, or certain other government pension benefits. Even older people who have not paid into the Social Security system are eligible for Medicare, subject to certain application and premium payment provisions.

It is less well known that Medicare is also available to people under the age of 65 who have become eligible to receive SSDI benefits. However, with rare exceptions for certain kidney problems, Medicare benefits for the disabled do not begin until an individual has been eligible to receive SSDI for 24 months. Because there is a five-month waiting period from date of disability before SSDI payments start, this means that Medicare actually does not begin for 29 months. This waiting period often created a gap in medical coverage between the time an employer's policy lapsed and Medicare began. Fortunately, the problem has lessened since the passage of the so-called COBRA law (Consolidated Omnibus Budget Reconciliation Act of 1985) and its later amendments, which mandate that most group health insurance benefits must continue for 29 months after a disabled employee has stopped working (18 months for nondisabled workers; 36 months for spouses and dependents). However, as with all COBRA benefits, a beneficiary may be required to pay premiums for this coverage that are significantly greater than those he paid as an employee. COBRA was amended in 1996 to extend group benefits for up to 29 months to qualified beneficiaries who become disabled within the first 60 days of COBRA coverage and to their nondisabled dependents.

Many misconceptions about Medicare may complicate your planning for medical costs. Although Medicare is not exactly comparable to the best group health insurance policies, its two parts, Part A, Hospital Insurance, and Part B, Medical Insurance (physician and outpatient services), are intended to function something like a comprehensive major medical plan. This model is now referred to as the "Original Medicare

Plan," or fee-for-service, to distinguish it from the recently created Part C or Medicare+Choice. However, despite being fee-for-service, both Parts A and B impose significant limitations on fees and services that can wreak havoc for the typical person with Parkinson's disease who has large, ongoing medical expenses, particularly for outpatient prescription drugs. Although legislative activity is under way to add an outpatient drug benefit, Medicare does not now pay for most prescription drugs except those provided when a patient is in the hospital. Neither does it pay the full cost of office visits to doctors or most other outpatient services; it generally reimburses 80 percent of the Medicare fee schedule amount, which varies somewhat depending on your geographic region.

Many services are not covered at all, including routine physical examinations. Some outpatient procedures of special interest to people with Parkinson's disease are limited in scope, payment, and duration. These include physical, speech, and occupational therapy, which are capped. Since 1997, Medicare caps the amount of outpatient physical and speech therapy services at $1,500 per year; occupational therapy at $1,500 per year. Many types of durable equipment are covered by Medicare within strict guidelines that usually include a doctor's certificate of medical necessity; other devices that are helpful to a person with Parkinson's disease are not covered, such as a raised toilet seat. Some types of services that are usually covered will not be if they are deemed medically unreasonable and unnecessary.

The Part B (Medical Insurance) premium was $45.50 per month in 1999; the deductible, $100 per year. Both premium and deductible are expected to rise in the near future. Unless you go to doctors or clinics that accept assignment of claims as their sole fee, the difference between what you are charged and what Medicare reimburses may be in excess of the general 80/20 percent copayment. However, Medicare limits the total fee that nonparticipating doctors (those who do not accept assignment) may charge to 115 percent of the approved fee. Nonparticipating doctors must also provide a written estimate of the costs of elective surgery over $500, or the patient is entitled to a refund of any payments that exceed the approved fee. Medicare beneficiaries sometimes discover that because Medicare often pays less than half the amount that many doctors charge their non-Medicare patients, they have trouble finding physicians, particularly nonspecialists, who will agree to take them on as new patients. In addition to fee limitations, some doctors simply believe it is too expensive and too aggravating to comply with Medicare's mandate that all providers must file claims on behalf of Medicare patients. Fortunately, those medical specialties that routinely deal with an elderly population, such as cardiologists and neurologists, and who have large Parkinson's disease practicesm are usually set up to handle Medicare patients efficiently.

Patients can also face problems with hospital costs, although acceptance of assignment is rarely an issue. Medicare Part A reimbursements are often less than those made by "third party payers" (insurance companies or employers). Benefits are limited: after the sixtieth day of confinement during a benefit period (which starts upon admission to a hospital and ends when the patient has not been an inpatient for sixty consecutive days), significant copayments without any stop-loss or coinsurance cap are required. If a new benefit period has begun (readmission after 60 days have elapsed), another deductible is charged; Medicare beneficiaries might conceivably have to pay several deductibles in a single calendar year. The deductible—$768 in 1999—is adjusted annually.

If you need help paying the cost of either Parts A or B and have little income and few assets, you may be eligible for the "Qualified Medicare Beneficiary" (QMB), "Specified Low-Income Medicare Beneficiary" (SLMB), or "Qualifying Individual" (QI) programs. You apply for these programs through Medicaid. Qualifying income limits are subject to change every year.

Medicare does pay for some home health care services, including skilled nursing, home health aides, and therapy services under a physician's plan of treatment, subject to qualifying criteria. However, these services are intermittent, part-time, and/or short-term.

You do not have to have had a prior hospitalization if you meet the eligibility requirements: (1) you need intermittent skilled nursing care, physical therapy, or speech therapy; (2) you are confined to your home; (3) your doctor determines that you need home health care and sets up a plan for such care; and (4) the services are provided by a Medicare-participating home health agency. Home health benefits can include the full cost of some services, including medical supplies, and 80 percent of the approved amount for durable medical equipment such as hospital beds, walkers, and wheelchairs. Remember that home health care does not include custodial care services.

Medicare also provides services in skilled nursing facilities, but again only in narrowly circumscribed situations. In the case of inpatient skilled care, services are available for a limited time—for up to 100 days in a benefit period after a prior three-day hopitalization—but are fully paid for only 20 days. In 1999 a beneficiary must pay up to $96 for the next 80 days of services and all costs thereafter. Medicare does not pay for long-term or custodial care either at home or in a skilled nursing facility.

Given its deficiencies, if you are a Medicare beneficiary with a chronic illness such as Parkinson's disease, what can you do to improve your chances of gaining access to the health care of your choice? First and foremost, educate yourself and your doctor(s), as necessary, about the annual changes in Medicare. It is impossible to follow the news without being aware that Medicare is always subject to changes, chief among them rising premiums, copayments, and deductibles, along with variations in health maintenance organizations (HMOs) and managed care options. For a person with Parkinson's disease, particular attention should be paid to changes in benefits, such as different requirements for therapies, payment for durable medical equipment, prescription drug coverage, and home health services. You cannot overestimate how important it is to keep abreast of current and proposed regulations! You can perhaps best acquire basic information in an easy-to-understand form through Medicare's own publications, especially the annually updated handbook, "Medicare and You," which also provides names, telephone numbers, and addresses of other resources. For a quick start at deciphering Medicare, call (800) Medicare (633-4227); on the Internet: http://www.hcfa.gov// and www.medicare.gov.

Don't overlook voluntary health organizations and their publications as well as your congressional offices, which can keep you informed on various topics if you tell them of your interests.

One example of a major recent change in Medicare benefits occurred when a new Part C, also known as Medicare+Choice, began in 1999. Part C is intended to offer expanded, standardized, alternative coverage, including managed care, to all Medicare beneficiaries, although Parts A and B will still remain for those who want their fee-for-service.

Before enrolling in a Medicare+Choice alternative, you need to study the program so that you are sure that you understand its risks and benefits versus original Medicare, including limited doctor and hospital selection, premium costs, copayments, and additional benefits, such as outpatient prescription drugs. You also need to understand how to enroll and, if you are not satisfied, how to get out of one plan without jeopardizing your health care coverage. One of the best features of the previously mentioned Medicare handbook is its worksheet for comparing Medicare health plans, including supplemental or Medigap insurance policies. Please note that not all the Medicare+Choice options are available everywhere.

Health Insurance

Whether Medicare-eligible or not, you need to become fully informed about all health insurance options because a diagnosis of Parkinson's disease will greatly complicate your ability to purchase private health insurance on the open market. You must protect whatever coverage you already have while investigating other possible sources of care. For example, you may find that you can continue some or all of your health benefits from your former employer. However, as health care costs increase, some employers are tempted to cut back or curtail promised benefits to former employees. There is ongoing litigation in this area, but as a practical matter—ensuring good health care today—you and your family must be willing to consider reasonable alternatives, such as choosing to be carried on a spouse's insurance plan if possible, even at extra cost. If the person with Parkinson's disease is still working, as a couple you may decide to "overinsure" through double coverage under both employer group plans, if available, to avoid the risk of gaps in coverage, Such stratagems are not always possible as group plans place more restrictions on spousal and dependent coverage, but they should be explored because these plans almost always offer the best benefits at the lowest cost.

Fortunately, changes in age discrimination statutes now require that employers with more than 20 employees who offer group health coverage must also offer the Medicare-eligible worker and/or spouse who is 65 years old or over the same coverage, under the same conditions (with certain exceptions) that are provided to younger workers and spouses. The employee and/or spouse have the right to decide voluntarily whether to have Medicare or the group plan act as primary payer, and, depending on what benefits are offered under the group plan—for example, payment for prescription drugs—this may help them secure more complete coverage. There are other important protections as well as limitations on pension, disability, and related employee benefits under age, tax, and labor statutes and their amendments, such as the Employee Retirement Income Security Act of 1974 (ERISA), which may affect insurance and financial planning. Because ERISA-qualified benefit plans are subject to certain disclosure requirements, an employed or retired worker can contact his plan's administrator and/or the U.S. Department of Labor Pension and Welfare Benefits Administration for information about his specific plan and his general benefit rights under ERISA.

You should also carefully investigate any insurance policy you are considering, even one from a fraternal or professional group with which you may be associated. Investigation means examining the actual policy itself, not simply the advertising brochures and applications. You should compare price and benefits and seek professional counsel from attorneys, doctors, or other knowledgeable advisors, as appropriate, before purchase. Depending on the state in which you reside, you might also consult the State Insurance Commission, which regulates the insurance industry. This agency should be able to provide at least basic information about other kinds of health insurance, Medicare-related or otherwise, that may be available to state residents who have special needs as a result of preexisting conditions or large medical expenses. At least in the case of Medicare, Congress attempted to lessen state-to-state differences through the aforementioned Medicare+Choice in 1999.

Another significant recent insurance reform is the Health Insurance Portability and Accountability Act of 1996 (HIPAA), which guarantees "portability" of group health insurance when you lose or change jobs, even if you have a preexisting medical condition or health history; it also covers dependents.

Insurers and employers cannot have different eligibility rules that discriminate against workers based on their health status or history. All workers who are eligible for a medical plan must be offered enrollment at the same price, irrespective of their health status.

The HIPAA limits exclusions for preexisting conditions for new enrollees to a maximun of 12 months for a condition that was treated or diagnosed in the six months before enrollment (newborns, adopted children, and pregnancies are exempt from a waiting period).

In general, workers who had health insurance at their previous job are immediately eligible for coverage at their next job if the new employer provides insurance. The 12-month waiting period must be reduced by the period of continuous coverage before their enrollment. Continuous coverage means coverage without a lapse of more than 63 days. Employers can still deny benefits during a probationary period, (e.g., 90 days). But continuous coverage can go on; the employer cannot use a probationary period to subject the new employee to a break in coverage and trigger a full 12-month waiting period.

The HIPAA also requires a special enrollment period for employees who declined the employer's plan because they had other coverage (e.g., through a spouse's plan). If that coverage ends, they have 30 days to enroll in the employer's plan.

With some exceptions, insurers who sell policies to small employers (those with two to 50 employees) in a state must offer group benefits to all small employers in that state. Insurers would have to renew the policies unless there was fraud or nonpayment of premiums.

The HIPAA provides some important protections for individuals who leave a group plan and want to purchase their own policy. Generally, insurers cannot refuse to cover eligible individuals or impose exclusions for preexisting conditions. An eligible individual is someone who has had 18 months of continuous coverage, most recently in a group plan; is not eligible for other group coverage; and has exhausted COBRA or other continuation coverage.

Insurers can limit the number of policies offered, but they have to be representative of those offered to other workers, not just individuals leaving group plans. In those states that have been certified by the Secretary of Health and Human Services to have guaranteed availability to individuals leaving group plans, such as state risk pools or open enrollment insurers such as Blue Cross/Blue Shield, insurers are not required to offer individual policies.

Contact your State Insurance Commission or Board of Insurance for information about what is available in your state. You should do this irrespective of whatever information you are given by your employer.

The HIPAA started a four-year trial period in 1997 for a limited number of individuals with high-deductible insurance plans (no lower than $1,500 for an individual; $3,000 for a family) to set up medical savings accounts (MSAs) using tax-deductible contributions. Money can be withdrawn from MSAs without tax penalties to pay for medical expenses, and you can save what is not spent. The trial population includes workers at companies with 50 or fewer employees, self-employed individuals, and the uninsured (who must buy catastrophic coverage). Medical savings accounts are also available to people on Medicare. Congress may vote to extend or amend eligibility requirements at the end of the four-year trial period. For more information, contact the U.S. Department of Labor at (202) 219-8776 or see www.dol.gov/dol/pwba.

Another possible source of treatment is the military health care system, which provides a variety of benefits, including long-term nursing care and adult daycare services, to active duty personnel, service veterans, retirees, spouses, ex-spouses, and children. Eligibility for particular benefits is dependent on such factors as a claimant's military status (veteran with a service-related disability versus nondisabled veteran or retiree), the type and location of the facility at which the treatment is sought (military versus civilian), and the availability of beds and/or staff. The Civilian Health and Medical Program of the Uniformed Services (CHAMPUS) is a medical plan for U.S. military retirees, spouses, certain ex-spouses, widows(ers), and children, among others. Although it is subject to many qualifications and restrictions, this program may be available even though a qualified (and registered) beneficiary has not used it for many years and/or has access to other sources of coverage. In most cases, CHAMPUS coverage ends when a person becomes eligible for Medicare; the previously mentioned protections of the age discrimination statutes do not apply for this program.

Medicaid

Medicaid is the federal/state health program intended for the very poor—not only mothers and children, but also the indigent aged, blind, and disabled. People who are eligible for SSI payments in most states are also entitled to receive Medicaid medical benefits and, unlike Medicare, there is no 29-month waiting period before coverage begins. Because eligibility standards and benefits vary from state to state, anyone who thinks he may be eligible must investigate the requirements for Medicaid in his state of residence. This might best be done by checking several sources because requirements change frequently, and even people who routinely deal with the program are often not always fully informed about current regulations. Sources include the state and/or local Medicaid offices, the offices of SSA, the national or regional offices of the Health Care Financing Administration (HCFA) (the federal agency that regulates both Medicare and Medicaid), voluntary health agencies that deal with the elderly and/or patients with Parkinson's disease, and state and local health or consumer advocacy groups. If you have questions that range beyond the strictly routine, you will have to go above the level of the clerical workers who take initial inquiries.

Medicaid provides many of the same benefits as Medicare, plus others, including eyeglasses and prescription drugs, depending on the state. The key benefit it offers that Medicare does not is nursing home care. Although some people with Parkinson's disease may be eligible for a wide range of Medicaid benefits because they are indigent, aged, and/or disabled, the more pressing concern for most is the possibility that they may need nursing home care.

Medicaid nursing home care is offered in every state, but not in every U.S. territory. As with all Medicaid services, you must have extremely low income and limited resources (assets) in order to be eligible. But the requirements for nursing home qualification are more generous than those for other Medicaid programs. There are also important exceptions to its income and asset rules.

Depending on the state, you may not have more than approximately $2,000 in assets and $1,500 in monthly income. This income threshold is based on a formula tied to SSI levels, which, depending on the state, may automatically change annually or may only be altered by action of the state's legislature. Income and asset rules for married couples are far more liberal as a result of the Medicare Catastrophic Coverage Act of 1988. Although most of this act was later repealed, the Medicaid portions, including the so-called spousal impoverishment provisions, continue in effect. Income attributed to the institutionalized spouse must meet state eligibility levels. In almost every state, however, the spouse who remains at home may keep his own income and, in some cases, a basic living allowance from the institutionalized spouse's income. This allowance is derived from a formula that, again, has some variation from state to state but is meant to bear a relationship to official poverty levels and family income and needs. The Act also expanded significantly the value of the assets a couple may keep and still qualify for Medicaid. They may now keep a minimum of $81,960 in assets.

In addition to these rules, states exempt outright certain kinds of income and property from eligibility consideration for both married and unmarried individuals. Exemptions commonly include the residence to which the institutionalized person expects to return (even when this is a remote possibility, although in some states this exemption is of limited duration only) or where the spouse resides, a certain amount of personal or household property, burial plots, some burial costs, wedding rings, and the limited value of a car (no limits in some cases). Other income can also be exempt: a monthly allowance for the institutionalized person for personal needs (at least a minimum of $30); the amount needed to pay for some medical expenses that are nonreimbursed from other sources (according to complicated formulas, this can help people "spend-down" or reduce income to Medicaid-qualifying levels); income received because a person is a member of a certain group (for example, particular American Indian tribes, Holocaust survivors receiving reparations from Germany); certain government services, allowances, and payments (housing, food, energy, emergency assistance, and so forth); and some income in cash or kind (e.g., food) produced from certain property. Again, such exemptions for either income or assets depend on a particular state's Medicaid regulations and can be much more extensive (or limited) than those listed.

Despite these exemptions, the fear of many people clearly remains that they and their spouses may be impoverished before they can qualify for needed long-term care. At the same time, because of inalienable pension benefits or other income that put them over their state's eligibility limits, some people fear that they may never be able to spend-down to qualifying levels; if they need nursing home care, they will have to find facilities that they can afford as private-pay residents. As a result of these requirements, many people have sought to devise a way to protect assets or, conversely, to lower income in order to qualify for Medicaid benefits. This has provoked some controversy in recent years.

People who would not hesitate to claim any tax deduction to which they are entitled often express outrage at the thought of Medicaid-eligibility planning, at least when they or their family members are not the ones doing the planning! Yet Medicaid rules governing assets do allow for some flexibility.

If there is a concern about income levels, sometimes retirement benefits can be structured so that, for example, benefits are paid in a lump sum, thereby giving the beneficiary more alternatives for future financial planning. Or income to one spouse may be lowered by electing to increase survivorship benefits to the other. These kinds of maneuvers are not possible with many retirement plans, and in any case they must be exercised in a timely manner, usually upon retirement. As earlier noted, according to Medicaid formulas, even people with "excess" income may still be able to spend-down to qualifying levels either permanently or for some period of time when they incur certain large medical expenses.

It is beyond the scope of this chapter to describe the various transfer and trust arrangements that might be used to preserve assets and qualify for government programs such as nursing home Medicaid. The warning must always be made that the rules governing these programs are subject to change. But it is also the case that you can often plan ahead to prepare for future needs. The best way to do this is to seek counsel from lawyers who are experienced in trust matters and disability. In addition to attorneys certified in trust and probate (check local and state bar association listings), another possible source of expertise is the National Elder Law Attorneys Association, Inc., at 1604 N. Country Club Rd., Tucson, AZ 85716, (520) 881-4005; http://www.naela.org, for attorneys in your state. This is important because Medicaid, a federal/state program, has some variation in requirements from state to state. Even in those states that have a strict income limit for eligibility, a knowledgeable practitioner may be able to structure your estate, for example, through the use of a Miller trust or a supplemental needs trust, so that you can in fact qualify to receive Medicaid nursing home care.

In general, transfers of property made within the so-called "look-back" period are subject to penalty, meaning Medicaid eligibility will be lost for a certain number of months according to formulas that vary from state to state based on average costs of private-pay nursing home care. The look-back period ends on the date a Medicaid application is filed and begins 60 months earlier for property transferred to or from most trusts; 36 months for all other transfers. There are many, many exceptions to these general rules, including, for example, transfer of a home to a spouse or permanently disabled child. Once again, expert counsel is essential. You should also consider whether Medicaid qualification is in your best interest based on your income, assets, and the availablility of other programs in your state such as community-based home care. That is, there may be other alternatives, government or private pay, that will give you the services you need without your having to undertake drastic qualifying measures.

Financial advisors may be able to offer some estate planning help. Be advised, however, that even agents who claim to be "independent" may in fact be selling something such as annuities, mutual funds, or insurance, and earning their fees through commissions.

Other people in addition to the recipient of nursing home Medicaid should be involved in any planning and implementation process. For example, your spouse may be involved in the transferring and restructuring of marital income and property by converting nonexempt assets into exempt assets. Health care professionals who deal with Parkinson's disease should also be informed of patient and family concerns and be able to offer advice about possible treatment and care needs. Because custodial care, either at home or in a facility, is often necessary as a result of this condition, you should make every effort to educate yourself and your doctors as early in the disease process as possible. This may mean you will have to change doctors if they do not seem knowledgeable or interested in your problems. It may also mean researching various sources of long-term care information such as local home health agencies, nursing homes, voluntary health organizations (e.g., the Parkinson's disease societies), support groups, the Internet, and the HCFA.

Can a person with a diagnosis of Parkinson's disease simply purchase a long-term care policy and thereby avoid the problem of Medicaid qualification altogether? Unfortunately, because it is a reasonable expectation that a person with Parkinson's disease may need such care, it is extremely unlikely that you could buy a policy, even one that specifically excludes the diagnosis. Once again, however, if you should have access to such a benefit through your employer, you must determine eligibility requirements and make sure that you do not lose any conversion rights if they exist. You should also make absolutely certain that Parkinson's disease is a covered condition; sometimes insurance companies try to avoid liability for conditions such as Parkinson's disease or Alzheimer's disease under policy exclusions for "organic brain syndrome" or similar diagnostic descriptions, This kind of benefit is still fairly unusual but not unheard of with some large employers and union contracts, especially those offering so-called cafeteria plans with a varied menu of benefits to choose from.

WILLS, TRUSTS, POWERS OF ATTORNEY, AND OTHER ESTATE MATTERS

People with Parkinson's disease and their families are not unique in having an interest in wills, trusts, powers of attorney, and other estate and probate matters. But because of the illness, as well as advancing age, these issues should assume greater importance to you. This is especially true if you are concerned about spend-down and Medicaid, competency, the use (or misuse) of heroic medical efforts, and the like. You and your spouse may never have gotten around to executing a will, or you may have questions about altering your wills in light of changed circumstances. Although the mere diagnosis of Parkinson's disease should not cause immediate alarm, there is no reason to procrastinate in resolving these matters. As with some of the issues already discussed, prudent planning can lessen future problems and quiet current worries.

No one is required to have a will; the laws of intestate succession dictate how property is to pass to heirs, and this is often exactly how people would divide their property anyway. A will is simply a formal plan of disposition of your estate that designates who will handle this transfer (the executor), how debts and taxes will be paid, and which beneficiaries will receive property from your estate. Upon your death, the will is filed with the probate court, which oversees the disposition. Despite misconceptions to the contrary, in most cases the probating of a will is neither costly nor complicated. As family circumstances change, you may want to set out different arrangements. Provisions in a will might include making a charitable bequest, leaving more or less property to certain individuals, or even removing some property from your estate so that it can be handled outside the probate system for tax or other reasons.

Although a will is probably the simplest and least expensive means for distributing your property, it is not the only one. Individual retirement accounts (IRAs), survivorship accounts, and life insurance are common examples of property that is beyond probate, meaning that it will automatically pass to the survivor or designated beneficiary with no court supervision.

If you have enough property to justify the expense of creation and administration, a trust may be an appropriate instrument for distributing your assets. There are many kinds of trusts that have various advantages and disadvantages, depending on individual circumstances. In addition to the costs of setting it up and running it, a trust may result in some tax liabilities. Contrary to popular misconceptions, a trust does not insulate its creator from creditors. But under the right circumstances, trusts can provide an effective means for accomplishing certain goals.

One kind of trust, a testamentary trust, is written into the will itself and comes into effect upon the testator's death. The property going into this kind of trust is handled according to the provisions contained in the will. The reasons for creating a testamentary trust may include certain tax advantages, a desire to carry out some charitable goal, or to provide a means by which to regulate the distribution of your property over time, for example, a spendthrift trust for irresponsible beneficiaries.

Another kind of trust is a lifetime trust. As the name suggests, it is created during the lifetime of the trustor (creator of the trust). The trustor may wish to maintain control over certain assets during his lifetime but still avoid probate or the effort and expense of a guardianship, for example, for a minor child's estate or that of an incompetent beneficiary. A lifetime trust may be set up to come into existence upon some future occurrence. One estate planning mechanism along these lines could be a revocable lifetime trust coupled with an appropriate power of attorney created in advance of a disabling event to allow the trustee (the person who is designated to manage the trust assets and income according to the terms of the trust) more flexibility than he would have with either instrument alone.

A trust may also be created to operate in the event of the incompetency of its trustor. This event might be anticipated by some patients with Parkinson's disease who do not want the expense, publicity, or difficulty of a guardianship where every action the guardian performs must be approved by the probate court. Of course, incompetency is not an inevitable outcome of Parkinson's disease, but some people with Parkinson's disease do become mentally incompetent as a result of drug side effects, the progression of the disease itself, or possibly some other unrelated medical condition. Some people may not suffer a cognitive or mental loss, but they may simply be too physically incapacitated to handle their business and personal affairs or to make decisions about their own medical care.

Issues of incompetency can be handled by a mechanism less complicated than a trust, namely, a power of attorney and/or a directive to physicians (sometimes referred to as an "advance" directive, but better known as a living will and regulated under a state right to die or natural death act). A power of attorney can designate another person to make business or financial decisions for its grantor. Depending on its provisions, the power to make these decisions can be very specific or very broad and may be written to become effective upon the grantor's physical or mental incapacity (a "durable" power of attorney).

In many states a power of attorney for health care may be available to allow another person to make certain health care decisions on behalf of the grantor under circumstances specifically defined by statute. A "directive" is somewhat similar to this in that the grantor instructs health care workers to provide (or withhold) some treatments when the grantor is unable to speak for himself, and usually only for terminal conditions. The appointment of a health care representative (sometimes called a health proxy) is another way to delegate the authority to make certain treatment decisions, subject to statutory requirements and the terms of the agreement granting the consent to health care. This kind of agreement, which is somewhat similar to both a directive and a power of attorney for health care, may be more commonly used for ordinary, as opposed to life-threatening, medical care. Like the health power, it is not recognized in every state and, depending on the jurisdiction, may need to be used in conjunction with other legal papers.

All of these documents can be canceled by the grantor. They are governed by statutes in each state, which, depending on the particular statute, may mean that they are invalid unless the grantor has strictly complied with all requirements—the proper witnessing, filing, disclosures, and so on. Even when valid, it is often difficult to have powers of attorney accepted by some third parties, such as banks, which may be concerned about their own liability if they act on them. Another point to consider is *where* the grantor of the powers expects them to be enforced. Because there is as yet no uniformity in the statutes from state to state, a power that complies with the law in one jurisdiction may be invalid if used in another, or it may have to comply with certain specific requirements if it is to be effective for control of some kinds of property, such as real estate.

Nevertheless, there is good reason for the person with Parkinson's disease to consider the use of powers of attorney and directives in certain situations. For example, if you plan to enter a hospital for extended treatment, you may want to have a directive and/or a durable power of attorney for health care properly drawn up, executed, and/or filed. There may be strictly defined "exceptions" to the need for written directives. For instance, you may make an oral or nonwritten directive (for example, eye blinking to indicate his desires), or a spouse or adult children or some other interested party as set out in the pertinent statutes may be permitted to make decisions for an incapacitated or incompetent person. Note that in all such situations, the statutes still require the proper witnessing and professional medical concurrence, Therefore, to avoid confusion and delay, the written "medical" powers may be ones to keep in place more or less permanently. Likewise, you may think you need to have a valid durable power of attorney on hand as well. In the case of incompetency coupled with nursing home confinement, this could allow the person designated in the power of attorney to begin to manage property immediately.

One must be of sound mind to create a valid power of attorney or living will. Under the recently enacted Patient Self-Determination Act of OBRA 1990, institutions that receive Medicare and/or Medicaid funding, including hospitals, HMOs, home health agencies, hospices, and nursing homes, are required to inform adult patients/residents about their right to limit treatment and care through the use of these documents. At the time they become subject to care, patients must be given both a written description of their state's laws governing these rights and the written policies of the health provider (providers without written policies will have to develop them). Providers will also have the responsibility of noting the patient's directive status in his medical records but cannot condition care on the basis of whether he has executed any particular document. Notwithstanding this law change, which seeks to create national procedures for patient consent to treatments, the problem still remains that by the time a person is admitted for care he may no longer possess the requisite mental capacity to execute any valid instrument. Therefore, you should at least begin to think about issues of incapacity and incompetency and how you can minimize some of the consequences.

Directives, powers of attorney, wills, and trusts are mostly governed by state laws. The statutory requirements are strictly construed, so that even a simple error can invalidate the whole document. For this reason, you should consult an attorney experienced in estate matters to answer your questions, advise on alternative planning strategies, and draft any documents. Simple wills, trusts, and powers should not be unduly expensive. But it is not wise to cut corners with mass-market form books or inexperienced counsel because the outcome may be unfortunate.

DEBT ISSUES

The costs of medical treatments, therapy, and, if necessary, long-term custodial care can become financially ruinous. In addition to these direct costs of Parkinson's disease, the normal expenses of life continue— housing, credit cards, auto payments, insurance, and personal obligations. Therefore, the standard advice for anyone to be prudent about your spending habits is made all the more compelling when the additional burden of chronic and progressive illness is added. With nursing home costs for private-pay patients now averaging well over $40,000 annually in many parts of the country, it is a rare family whose financial position is invulnerable, even if your assets are substantial. Your family should begin to organize its financial affairs soon after diagnosis. This can be simply tallying assets and liabilities and devising a monthly budget, or it may include seeking professional advice for investment and tax planning.

Sometimes dealing with debts is the major financial issue for a person with Parkinson's disease and his family. This is especially true if, for example, one spouse has had to stop working because of the disease or if medical or other personal expenses have grown out of control. Fortunately, you can take steps to manage your debts. These include such basic actions as discussing payment problems with creditors and, if possible, working out new payment procedures. You can also use the services of

professional debt counselors or attorneys to create a payment plan or creditor's arrangement.

Such an arrangement is not always possible. A creditor may attempt
to repossess secured property—a house or car—or may file suit for collection of a delinquent debt. There may be defenses to such an action, but
the key point is not to ignore your obligations and thereby risk com-
pounding your problems. You are not required to retain an attorney to
handle such disputes, but you will be at a severe disadvantage if you do
not have representation. Even if a creditor obtains a judgment against you
or forecloses on property, you are not without some protections. These
differ from state to state, and some states are more lenient to debtors. In
no state may you be jailed for debts (with a limited exception for parents
who do not pay child support). In all states, however, garnishment can
occur for some kinds of obligations. This is a legal procedure whereby a
debtor's property that is in the hands of a third party is taken by a creditor to satisfy a debt. Many states also allow garnishment for child
support and other kinds of debts, including consumer debts, although
there are varying limits on the percentage of a paycheck that may be
seized.

Certain of your property is exempt from some collection efforts. In
many states the homestead (your home) may not be taken to satisfy a debt
(with the exception of the mortgage or other obligations for which the
house and land are collateral). In general, pensions, including disability
pensions, cannot be taken by a creditor. IRA accounts are also protected
from seizure. The Internal Revenue Service can seize almost any property,
however, and state and local governments can also get judgments against
a person who owes taxes and fees and can take homestead property to
satisfy such debts.

If debt problems threaten to become overwhelming, you may need
to seek the protection of the federal bankruptcy laws. A Chapter 7 is a liq-
uidation of assets. You can choose homestead exemptions but give up
nonexempt assets, with the proceeds being paid to creditors under the
direction of the court. Most debts can be discharged. One common reason
for choosing a Chapter 7 is the size of the unsecured debt—extremely
large medical bills, for example.

Chapter 13 allows you to pay your debts in monthly installments.
You must have a regular income so that you will be able to make consis-

tent payments under the repayment plan. By this definition, even an individual operating a small business or a person receiving welfare or other "nonwage" income can qualify. Spouses can file separately or jointly. There is also a debt ceiling for people who file a Chapter 13; for an individual or spouses filing jointly, the unsecured debt total cannot exceed $250,000; the secured debt, $750,000.

You are protected, with some qualifications, from collection efforts of creditors while the plan of repayment is in effect. You submit a part of your future income to the bankruptcy trustee under the repayment plan approved by the bankruptcy court.

Although some plans provide for 100 percent repayment to creditors, many do not. There is often a guideline percentage that the court follows in approving plans—approximately 70 percent in some bankruptcy districts—but there is some variation based on the financial circumstances of each debtor. At the end of the plan, the debtor will be discharged (released) from most debts.

Certain debts are not discharged by bankruptcy. Alimony, spousal maintenance, child support, and most taxes are not dischargeable, although under a Chapter 13 plan some of this past debt may be paid over an extended period. Debts arising through fraud or the false representations of the debtor are not dischargeable. Debts arising from a debtor's malicious, willful, or tortious misconduct are not dischargeable. Debts that are unscheduled, that is, not listed in the bankruptcy papers, are usually not discharged.

Filing bankruptcy automatically stops collection activity by creditors except through the bankruptcy court. Even short of filing bankruptcy, you can be protected from extreme harassment by creditors. Debt collection practices are regulated by both federal and state laws, principally by the federal Fair Debt Collection Practices Act and individual state statutes. These laws apply mostly to consumer debts, as does the federal law. The federal act regulates collection agents and their practices. Common law tort theories relating to privacy, defamation, and infliction of mental distress may apply to unfair collection practices.

Some of the prohibited practices under these acts are threats of criminal action if the debt is not paid, calling employers and discussing the debtor's debt with them, phoning or visiting the debtor at odd hours, making abusive, harassing calls to the debtor or his family, or continuing to harass the debtor personally after the creditor or his agent has been advised that a debt is in dispute. These acts provide penalties for violators, including costs, attorney's fees, and, in some cases, cancellation of the debt itself.

TAXES AND TAX PLANNING

Parkinson's disease provides no dispensation from concerns about taxes, and you should begin to think carefully about the tax consequences of changes that may occur in your financial and medical situation as a result of the illness.

As long as you continue to work, the earned income from your job will be taxed as it always has been. Likewise, temporary or permanent private disability pension income will also be taxed with the following exception: in some cases, disability income from an employer-provided plan for which the beneficiary has paid some premiums may be all or partially tax-free. SSDI payments are not taxable unless income from other sources—a spouse's job, income from investments, and so forth—brings an individual's total income to more than $25,000 a year; $32,000 for a couple. After this point, up to 85 percent of these payments are taxed for an individual with income over $25,000; $34,000 for a couple. A recipient of either private or government disability income pays no Social Security taxes (FICA) on these benefits.

The costs of medical care, whether directly related to Parkinson's disease or not, may be eligible for a tax deduction after total medical expenses exceed 7.5 percent of adjusted gross income—that is, the individual's or family's total income less certain deductions such as IRA contributions, but before considering itemized deductions, such as home mortgage interest or charitable contributions.

The practical effect of this limit, especially for someone with Parkinson's disease who is still working or who has a working spouse, can be that little or no tax benefit results because the deduction is based only on those costs that are not reimbursed by insurance. For example, if you and your spouse together have an income of $30,000 a year, you could itemize only that portion of your medical bills above $2,250 that was not covered by insurance. This medical deduction is available only if total itemized deductions are more than a base amount—including not only medical expenses over this 7.5 percent limit but also others, such as interest and/or charitable contributions. In 1998 this base amount was $7,100 for a married couple.

Notwithstanding these limitations, there are several significant ways that you can get some tax relief by planning ahead. First, the limits just described are set on an annual basis; the taxpayer receives the deduction for allowable medical expenses paid in a given year. Therefore, if you can choose the year in which a bill is to be paid, you should try to pay it in a year when you will have other medical costs that can be lumped together to exceed the minimum limits. This can best be illustrated with doctor or hospital bills that occur around the end of one year or at the beginning of the next year. You would be well advised in this situation to discuss with your doctor(s) and hospital business office the possibility of scheduling payments so as to provide the maximum tax benefit. For tax purposes "payment" means writing a check to the health care provider. If you borrow money to pay your medical bills or pay by credit card, the deduction occurs in the year in which the original bill is settled, not when the debt is paid to the bank or credit card company. If you later receive an insurance reimbursement for a bill you paid and for which you took a deduction, you may have to pay tax on the reimbursement in the year you receive it.

Many people are not aware that they are entitled to deductions for the reasonable costs of treating their medical conditions, not just the direct and obvious costs like doctor or hospital expenses. These costs may include prescription drugs (there is a separate limit), some of the premiums for medical insurance, and transportation costs in seeking health care, including auto mileage. Of particular importance if you must travel out of town to receive specialized treatment, these costs could include airfares, hotels, and other related travel expenses.

Medical equipment, such as wheelchairs, scooters, crutches, and so on, and home improvements, including ramps, guardrails, and special bathroom fixtures that help you deal with your condition, may be deductible. More expensive improvements, such as an elevator or a swimming pool for physical therapy, may also be deductible. However, in the case of such major improvements, you and your doctor must agree that there is medical justification for the expenditure. The amount of the tax deduction for some types of improvement will be reduced by any increase in the resale value of your home. Cosmetic embellishments, such as land-scaping, repainting, and redecorating, cannot be deducted. To help support the claimed deduction, you are well advised to seek a written estimate by an experienced realtor or appraiser as to any increase in resale value.

Another area for medical deduction is nursing care provided in the home. This may be deductible even if it is not provided by a full-time registered nurse. Maid service is not deductible, but it is legitimate to deduct a portion of the cost if the person who provides housekeeping services also performs nursing care.

Sometimes people are concerned that taking what they perceive to be large or unusual deductions will increase the odds of a tax audit. Although this is possible, medical deductions are not considered to be especially risky by many tax professionals because taxpayers generally have good proof in the form of bills, canceled checks, and health records. If you and/or your health provider have concerns about the validity of a deduction, you should seek the counsel of a CPA or tax attorney before incurring a large expense. Your accountant or attorney should be able to offer advice on the proof required and, as appropriate, how to structure payment.

Although no amount of knowledge or planning can ensure a perfect solution to all the nonmedical problems of an illness such as Parkinson's disease, it is a rare problem indeed that cannot be managed more effectively if you have some foresight, coupled with good and timely professional help.

PART IV

Epilogue

Past Perspectives
and Future Horizons

The history of Parkinson's disease is one of the best illustrations of the multitude of paths to scientific discovery and advancement. The gradual development of ideas combined with laborious observation and experimentation over many years, unusual insights leading to sudden leaps, natural experiments, and accidental discovery, have all marked the history of the disorder and have played a role in our current knowledge. Because past achievements mold the shape of future advances, we outline here the major landmarks before moving on to consider what promise future research horizons hold.

THE HISTORY OF PARKINSON'S DISEASE

References to the symptoms of the illness in ancient texts suggest that Parkinson's disease has probably existed for centuries. However, it was not until 1817 that the various symptoms were described together as forming a single illness by James Parkinson.

The first of the six children of John and Mary Parkinson, James was born in 1755. His father was a pharmacist and surgeon who worked in Shoreditch, then a village near London, where the family also lived. James studied medicine and then joined his father as a general practitioner, and he too both lived and worked in Shoreditch. He married Mary Daler, with whom he had six children, four of whom survived, and one who became a physician. Besides his essay on the "shaking palsy," the name for Parkinson's disease at the time, he produced a number of other publications. He was also a political activist and is described as a social reformer. He died in 1824.

An Essay on the Shaking Palsy, which was 66 pages long, was published in 1817. In the first chapter, the history of the illness is outlined, a definition is given, and six patients are described, not all of whom had been personally examined by Parkinson. The symptoms are described in more detail in Chapter II. Chapter III deals with distinguishing the "shaking palsy" from other disorders, and Chapters IV and V, respectively, cover possible causes and the methods of treatment.

Parkinson had the mark of a true scientist. In the preface, acknowledging the hypothetical nature of his statements about the illness, he wrote that "mere conjecture takes the place of experiment." Two of Parkinson's major achievements are evident from the essay. The first is the fact that, as already mentioned, although the disorder may have existed for many years, it was not recognized as a separate disease until the publication of the essay, at the beginning of which he wrote that the illness "has not yet obtained a place in the classification of nosologists; some have regarded its characteristic symptoms as distinct and different diseases, and others have given its name to diseases differing essentially from it." Second, Parkinson was an astute observer, and his descriptions of the age of onset, the slow mode of onset, and the progressive and chronic nature of the disorder, as well as of the symptoms, are still valid today. This is remarkable because he had at his disposal none of the medical tools or tests that are now commonly used.

Parkinson mainly concentrated on describing tremor. The other main symptoms—bradykinesia, rigidity, balance difficulties, and walking problems—were highlighted by Jean-Martin Charcot, the first professor of neurology at the Salpêtrière hospital in Paris. In the course of his famous Tuesday lectures, which were published in 1877, Charcot stated that the term *paralysis agitans,* or *shaking palsy,* was inadequate because the shaking or tremor was absent in some cases and there was no evidence of palsy or paralysis in any case. He proposed that instead, since James

Parkinson had provided the first detailed description of it as a separate illness, it should be known as the *maladie de Parkinson*, or Parkinson's disease.

Paralysis agitans was also considered in detail in William Gowers's *Manual of Diseases of the Nervous System,* which was published in 1886. Gowers, the prominent British neurologist working at the time at what is now the National Hospital for Neurology and Neurosurgery, included in his observations on the amplitude and frequency of tremor the fact that tremor could remain confined to one side of the body for many years but then spread to the other. Problems with balance and walking were also reviewed. However, Gowers placed more emphasis on rigidity, the monotonous speech, and the expressionless face.

The epidemic of *encephalitis lethargica* in 1918, which lasted until 1926, gave rise to a large number of chronically disabled people with parkinsonism. As described earlier, the illness started with flulike symptoms, sleepiness, paralysis of eye movements, rigidity, slowness of movement, and behavioral changes. Approximately 40 percent of sufferers died in the acute phase. Those who survived recovered to some extent, but after some years they entered the chronic phase, with all the predominant symptoms of parkinsonism. These showed some similarities to, as well as differences from, those of Parkinson's disease as described by Parkinson, Charcot, and Gowers. This suffering on a vast scale served to demonstrate that parkinsonian symptoms could have more than one cause, creating the concept of parkinson*ism* and paving the way for the distinction between classic Parkinson's disease and secondary parkinsonism, and the subsequent refinement of diagnostic categories from the 1960s onward.

Neither Parkinson nor Charcot knew precisely which area of the brain was affected in Parkinson's disease and, as noted earlier, it was not until postmortem examinations of the brain became possible that any progress was made. In 1893 in Paris, a patient with unilateral Parkinson's disease was found to have a small tumor pressing on the basal ganglia. So attention now focused on the basal ganglia as a possible site of damage in Parkinson's disease. A year later Édouard Brissaud, a French professor of neurology, suggested that damage to the substantia nigra in the brainstem, which has many close connections with the basal ganglia, might cause

Parkinson's disease. The first major discovery confirming this was made by Tretiakoff as part of his doctoral thesis. On the basis of the postmortem examination of nine patients with Parkinson's disease, Tretiakoff confirmed the loss of pigmented cells of the substantia nigra and the presence of the spherical bodies previously described by Frederick Lewy (Lewy bodies) in those cells that remained.

In 1957 Montagu discovered the neurotransmitter dopamine in the brain. During 1957–1959 the Swedish professor Arvid Carlsson demonstrated that dopamine was concentrated in the areas of the brain considered to be affected in Parkinson's disease. In experiments with rats, injections of the drug reserpine resulted in signs of parkinsonism and the reduction of a number of neurotransmitters, including dopamine, in their brains. When the rats were injected with levodopa, the symptoms of parkinsonism disappeared. In 1960 Ehringer and Hornykiewicz demonstrated the depletion of dopamine in the basal ganglia of the brains of people with Parkinson's disease. This was followed in 1961 by the administration of levodopa to patients by Birkmayer and Hornykiewicz as well as Barbeau, which started a new era in the medical treatment of the disorder. However, it was not until 1967 and the publication of George Cotzias's results of administering levodopa in larger doses that the therapeutic revolution started.

As described in Chapter 3, the first drawback of levodopa therapy was that many people developed nausea and vomiting because of dopaminergic stimulation of the vomiting centers in the brain. The development and introduction of selective peripheral decarboxylase inhibitors such as carbidopa (in Sinemet) and benserazide (in Madopar) overcame this problem in most cases. The next therapeutic advance was the designing of synthetic directly acting dopamine agonists such as bromocriptine, pergolide, and lisuride. Later, more specific dopamine agonists (i.e., pramipexole and ropinirole) were developed and approved for general use. This was followed by medication such as selegiline hydrochloride (Deprenyl), aiming to prolong the duration of dopamine action in the brain by inhibiting monoamine oxidase B, which causes the breakdown of dopamine.

The 1950s also saw another revolution: the development and use of neuroleptic medication for the treatment of the more severe mental disorders such as schizophrenia and manic-depressive psychosis. Although this class of medication effectively controlled the target mental illness, a frequent side effect was the development of parkinsonism, which could be reversed by withdrawing the medication. The report of such chemically induced and reversible parkinsonism led to predictions that the cause of Parkinson's disease would soon be discovered.

In the late 1970s and 1980s the "MPTP story" unfolded, and from that "natural experiment" a number of significant ideas have emerged:

❖ Using MPTP (1-methyl-4-phenyl-1,2,3,6-tetrahydropyridine) an "animal model" of parkinsonism has been developed: by inducing parkinsonism in animals it is possible to conduct controlled experiments and trials of new medications before their use in clinical trials on patients.

❖ As described in Chapter 1, the MPTP story has opened up a whole new approach to the study of the possible causes of Parkinson's disease. It focused attention on impairment of mitochondrial mechanisms and the possible causal role of environmental or endogenous toxins.

❖ The protective effect of certain types of monoamine oxidase inhibitor medication against MPTP in laboratory animals led to the study of the possible neuroprotective effect of this class of medication in Parkinson's disease.

The MPTP story illustrates the fact that scientific advance does not necessarily occur at a steady pace, but may take the form of occasional harelike leaps interspersed with periods of crawling.

THE WAY AHEAD

This short history of Parkinson's disease is convincing evidence that we have come a long way since 1817, when James Parkinson published his essay. In fact, Parkinson's disease is unique among neurologic disorders in that during the last 30 years research has revolutionized our understanding of the disorder and its treatment. The landmarks in this route of discovery were:

1960s   the discovery of the degeneration of dopamine-producing cells in the substantia nigra as the cause of the symptoms of Parkinson's disease

1970s   the discovery of dopamine replacement therapy with levodopa

1980s   the battle against the long-term complications of levodopa therapy

What will the 1990s be remembered for? We can spot important landmarks: brain implantation of fetal tissue, preventive therapy, important research into the causes of the disease, and the development of diagnostic testing equipment such as by positron emission tomography (PET) to detect the illness before the symptoms become manifest. What is particularly reassuring is that research into Parkinson's disease is at the top of the agenda in many fields of neuroscience. This is partly because progress in Parkinson's disease research also constitutes pioneering work in relation to our understanding of brain function. It is said that nothing succeeds like success! As a consequence of the relatively steady progress in unraveling the mysteries of the disorder that has occurred in the last 30 years, research into Parkinson's disease attracts a large number of first-rate scientists from a variety of disciplines. Research now and in the near future will take many different routes, and the journey along several of them is likely to prove fruitful.

The Search for the Cause

The foremost question in the mind of every person with Parkinson's disease is "Will there be a cure in my lifetime?" To find a cure, we have to find the cause. In the search for the cause, the main question posed by scientists is "What causes the degeneration process in Parkinson's disease?" Two sets of theories are currently dominant, and research effort centers on these. The first is the possibility that Parkinson's disease may be the result of a slow-acting viral infection; the second concerns the possible role of exposure to an environmental toxin.

If we knew what starts the degeneration process that results in dopamine deficiency in Parkinson's disease, it might be possible to halt it or even prevent it from occurring in the first place. Therefore, research into the cause of the disease goes hand in hand with finding ways to detect presymptomatic or early Parkinson's disease and the development of neuroprotective therapy to halt its progression.

Elderly people often exhibit in mild form some of the symptoms that are reminiscent of Parkinson's disease, such as slowness of movement, stooped posture and shorter strides, and a greater number of falls. Given that some of the pathologic and chemical changes that occur in the brain in the process of aging are similar to those found in Parkinson's disease, and because age is the most definite predisposing factor for the disorder, research to explore the hypothesis that Parkinson's is an accelerated aging process may also be worthwhile.

The Search for Presymptomatic and Diagnostic Markers

From research findings, we know that symptoms of Parkinson's disease become evident only after striatal dopamine is depleted by approximately 80 percent. This means that a number of years intervene between the start of the degenerative process and the first appearance of the symptoms. In light of this gradual process of dopamine depletion, scientists have been eager to develop tests that would allow them to identify the presymptomatic state. This has been coupled with efforts to develop tests that would allow reliable diagnosis of classic Parkinson's disease once the symptoms have become manifest.

The search for presymptomatic and diagnostic markers is important for several reasons:

❖ A diagnostic marker would permit a definitive diagnosis of Parkinson's disease and the certainty of being able to differentiate it at an early stage from other related disorders. This is particularly important when enrolling patients for drug trials; erroneous diagnoses can confound the resulting data.

❖ It would also serve as a measure of the underlying disease process— as a useful index of the severity of the illness and of the changes that occur as it progresses. In addition, it would provide a means of assessing the effectiveness of the various forms of treatment.

❖ With diagnostic markers, it might be possible to detect the disease before the symptoms become fully expressed, which in turn might make it possible to instigate preventive measures, such as neuroprotective therapy, that would halt or slow progression of the disease.

A number of tests have been explored as potential diagnostic markers, to do with reduced sense of smell, abnormalities in visual evoked potentials, and fluorodopa uptake patterns assessed with PET. However, none of these changes has proved to be specific to Parkinson's disease, and so none has been particularly useful as a marker. But although no single useful diagnostic marker has yet emerged, a number of lines of enquiry hold particular promise. Research into mitochondrial abnormalities in Parkinson's disease is a most exciting area, and abnormalities in the metabolism of particular substances in the brain are also being pursued as potential biological markers. More sensitive PET scanning to detect subclinical levels of dopamine deficiency in the putamen, insufficient to produce overt symptoms, can also be useful in identifying the presymptomatic state. Other approaches to early diagnosis include the search for immunologic markers of Lewy body degeneration in the cerebrospinal fluid, the assessment of extracerebral dopamine metabolism—changes induced by dopamine outside the cerebral cortices—as an index of what is happening in the brain, and the possible detection of Lewy bodies in extracerebral tissues.

The Search for Preventive Therapy

The focus of the search for preventive therapy is on two particular areas. First, the development and use of medication that will slow down, and others that may halt, the progression of the disease process altogether. The results of the DATATOP and other studies have demonstrated that selegiline delays the need to start levodopa therapy. As selegiline produces a mild symptomatic benefit, it is unclear whether its effects are due to protective (slowing down progression of the illness) or symptomatic (simply improving symptoms) mechanisms. Research into the use of other monoamine oxidase B inhibitors to slow the progression of Parkinson's disease continues. The second focus of research in this area has been on the development of methods of protecting against the damage caused by free radicals and other agents that increase "oxidative stress," assuming that may be involved in the degeneration process. The use of growth factors that may promote sprouting in dopamine-producing neurons and antioxidant agents are also being explored.

The discovery of such neuroprotective therapy will, of course, have personal significance for those who have just developed the illness. Moreover, the search for preventive therapy is well justified in terms of health economics. It has been estimated that if a hypothetical drug slowed down the progression of Parkinson's disease by approximately 10 percent, it would produce annual savings of $520 million for the U.S. health care system. This figure is based on the prolongation of employment of people with Parkinson's disease and their continued payment of income tax, decreased disability payments, and the postponement of the need for hospitalization and residential care.

The Search for Effective Treatments

The focus of the search for effective treatments is on finding medications that offer the benefits of levodopa but with longer-lasting effects and without levodopa's long-term complications. This could be achieved in several ways. First, by developing better means of delivering dopamine to the brain. Second, by using drugs that would prolong the effects of dopamine, such as monoamine oxidase inhibitors and catechol-O-methyl-transferase. Third, by exploring neurotransmitter systems other than the dopaminergic one in treating the symptoms.

Many of the side effects of levodopa arise from the fact that, in the course of its conversion to dopamine, levodopa indiscriminately stimulates all types of dopamine receptor. The future development of dopamine agonists that selectively stimulate subpopulations of dopamine receptors may reduce these side effects. The development of new drug-delivery systems such as controlled-release pills, subcutaneous infusions, and skin patches may also prove to be worthwhile by maintaining steadier levels of dopamine. Some symptoms of Parkinson's disease, which may be related to the impairment of other neurotransmitter systems in the brain, do not respond to dopaminergic medication, so classes of drugs other than dopaminergics may be of value in treating them.

The further development of brain implantation techniques may improve the efficacy of this treatment. But many questions about the procedure remain to be addressed. With much more basic and applied research, brain implantation technology may advance to the point where it becomes possible to reverse the degeneration of neurons in the substantia nigra and the resulting dopamine deficiency by neural implants that take on the role of dopamine production. Further refinement of other surgical procedures such as pallidotomy and thalamotomy, and pallidal, subthalamic nucleus and thalamic stimulation, will continue to provide better symptomatic relief in cases with severe rigidity or tremor.

The Search for Improved Service Provision

Medicine is a biologic science, but healing is an art. The technologic advances that have occurred in most fields of medicine during the last 100 years have somewhat distanced it from what should be its primary concern—ensuring people's health and well-being and preventing disease. In the course of present-day high-tech medicine, technology sometimes takes precedence and the human approach is overshadowed and forgotten during medical consultations. Furthermore, as we noted in Chapter 4, the "acute model" of illness—according to which the individual falls ill, seeks medical treatment, and is then cured—prevails in much of medicine. This model is applicable to illnesses such as Parkinson's disease, whose progressive nature must be a major concern in its medical management. Of prime consideration here must be a good "quality of life," which depends not only on optimal symptomatic control but also on the introduction of methods for promoting good coping and emotional and practical adjustment to the illness.

In standard neurologic practice, the psychosocial needs of patients with chronic neurologic illness are rarely addressed. To overcome some of the shortcomings, contact with key workers trained in nursing, social work, or physical, occupational, or speech therapy can be valuable for people with Parkinson's disease.

It is also necessary to introduce steps to address the needs of people with chronic illnesses such as Parkinson's disease. One way to do this would be through the nationwide development of key worker services aimed at improving the quality of life for people with Parkinson's disease and their families. Unfortunately, with the restricted resources available, all services need to be justified in terms of cost. It is difficult to quantify improvements in "quality of life" in financial terms. But although employing key workers may be more costly in the short term, in the long term, if the need for hospitalization or institutional care can be avoided or delayed, it is likely to lead to substantial savings for health services.

You Could Help

What we know about Parkinson's disease and its treatment is based on many years of research around the world on many thousands of people with the illness. The search for the cause, for prediagnostic and diagnostic markers, for effective treatments, for preventive therapy, and for improved service provision will require many more years of dedicated and creative research by scientists and clinicians, as well as the willing participation of many thousands more patients in these studies. If you feel up to it, both patient and caregiver can contribute to this process of discovery in a number of ways:

❖ by giving up a few hours of your time every year to volunteer to participate in research studies

❖ by considering whether, after your death, you would be willing to donate your brain tissue to a brain bank—brain banks are at the forefront of the search for a cause of Parkinson's disease

❖ by spending time in fund-raising activities for PD organizations—the money collected partly funds research studies.

In most research projects, including those that involve the donation of tissue to a brain bank, the participation of the caregiver is equally appreciated, as it provides information on healthy individuals that can be compared with the information obtained from people with the disease. With such a comparison it is possible to assess the type and extent of change from normal.

What does all this mean for the person who has had Parkinson's disease for the last 5, 10, 20, or 30 years, or for the person who has just been diagnosed as having it? Will a cure become available in time for them—a cure in the sense that a cough can be cured, with complete restoration to normal health? This is certainly a prospect for the future, if not on the immediate horizon. But effective treatments that may be as good as a cure *are* feasible and within sight. More important, service provision can certainly be improved so as to ensure a high quality of life for everyone with Parkinson's disease and their caregivers and families.

We end on a note of optimism by quoting the man whose powers of observation gave his name to the disease: "There appears to be sufficient reason for hoping that some remedial process ere long be discovered."

APPENDIX I

Drug Finder

The most commonly prescribed antiparkinson drugs are listed in Tables 1 and 2, with a brief description of doses and formulations.

Most tablets and capsules have distinctive shapes, markings, coloring, and code numbers to facilitate identification. The letters and numbers are often very small, and a magnifying glass may be needed to read them. Some manufacturers impress the company name on their tablets and capsules. The DuPont name appears on the red Symmetrel (amantadine) capsule, and the Roche name on the Madopar (benserazide/levodopa) capsule. Other manufacturers print an initial or an identifying trademark or logo on their products. Lederle Laboratories, for example, has an L in script on the front of each tablet. Merck, Sharp & Dohme products have the letters MSD in boldface above an identifying three-digit number, and Sandoz marks an S within a triangle. Tablets are usually scored on the reverse side so that they can easily be broken in half for smaller doses. The pattern of the scoring is often distinctive.

Despite all these identifying features, some pills may be difficult to identify. If there is any doubt about the identity of a forgotten bottle of pills, discard it or consult a pharmacist before using the drug.

Table 1. Commonly prescribed antiparkinson drugs

Brand (trade) name	Generic name	Formulations
Anticholinergics		
Akineton	Biperiden	2 mg white tablet
Artane	Trihexyphenidyl	2 and 5 mg white tablets and 5 mg long-acting capsules
Cogentin	Benztropine	0.5 and 2 mg round white tablets and 1 mg long elliptical white tablets
Kemadrin	Procyclidine	2 and 5 mg white tablets
Symmetrel	Amantadine	100 mg bright red capsule
Dopamine receptor agonists		
Dopergine[a]	Lisuride	0.2 mg, 0.5 mg, 1 mg white scored tablets
Parlodel	Bromocriptine	2.5 mg white tablets and 5 mg capsules, caramel and white
Permax	Pergolide	0.05 mg ivory; 0.25 mg green, and 1 mg pink tablets; rectangular scored
Mirapex	Pramipexole	0.125, 0.25, 0.5, 1.0, and 1.5, all white
ReQuip	Ropinirole	0.25 white, 0.5 yellow, 1.0 green, 2.0 pink, and 5.0 blue
Type B monoamine oxidase inhibitors		
Eldepryl	Selegiline (deprenyl)	5 mg white triangular scored tablets

[a]Not available in the United States.

Levodopa-decarboxylase inhibitor combinations		0.5 gram (pink)
Madopar[c]	Benserazide/ levodopa	Capsules
		25/100 mg (pink and blue)
		50/200 mg (caramel and blue)
		Dispersible tablets
		"625" 12.5/50 mg (pink tablets)
		"125" 25/100 mg (pink tablets)
Madopar[c] HBS[b] 125	Benserazide/ levodopa	Capsules 25/100 mg (blue and black)

| Sinemet | Carbidopa/ levodopa | Elliptical tablets, scored 10/100 mg (dark dapple blue) 25/250 mg (light dapple blue) 25/100 mg (yellow) |
| Sinemet CRI | Carbidopa/ levodopa | 50/200 mg (peach) 25/100 mg (pink, not scored) |

ªNote: 0. 1 gram = 100 mg; 0.25 gram = 250 mg; and 0.5 gram = 500 mg.
ᵇThese preparations of Madopar and Sinemet are sustained-release (also called controlled-release or slow-release) formulations.
ᶜAvailable in Canada but not in the United States.

Resources

* Modified from Biziere KE, Kurth MC. *Living with Parkinson's Disease.* New York: Demos, 1997.

Voluntary Organizations for People with Parkinson's Disease

Several nonprofit voluntary organizations in the United States and Canada provide patient services and research support in the field of Parkinson's disease. The major voluntary ones are:

The Parkinson's Disease Foundation, Inc.
Robin Anthony Elliott, Executive Director
William Black Medical Building
Columbia-Presbyterian Medical Center
710 West 168th Street
New York, NY 10032-9982
Tel: (212) 923-4700; (800) 457-6676
Fax: (212) 923-4778
E-mail: info@pdf.org
Web Site: http://www.parkinsons-foundation.org

The 1999 merger of the Parkinson's Disease Foundation with the Chicago-based United Parkinson Foundation created a single national organization that provides patients and their families and the general public with the information required to understand Parkinson's disease, as well as an increased basic science/clinical research program that is world-wide in scope. The Foundation supports research at three major Parkinson's disease centers: Columbia Presbyterian Medical Center and Cornell University in New York and Rush-Presbyterian–St. Luke's in Chicago. Patients and/or families may request printed information as well as referrals to knowledgeable neurologists at both the New York and the Chicago (Midwest branch) offices, the latter at 833 West Washington Boulevard, Chicago, IL 60607; telephone: (312) 733-1893, fax: (312) 733-1896, E-mail: PDFCHGO@enteract.com. The PDF presently publishes a quarterly newsletter and a quarterly science bulletin for those who want to keep abreast of scientific research accomplishments. Additionally, the Chicago office has numerous booklets available and a reading list referring to nearly 100 individual essays on various topics of interest to patients and families. All materials were reviewed before publication by the Foundation's eminently qualified Medical Advisory Board.

The American Parkinson Disease Association, Inc.
Joel Gerstel, Director
1250 Hylan Boulevard
Staten Island, NY 10305
Tel: (718) 981-8001; (800) 223-2732
Fax: (718) 981-4399
Web Site: www.apdaparkinson.com

The APDA supports a national program of patient service, including clinics and information centers throughout the United States. Local chapters organize patient education symposia featuring presentations by leading investigators in the field of Parkinson's disease. The association publishes a quarterly newsletter, booklets, and other informational materials. The APDA also sponsors basic and clinical research programs conducted at academic institutions throughout the country.

The National Parkinson Foundation, Inc.
Julian Pearson, Director
1501 Ninth Avenue/Bob Hope Road
Miami, FL 33136
Tel: (305) 547-6666
Information lines: (800) 327-4545; in Florida (800) 433-7022
Fax: (305) 243-4403
Web Site: www.parkinson.org

The National Parkinson Foundation (NPF) awards research grants to investigators throughout the United States; identifies and supports centers of excellence for Parkinson's disease research in the United States, Europe and Japan; sponsors international symposia on Parkinson's disease and publishes the proceedings; and publishes a quarterly newsletter for patients and their families as well as several informational pamphlets.

Parkinson's Action Network
840 Third Street
Santa Rosa, CA 95404
Tel: (707) 544-1994; (800) 850-4726
Fax: (707) 544-2363
E-mail: info@parkinsonaction.org
Web Site: www.parkinsonaction.org

The Parkinson's Action Network was established to provide a "unified, national voice for the Parkinson's community"; its aim is to promote research leading to effective treatment and a cure through a congressional lobbying efforts.

The Parkinson Foundation of Canada
Blair McRobie, CEO
390 Bay Street, Suite 710
Toronto, Ontario, Canada M5H 2Y2
Tel: (416) 366-0099; (800) 565-3000 (Canada only)
Fax: (416) 366-9190
E-mail: alicia.pace@parkinson.ca
Web Site: www.parkinson.ca

The The Parkinson Foundation of Canada operates through a network of local chapters and self-help groups to assist patients and their families. The foundation also funds several research grants to scientists working on Parkinson's disease in Canada.

Where to Obtain Information About Ongoing Clinical Trials in Parkinson's Disease

Unlike what exists for diseases such as AIDS and cancer, there is no computerized, on-line listing of ongoing clinical trials in Parkinson's disease. Information on some of the trials can be obtained from the National Institute of Neurological Disorders and Stroke (NINDS) or from the Parkinson's Disease Foundation.

National Institute of Neurological Disorders and Stroke (NINDS)
National Institutes of Health
9000 Rockville Pike
Bethesda, MD 20892,
Tel: (301) 496-6609
Web Site: nih.gov/science/campus

The NINDS conducts research on Parkinson's disease in its own research laboratories and maintains an active program of clinical research at the clinical center, a large hospital located in Bethesda. Its Experimental Therapeutics Branch (ETB) actively searches for new symptomatic treatments for Parkinson's disease and tests new drugs in animals and in patients. They will provide information concerning clinical trials conducted at ETB. Patients who are interested in participating in clinical trials will usually be asked to have their physicians send or fax letters of referral and case summaries to the ETB.

Parkinson Study Group (PSG)
Clinical Trials Coordination Center
The Mount Hope Professional Building
1351 Mount Hope Avenue
Rochester, NY 14620
Tel: (716) 275-7311; fax (716) 461-3554

The PSG is a consortium of 38 physicians in the United States and Canada devoted to conducting multicenter clinical trials in Parkinson's disease. This is the group that conducted the now famous DATATOP study to examine whether selegiline (Deprenyl) could slow the progression of Parkinson's disease. The PSG members continue to study the effects of new drugs in patients with Parkinson's disease. Information about ongoing clinical trials can be obtained by calling the PSG Coordination Center in Rochester, New York.

Where to Find Information on Research in Parkinson's Disease

At the beginning of each calendar year the NINDS makes available an annual summary of research on Parkinson's disease. Copies can be obtained by writing to the Office of Scientific and Health Reports, NINDS, Building 31, Room 8A16, National Institutes of Health, Bethesda MD 20892; tel: (301) 496-5751. Similar information can be derived from the PDF's Science Bulletin (see PDF).

The Parkinson's Web (http://neuro-chief e.mgh.harvard.edu/parkin-sonsweb/Main/PDmain.html.) is an international nonprofit effort to use the Internet as an on-line archive of information on Parkinson's disease, its treatment, strategies for coping and research news. It is intended for patients, their families, and friends. Further information can be obtained from Ken Bernstein, President of the Young Parkinson's Chapter of Massachusetts and coordinator of the Parkinson's Web; tel: (617) 527-2803; fax (617) 527-2077; or E-mail cocosolo@aol.com.

"Parkinson's Disease Update" is a monthly newsletter devoted to bringing information on the most current medical, social and psychologic aspects of Parkinson's disease. Its publisher firmly believes in the value of disseminating research news on the disease as quickly as possible, to bring relief to all those who suffer from the disease and also to help find a cure. More information and costs can be obtained from the Medical Publishing Company, P.O. Box 450, Huntingdon Valley, PA 19006; tel: (215) 947-6648; fax: (215) 947-2552.

For Spouses of Individuals with Parkinson's Disease

The Well Spouse Foundation
610 Lexington Avenue, Suite 814
New York, NY 10022-6005
(212) 644-1241; (800) 838-1338

The Well Spouse Foundation is a national self-help organization of spouses/partners of people who are chronically ill or disabled. Its goal is to provide emotional support to well spouses via local support groups, a newsletter, conferences and other activities.

Index

The following titles of interest are available from Demos Medical Publishing, Inc.:

Living with Parkinson's Disease
Kathleen E. Biziere, M.D., and Matthias C. Kurth, M.D.

Insurance Solutions: Plan Well, Live Better
A Workbook for People with Chronic Disease and Disabilities
Laura D. Cooper

Health Insurance: How to Get It, Keep It, or Improve What You've Got
Robert Enteen

Tax Options and Strategies for People with Disabilities, 2nd edition
Stephen B. Mendelsohn

To receive additional information on these or any of our other titles, call our
toll-free number:

(800) 532-8663.
Demos Medical Publishing, Inc.
386 Park Avenue South
New York, NY 10016
Phone (212) 683-0072
Fax (212) 683-0118
E-mail: orderdept@demospub.com